NEUROPEPTIDES AND NEURAL TRANSMISSION

International Brain Research Organization
Monograph Series
Volume 7

INTERNATIONAL BRAIN RESEARCH ORGANIZATION MONOGRAPH SERIES

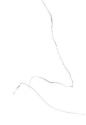

INTERNATIONAL BRAIN RESEARCH
ORGANIZATION MONOGRAPH SERIES
Volume 7

Neuropeptides and Neural Transmission

Edited by

Cosimo Ajmone Marsan, M.D.
EEG Laboratories
University of Miami
Jackson Memorial Medical Center
Miami, Florida

Wladyslaw Z. Traczyk, M.D.
Department of Physiology
School of Medicine in Lodz
Lodz, Poland

Honorary President

Ulf S. von Euler, M.D.
Department of Physiology
Karolinska Institutet
Stockholm, Sweden

Raven Press ■ New York

Raven Press, 1140 Avenue of the Americas, New York, New York 10036

The material contained in this volume was submitted as previously unpublished material, except in the instances in which credit has been given to the source from which some of the illustrative material was derived.

Great care has been taken to maintain the accuracy of the information contained in the volume. However, Raven Press cannot be held responsible for errors or for any consequences arising from the use of the information contained herein.

Library of Congress Cataloging in Publication Data

Main entry under title:

Neuropeptides and neural transmission

(Monograph series-International Brain Research
Organization; v. 7)
Proceedings of a UNESCO-IBRO symposium held at
the Polish Academy of Sciences, Jablonna, June 2-4,
1979.
Includes bibliographical references and indexes.
1. Neurotransmitters--Congresses. 2. Neural
transmission--Congresses. 3. Peptide hormones--
Congresses. I. Ajmone-Marsan, Cosimo.
II. Traczyk, Wladyslaw, 1928-
III. United Nations Educational, Scientific and
Cultural Organization. IV. International Brain
Research Organization. V. Series: International
Brain Research Organization. Monograph
series-International Brain Research Organization
v.7. (DNLM: 1. Peptides--Physiology--Congresses.
2. Neural transmission--Congresses. W1 1N7IS
v.7/QU68 N4945 1979)
QP364.N45   599.01'88   80-18766
ISBN 0-89004-501-1

Preface

In the last decade since the isolation of active peptides from hypothalamus and determination of their chemical structure, there has been much development in research concerning their physiological role not only in the anterior pituitary control but also in the neural processes in the whole brain. Taking this into consideration, the Executive Committee of the International Brain Research Organisation during its meetings in July 1977, and April 1978, decided to contribute an official IBRO symposium in 1979 on the role of neuropeptides in neural processes. The organization of the Symposium was entrusted to the Polish members of IBRO.

The purpose of the Symposium was to bring together the most distinguished scientists specializing in various aspects of neuropeptide action. The general topic of the Symposium was *Neuropeptides and Neural Transmission,* so it would be understood that several neuropeptides were to be discussed during the meeting. This multidisciplinary approach, appears to have been very fruitful, and in agreement with the aims of IBRO, in pooling together the scientists of different disciplines in the common goal of brain research.

During the Symposium in which 62 scientists from 15 countries participated, the presented papers dealt with the role of neuropeptides in the brain, evidence for their activity in neurotransmission, electrophysiological and behavioral effects, and correlation with other central transmitter mechanisms. This volume contains the proceedings of the Symposium.

The Symposium successfully took place on June 2–4, 1979, in Jablonna near Warsaw, Poland, thanks to the very kind support of the Secretary General of IBRO, Dr. Mary Brazier, previously Director of IBRO Symposia, and was made possible by financial support of the Division of Scientific Research and Higher Education of the United Nations Educational, Scientific and Cultural Organization; the International Brain Research Organisation; Lilly Research Laboratories, the Polish Academy of Sciences; the Polish Physiological Society; and the School of Medicine in Lodz. Gratitude is extended toward all who supported the Symposium either financially or in other ways, and especially to the staff of the Department of Physiology, School of Medicine in Lodz.

Cosimo Ajmone Marsan
Władysław Z. Traczyk

Address by the President of the Polish Academy of Sciences

The Polish Academy of Sciences had the pleasure in the past to be the host of the International Brain Research Organisation Symposia. Jablonna is for the third time the site of an IBRO Symposium in about twenty years of IBRO activities. This time we have gathered to discuss the role of neuropeptides in brain function.

I hope that new data presented at this Symposium will further reduce the gap between the notion of mind versus brain function. Some neural processes occurring in the brain, including pain sensation, learning, and memory, will be better understood. I also hope that the discussions during the Symposium will offer new ideas for further fruitful research work on the role of neuropeptides in brain function. I wish you successes in this field at the present Symposium and further achievements which, I hope, will prove helpful for all of mankind.

Witold Nowacki

Contents

ix

Part II—Neurotensin, Enkephalins, and Endorphins

Contributors

M. G. Airapetjanz
Academy of Sciences of the USSR
Institute of Higher Nervous Activity and
Neurophysiology
Moscow, USSR

E. Arnauld
Institut National de la Santé
et de la Recherche Médicale
Unité de Recherches
de Neurobiologie des Comportements
rue Camille Saint-Saëns
33077-Bordeaux-Cedex, France

A. Balfe
Endocrine Department
Mater Misericordiae Hospital
Dublin 7, Ireland

J. L. Barker
Laboratory of Neurophysiology
National Institute of Neurological and
Communicative Disorders and Stroke
National Institutes of Health
Bethesda, Maryland 20205

T. Barth
Institute of Organic Chemistry and Bio-
chemistry
Czechoslovak Academy of Science
166 10 Prague 6, Czechoslovakia

K. Betschen
Institut für Physiologie
Medizinische Akademie Magdeburg
DDR-301 Magdeburg
Leipziger Strasse, GDR

N. Bhargava
Department of Pharmacognosy and Phar-
macology
University of Illinois at the Medical Center
Chicago, Illinois 60612

R. M. Buijs
Netherlands Institute for Brain Research
IJdijk 28
1095 KJ Amsterdam, The Netherlands

A. Burlet
Laboratoires d'Histologie
Facultè de Médecine
Avenue de la Forêt de Haye
B.P. 1080
54019 Nancy Cedex, France

D. Cannon
Endocrine Department
Mater Misericordiae Hospital
Dublin 7, Ireland

D. Chang
Institute for Biomedical Research
University of Texas at Austin
Austin, Texas 78712

M. Chateau
Laboratories d'Histologie et de Physiologie
Faculté de Médecine
Avenue de la Forêt de Haye
B.P. 1080
54019 Nancy Cedex, France

T. L. Chruściel
Institute for Drug Research and Control
Chełmska 30/34
00–725 Warsaw, Poland

J. R. Couch
Department of Medicine
Southern Illinois University
College of Medicine
Springfield, Illinois 62708

A. Członkowski
Department of Pharmacology and Phar-
macodynamics

Institute of Physiological Sciences
School of Medicine in Warsaw
Krakowskie Przedmieście 26/28
00–927 Warsaw, Poland

J. Dogterom
Netherlands Institute for Brain Research
IJdijk 28
1095 KJ Amsterdam, The Netherlands

F. Dreyfuss
Laboratoires d'Histologie et de Physiologie
Faculté de Médecine
Avenue de la Forêt de Haye
B.P. 1080, 54019 Nancy Cedex, France

L. Erdélyi
Attila József University of Sciences
Department of Comparative Physiology
6726 Szeged
Középfasor 52, Hungary

U. S. von Euler
Department of Physiology
Karolinska Institute
Solnavägen 1
S-104 01 Stockholm 60, Sweden

D. Felix
Institute of Pharmacology and Brain Re-
    search Institute
University of Zürich
CH-8006 Zürich, Switzerland

K. Folkers
Institute for Biomedical Research
University of Texas at Austin
Austin, Texas 78712

R. C. A. Frederickson
Lilly Research Laboratories
Eli Lilly and Company
Indianapolis, Indiana 46206

R. Gamse
Institute of Experimental and Clinical
    Pharmacology
University of Graz
Universitätsplatz 4
A-8010 Graz, Austria

P. D. Gesellchen
Lilly Research Laboratories
Eli Lilly and Company
Indianapolis, Indiana 46206

Ch. Gramsch
Department of Neuropharmacology
Max-Planck-Institut für Psychiatrie
Kraepelinstrasse 2
D-8000 München 40, FRG

W. Gumułka
Department of Pharmacology and Phar-
    macodynamics
Institute of Physiological Sciences
School of Medicine in Warsaw
Krakowskie Przedmieście 26/28
00–927 Warsaw, Poland

J. W. Guzek
Department of Pathophysiology
Institute of Pathology
School of Medicine in Lodz
Narutowicza 60
90–136 Lodz, Poland

K. Hecht
Department of Neuropathophysiology of
    Clinic of Psychiatry
/Charité/ Humboldt-University
104 Berlin
Schumanstrasse 20/21, GDR

D. P. Henry
Lilly Research Laboratories
Eli Lilly and Company
Indiana Indianapolis 46206

A. Herz
Department of Neuropharmacology
Max-Planck-Institut für Psychiatrie
Kraepelinstrasse 2
D-8000 München 40, FRG

R. G. Hill
Department of Pharmacology
The Medical School
University of Bristol
University Walk
Bristol BS8 1TD, United Kingdom

H. Hilse
Institute of Drug Research
Academy of Sciences of GDR
Alfred-Kowalke-Strasse 4
DDR-1136 Berlin-Friedrichsfelde, GDR

M. L. Hoddinott
Department of Pharmacology
The Medical School
University of Bristol
University Walk
Bristol BS8 1TD, United Kingdom

V. Höllt
Department of Neuropharmacology
Max-Planck-Institut für Psychiatrie
Kraepelinstrasse 2
D-8000 München 40, FRG

P. Holzer
Institute of Experimental and Clinical
  Pharmacology
University of Graz
Universitätsplatz 4
A-8010 Graz, Austria

P. Janicki
Department of Pharmacology and Phar-
  macodynamics
Institute of Physiological Sciences
School of Medicine in Warsaw
Krakowskie Przedmieście 26/28
00–927 Warsaw, Poland

F. Joó
Institute of Biophysics
Biological Research Center
Hungarian Academy of Sciences
Odesszai KRT 62
P.O.B. 521
H-6701 Szeged, Hungary

C. C. Jordan
Department of Pharmacology
University College London
Gower Street
London WC1E 6BT, United Kingdom

K. Jošt
Institute of Organic Chemistry and Biochemistry

Czechoslovak Academy of Science
166 10 Prague 6, Czechoslovakia

E. Kacprzak
Department of Physiology
Institute of Physiology and Biochemistry
School of Medicine in Lodz
Lindleya 3
90–131 Lodz, Poland

E. Kasafírek
Research Institute for Pharmacy and Biochemistry
U Elektry 8
194 04 Prague 9, Czechoslovakia

P. M. Keen
Department of Pharmacology
The Medical School
University of Bristol
University Walk
Bristol BS8 1TD, United Kingdom

K. Kmieć
Department of Pathophysiology
School of Medicine in Lodz
Narutowicza 60
90–136 Lodz, Poland

I. A. Kolemetseva
Academy of Sciences of the USSR
Institute of Higher Nervous
  Activity and Neurophysiology
Moscow, USSR

S. Konishi
Department of Pharmacology
Faculty of Medicine
Tokyo Medical and Dental University
Yushima, Bunkyo-ku
Tokyo 113, Japan

H. W. Kosterlitz
Unit for Research on Addictive Drugs
Marischal College
University of Aberdeen
Aberdeen AB9 1AS, United Kingdom

G. L. Kovács
Institute of Pathophysiology
University of Szeged School of Medicine
6701 Szeged, Pf. 531, Hungary

I. Krejcí
Research Institute for Pharmacy and Biochemistry
U Elektry 8
194 04 Prague 9, Czechoslovakia

W. A. Krivoy
National Institute on Drug Abuse
Addiction Research Center
Lexington, Kentucky 40583

B. Kupková
Research Institute for Pharmacy and Biochemistry
U Elektry 8
194 04 Prague 9, Czechoslovakia

F. Lembeck
Institute of Experimental and Clinical
Pharmacology
University of Graz
Universitätsplatz 4
A-8010 Graz, Austria

J. Libich
Department of Pharmacology and Phar-
macodynamics
Institute of Physiological Sciences
School of Medicine in Warsaw
Krakowskie Przedmieście 26/28
00–927 Warsaw, Poland

W. Lichtensteiger
Institute of Pharmacology and Brain Re-
search Institute
University of Zürich
Gloriastrasse 32
Ch-8006 Zürich, Switzerland

I. P. Lyovshina
Academy of Sciences of the USSR
Institute of Higher Nervous
Activity and Neurophysiology
Moscow, USSR

M. Łuczyńska
Department of Physiology
Institute of Physiology and Biochemistry
School of Medicine in Lodz
Lindleya 3, 90–131 Lodz, Poland

J. F. MacDonald
Helen Scott Playfair Neurobiology Unit
University of Toronto
Toronto, Canada

M. L. Mashford
University of Melbourne
Department of Medicine
St. Vincent's Hospital
Fitzroy 3065, Australia

N. Mayer
Institute of Experimental and Clinical
Pharmacology
University of Graz
Universitätsplatz 4
A-8010 Graz, Austria

M. J. Millan
Department of Neuropharmacology
Max-Planck-Institut für Psychiatrie
Kraepelinstrasse 2
D-8000 München 40, FRG

A. Molnar
Institute of Experimental and Clinical
Pharmacology
University of Graz
Universitätsplatz 4
A-8010 Graz, Austria

E. Morgenstern
Pharmacological Research Institute
of the Pharmaceutical Industry
Berlin, GDR

P. Oehme
Institute of Drug Research
Academy of Sciences of GDR
Alfred-Kowalke-Strasse 4
DDR-1136 Berlin-Friedrichsfelde, GDR

H. Osborne
Department of Neuropharmacology
Max-Planck-Institut für Psychiatrie
Kraepelinstrasse 2
D-8000 München 40, FRG

M. Otsuka
Department of Pharmacology
Faculty of Medicine

Tokyo Medical and Dental University
Yushima, Bunkyo-ku
Tokyo 113, Japan

L. Piesche
Institute of Drug Research
Academy of Sciences of GDR
Alfred-Kowalke-Strasse 4
DDR-1136 Berlin-Friedrichsfelde, GDR

B. Pernow
Department of Clinical Physiology
Karolinska Institutet
S-104 01 Stockholm 60, Sweden

M. Poppei
Department of Neuropathophysiology
  of Clinic of Psychiatry
/Charité/ Humboldt-University
104 Berlin, Schumanstrasse 20/21, GDR

D. Poulain
Institut National de la Santé
et de la Recherche Médicale
  Unité de Recherches
de Neurobiologie des Comportements
rue Camille Saint-Saëns
33 077-Bordeaux-Cedex, France

D. Powell
Endocrine Department
Mater Misericordiae Hospital
Dublin 7, Ireland

R. Przewłocki
Institute of Pharmacology
Polish Academy of Sciences
Smętna 12
31–343 Cracow, Poland

J. M. van Ree
Rudolf Magnus Institute for Pharmacology
Vondellan 6
3521 GD Utrecht, The Netherlands

R. F. Ritzmann
Department of Physiology and Biophysics
College of Medicine
University of Illinois
The Medical Center

P. O. Box 6998
Chicago, Illinois 60612

Å Rökaeus
Department of Pharmacology
Karolinska Institutet
Solnavägen 1
S-104 01 Stockholm 60, Sweden

S. Rosell
Department of Pharmacology
Karolinska Institutet
Solnavägen 1
S-104 01 Stockholm 60, Sweden

A. Saria
Institute of Experimental and Clinical
  Pharmacology
University of Graz
Universitätsplatz 4
A-8010 Graz, Austria

H. Schulz
Institute of Physiology
Medical Academy in Magdeburg
Leipziger Strasse 44
DDR-301 Magdeburg, GDR

H. Schwarzberg
Institute of Physiology
Medical Academy in Magdeburg
Leipziger Strasse 44
DDR-301 Magdeburg, GDR

P. Skrabanek
Endocrine Department
Mater Misericordiae Hospital
Dublin 7, Ireland

R. C. A. Frederickson
Lilly Research Laboratories
Eli Lilly and Company
Indianapolis, Indiana 46206

J. Soós
Institute of Biophysics
Biological Research Center
Hungarian Academy of Sciences
Odesszai KRT 62
P.O.B. 521
H-6701 Szeged, Hungary

J. M. Stewart
Department of Biochemistry
University of Colorado
School of Medicine
Denver, Colorado 80262

E. Strumiłło-Dyba
Department of Physiology
Institute of Physiology and Biochemistry
School of Medicine in Lodz
Lindleya 3, 90–131 Lodz, Poland

T. Suzue
Department of Pharmacology
Faculty of Medicine
Tokyo Medical and Dental University
Yushima, Bunkyo-ku
Tokyo 113, Japan

I. Szczepańska-Szyburska
Department of Pathophysiology
Institute of Pathology
School of Medicine, in Lodz
Narutowicza 60, 90–136 Lodz, Poland

Z. Szreniawski
Department of Pharmacology and Pharmacodynamics
Institute of Physiological Sciences
School of Medicine in Warsaw
Krakowskie Przedmieście 26/28
00–927 Warsaw, Poland

G. Telegdy
Institute of Pathophysiology
University of Szeged School of Medicine
6701 Szeged, Pf 531, Hungary

K. Thor
Department of Pharmacology
Karolinska Institutet
Solnavägen 1
S-104 01 Stockholm 60, Sweden

W. Z. Traczyk
Department of Physiology
Institute of Physiology and Biochemistry
School of Medicine in Lodz
Lindleya 3, 90–131 Lodz, Poland

D. H. G. Versteg
Rudolf Magnus Institute for Pharmacology
Vondellaan 6
3521 GD Utrecht, The Netherlands

J. D. Vincent
Institut National de la Santé
et de la Récherche Médicale
Unité de Recherches
de Neurobiologie des Comportements
rue Camille Saint-Saëns
33077-Bordeaux-Cedex, France

E. S. Vizi
Department of Pharmacology
Semmelweis University of Medicine
Ulloi ut 26
H-1445 Budapest, Hungary

V. Volbekas
Department of Pharmacology
Semmelweis University of Medicine
Ulloi ut 26
H-1445 Budapest, Hungary

R. Walter
Department of Physiology and Biophysics
University of Illinois
at the Medical Center,
Chicago, Illinois 60612

D. de Wied
Rudolf Magnus Institute for Pharmacology
Medical Faculty
University of Utrecht
Vondellaan 6
Utrecht 3521 GD, The Netherlands

Tj. B. van Wimersma Greidanus
Rudolf Magnus Institute for Pharmacology
Medical Faculty
University of Utrecht
Vondellann 6
3521 GD Utrecht, The Netherlands

M. Yanagisawa
Department of Pharmacology
Faculty of Medicine
Tokyo Medical and Dental University
Bunkyo-ku
Tokyo 113, Japan

E. Zimmermann
Department of Anatomy
and Brain Research Institute
University of California
School of Medicine
Los Angeles, California 90024

Neuropeptides and Neural Transmission,
edited by C. Ajmone Marsan and W. Z. Traczyk.
Raven Press, New York © 1980.

Introduction

U. S. von Euler

Physiology Department, Karolinska Institute, S-104 01 Stockholm, Sweden

The peptide history may be said to begin with the discovery of renin by Tigerstedt and Bergman in 1898. The true mechanism by which renin exerted its pressor action was not revealed however, as we know, until some 40 years later when Page in the USA and Braun-Menendez in Argentina and their groups found that renin needed a substrate to form the active peptide via precursors in the blood.

Only a short time after the turn of the century the peptide hormones entered the stage. More correctly one should perhaps say that the term "hormone" was introduced for an active compound which later turned out to be a peptide. I am referring to the secretin of Bayliss and Starling, discovered in 1902, and designated 'hormone' in 1906. Secretin resisted the attempts to reveal its nature and chemical composition for a long time, actually until 1962. It must be remembered that the purification, separation, and isolation techniques at that time—in the 1930s and 1940s—were not so well developed as nowadays. Chromatography was just developing and Craig's counter current distribution was available, but otherwise the techniques were very limited.

However, the chemical study of biologically active peptides was proceeding rapidly. Insulin was recognized as a peptide and so were the anterior pituitary hormones, characterized and isolated by Evans and Li in California. Kallikrein was described and turned out to be a case analogous to that of renin, an enzyme forming a peptide kallidin by acting on a suitable substrate.

The history of the posterior pituitary extracts reveals the difficulties that were encountered both in the characterization of their biological actions and with regard to their chemical nature. The vasoconstrictor effect of pituitary extracts was indeed observed by Oliver and Schäfer in 1895, almost at the same time as the pressor effect of suprarenal extracts, but another 10 years elapsed before Dale discovered the oxytoxic effect of fresh pituitary extracts in 1906. The only effect of the kidney discussed at that time was a diuretic action.

It is interesting to note that in 1906 Schäfer and Herring exposed their pituitary extracts to tryptic digestion but were unable to find any effect of this treatment. Dale repeated these experiments, which he published in 1909, and found that commercial trypsin and "pure pancreatic juice obtained by secretin" completely annulled the action of the pituitary extract. He added: "It may be suggested . . . that Schäfer and Herring were using an inactive preparation of trypsin: at least it is clear that the tryptic preparations used by me contained something which was not present in theirs." What a civil and delightful way to comment on a difference in results.

However, Dale apparently did not pay special attention to the peptide nature of the active compound in his extracts; thus it is not mentioned in the summary of the publication of 1909. I shall not go further into the sometimes heated discussion as to whether the different actions observed with posterior pituitary extracts were due to one or more substances. Actually, it wasn't until 1920 that Dudley succeeded in separating the pressor and oxytocic effects. Only gradually did the concept of the peptide nature of the pituitary hormones become fully realized and it wasn't until around 1930 that this fact became more generally recognized. Meyer and Gottlieb in their textbook *Experimentelle Pharmakologie* (1933) stated that vasopressin could not be a simple base, but was a complex compound.

However, at this time a number of other hormone-like biologically active compounds of peptide character became known. Collip (1925) characterized the parathyroid hormone as an "albumose." Mellanby studied secretin and referred to the purified compound as a polypeptide (1926). Cholecystokinin and gastrin were also considered to be secretin-like compounds and thus peptides. That insulin was inactivated by tryptic digestion was known even before that time.

I presume that the reason why I have been so kindly invited to write this introduction is my contribution to the brain peptides in the form of Substance P (SP). This compound was actually discovered in extracts of intestine when I worked in Henry Dale's Institute in London, but in the subsequent work with Gaddum we found it also in the brain. We had no other proof of its identity in the two organs besides the agreement in biological activity of the extracts and some general properties like solubility and stability in different media under various conditions. Certainly at that time we did not know that it was a peptide. It was readily dialysable, and quite active solutions could be obtained from extracts with ethanol and acetone in relatively high concentrations. Later, in 1936, it was shown to be salted out by ammonium sulphate, which provided a simple way of purification. Incubation with trypsin destroyed the biological activity, which confirmed our suspicion that SP was a peptide.

A big step forward was taken by Bengt Pernow in 1953 who found an efficient method of purification by adsorption chromatography and also demonstrated its distribution in the brain and peripheral nerves and the preponderance of SP in hypothalamus and basal ganglia.

Time does not allow me to go into the excellent work leading to isolation, chemical characterization, and synthesis of SP by Susan Leeman and her group, except that I would like to mention that it was her keen observation that a hypothalamic extract caused salivation in rats which lead her on the right track.

SP was probably the first peptide with a wide distribution in the brain to be described, suggesting that it might exert actions of a more general kind. The development of the radioimmunoassay method by Berson and Yalow meant a breakthrough in the studies of SP as well as other peptides in the CNS. From these studies (Powell, Hökfelt, Nilsson, Iversen, and others) it became evident that SP occurs in specific neurons, not only in various parts of the brain and in the dorsal roots but also in the intestinal nerve plexus and in single neurons in many places. SP shares this peculiar distribution in CNS and in the intestine with endorphins, enkephalin, vasoactive intestinal peptide (VIP), discovered in 1970, and even with other peptides such as somatostatin and gastrin. It would seem that these peptides have a modulating function both in the gut and in the CNS.

Is SP a neurotransmitter? This is in part a semantic question. Even if SP occurs intraaxonally in the neurons it still does not follow that it is a neurotransmitter proper. Its occurrence in dorsal roots led Lembeck as early as 1953 to assume that it could be the neurotransmitter of primary sensory neurons. This assumption was later supported by the experimental findings by Otsuka and his group. The strong reinforcing effect observed with SP both on the peristaltic reflex (Gernandt, 1942) and the twitch response to nerve stimulation in the vas deferens suggests that it could serve as an important modulator of nerve effects. This is true also for ganglionic transmission and for synaptic transmission elsewhere (Krivoy).

A question of interest is of course how SP or any other intraaxonal peptide is stored and released. The presence of SP in subcellular particles was shown by Lembeck and Holasek (1960), by Inoye in the brain, and by ourselves in peripheral nerves such as vagus and splenic nerves. It was also shown by Andrews and Holton (1958) that after section of a peripheral nerve the SP content decreased in the peripheral part and accumulated in the proximal part, suggesting that SP travelled down the axon, in a way similar to that of noradrenaline in adrenergic nerves. This would be in agreement with binding to granules. Apparently SP is stored in a protected or loosely bound form in the granules. Granules isolated from the vagus nerve of the dog did not release SP when suspended in Tyrode solution, whereas on subjecting the granules to hyposmotic lysis or acid treatment the full biological activity appeared in the solution. Activity faded, however, in a relatively short time, suggesting breakdown by some component in the granule suspension, presumably a peptidase.

Other questions which are still largely unanswered are the mechanisms for formation, storage, and release. In order to understand the physiological conditions under which the brain peptides exert their actions, more light has to be shed on these events. By analogy one might speculate that specific enzymes—as in the case of renin and kallikrein—are present in the peptide neurons, splitting off the active compounds from suitable precursors among the protein macromolecules.

For a number of the hypothalamogastrointestinal peptides a localization to endocrine cells in the gastrointestinal area has also been described. This leads to another field which has been discussed especially by Pearse who coined the term "APUD cells" (amine-precursor uptake and decarboxylation cells). Pearse and Polak described in 1975 the presence of SP not only in the cell bodies and processes in the plexuses of Auerbach and Meissner but also in the cytoplasm of basogranular endocrine cells in the intestinal mucosa. These cells, which occur mostly in the duodenum, have been identified tentatively as enterochromaffin. From these observations Pearse suggests that the possession by the enterochromaffin cell of the amino acid sequence of an established neurotransmitter peptide supports its identification as a cell of neuroectodermal origin. This hypothesis might then apply for a number of peptides occurring both in certain cells in the gastrointestinal area and in the CNS. The two groups within the APUD series thus comprise central neuroendocrine and peripheral neuroendocrine cells. The effort to bring some systematization in the amine- and peptide-producing cells seems commendable, and we can see now an analogy between the amine system in chromaffin cells and in neurons, and the peptide system. The full significance of the simultaneous occurrence of an amine, like 5-HT (5-hydroxytryptamine), and a peptide like SP in the same cell has not yet been elucidated, however.

The historical development of our knowledge of the occurrence and the physiological significance of the numerous peptides occurring both in the CNS and in the peripheral nervous system has perhaps taught us not to make such a sharp distinction between the systems. Historically, I think this first became evident when the CNS was found to possess a number of amine systems, which were revealed largely through the availability of the Falck-Hillarp histological method, and largely clarified by the systematic work of Fuxe and Hökfelt and their associates.

For the speculative mind it is hard to overlook the fact that peptide chains represent an almost inexhaustable source of specific messengers, derived from protein material. Perhaps the CNS utilizes a whole family of more or less specific peptides to maintain the intricate balance within the system. One might speculate that the true transmitter action is of all-or-none character—a "detonator" action—whereas the delicate tuning is mediated by a number of chemicals formed and released locally.

Several peptides are associated with behaviour and also memory and learning as, for example, vasopressin. Behavioural and neurological effects have also been noted in such peptide hormones as adrenocorticotropic hormone and beta-melanocyte-stimulating hormone. This important branch of behavioural studies was initiated by de Wied and his colleagues in Utrecht and has led to a large number of interesting observations.

It does not seem unlikely that peptide hormones in the brain may exert a modulating effect on neural activity by determining or influencing the background or "climate" on which the specific actions are projected. Such a concept would not preclude specific and localized actions, but would broaden the field of action of this group of neuroactive compounds.

Neuropeptides and Neural Transmission,
edited by C. Ajmone Marsan and W. Z. Traczyk.
Raven Press, New York © 1980.

Morphological and Functional Aspects of Substance P

Bengt Pernow

Department of Clinical Physiology, Karolinska Institute, Stockholm, Sweden

In 1931 von Euler and Gaddum (8) discovered in extracts from the equine brain and gut a smooth muscle-stimulating and hypotensive factor, called Substance P (SP). Extensive studies especially in the 1950s and 1970s have clarified both the occurrence of SP in the body and its pharmacological actions. It is now known that SP is a normal constituent of most organs, particularly connected to the nervous structures. Besides the effect on smooth muscle, SP has been found to exert numerous pharmacological actions in various organs, such as excitation of spinal motoneurons, secretion in salivary and pancreatic glands, diuresis, natriuresis, and anticholeresis, and to be involved in pain mechanisms. Furthermore, the release of SP from both central and peripheral nerve terminals is now well documented. All these findings have promoted an increasing interest in the function of this compound although, because of the wide distribution and variety of pharmacological effects, no conclusive evidence has so far been given for a specific physiological role for SP.

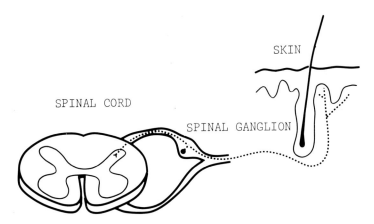

FIG. 1. Schematic drawing of a primary sensory neuron. The cell body is located in the spinal ganglion; its peripheral branch terminates in the skin and its central branch in the dorsal horn of the spinal cord.

By 1953 Lembeck (30) had already proposed a transmitter function of SP in the first sensory neuron, and recent electrophysiological and neurochemical studies (18,39,52) have given strong support for this theory. This proposed functional role of SP might explain both its widespread distribution in the periphery and several of its pharmacological actions, such as the circulatory, pain producing, and smooth muscle stimulating effects. This chapter reviews some of our present knowledge of SP in connection to sensory neurons (Fig. 1).

PRIMARY SENSORY NEURON

In 1953 Hellauer (17), Lembeck (30), and Pernow (43) had independently identified the presence of SP in the spinal cord with much higher concentrations in the dorsal than in the ventral roots. This observation was confirmed and extended some 20 years later with immunohistochemical and radioimmunological techniques.

Immunohistological Localization

Spinal Cord

A dense network of SP-positive fibers are found in the dorsal horns of the spinal cord, where the highest concentrations are observed in the Lissauer's tract and in laminae I and II with a decreasing number of fluorescent fibers in the ventral direction. Thus, the central part of lamina III and the whole lamina IV almost lack a specific immunofluorescence, whereas the ventral horns and the area around the central canal contain a network of moderate density (20,24,25,33) (Fig. 2).

Spinal Ganglia

In the rat spinal and trigeminal ganglia several SP-positive cell bodies and fibers are present at all levels. These cell bodies are mainly of a small size (B type) and between them SP fluorescence is found in fibers of fine caliber, probably unmyelinated axons. Roughly estimated, the SP neurons may constitute about 20% of all neurons in the spinal ganglia (21) (Fig. 2).

Peripheral Tissues

SP-positive fibers are found in most peripheral tissues, sometimes in relation to blood vessels, secretory cells, and ducts. In the skin the SP immunoreactive fibers are found both along blood vessels and as apparently free nerve endings. In the skin of the cat hind paw these axons are running in the connective tissue just beneath, and occasionally penetrating into, the epithelium (20,25)

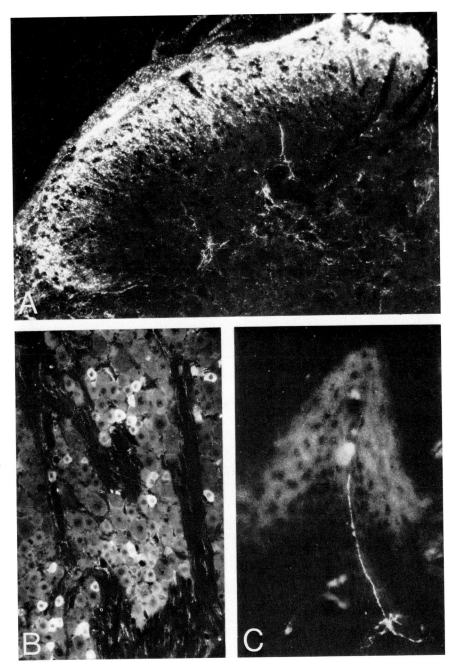

FIG. 2. Immunofluorescence micrographs of the spinal cord **(A)**, a spinal ganglion **(B)**, and the skin **(C)** after incubation of antiserum to SP. A dense plexus of SP immunoreactive fibers is seen in the superficial laminae of the dorsal horn **(A)**. In spinal ganglia several cells are SP immunoreactive **(B)**. A single SP immunoreactive fiber is seen in the skin penetrating into the epithelium **(C)**. A, ×140; B, ×120; C, ×240. From Hökfelt et al., ref. 23, with permission.

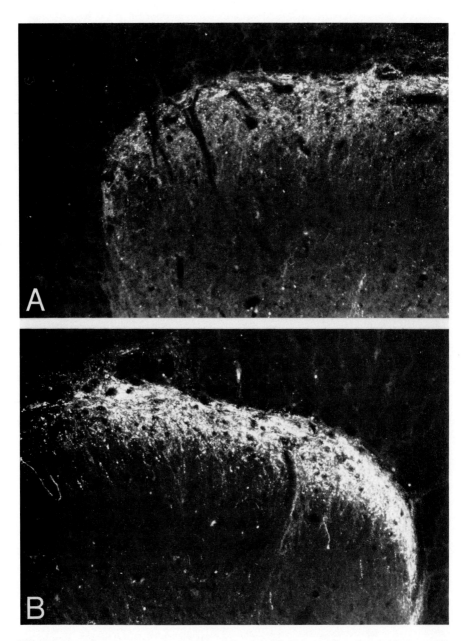

FIG. 3. Immunofluorescence micrographs of the cat dorsal horn after dorsal rhizotomy **(A),** and of control side **(B)** after incubation with SP antiserum. A marked decrease in the number of immunoreactive fibers can be seen on the operated side. ×140. From Hökfelt et al., ref. 25, with permission.

(Fig. 2). In all probability these fibers represent the peripheral branches of primary afferent neurons.

Using lesion technique to establish the connection between cell body groups and nerve terminal areas, SP-positive pathways in the primary sensory neuron have been studied. Thus, after unilateral transection of all dorsal roots below the L4 segment in the cat a marked decrease in SP immunoreactivity was observed in the dorsal, but not in the ventral, horn of the lesion side (Fig. 3). After constriction of peripheral nerves a marked accumulation of SP immunoreactivity was seen on the central side of the lesion (Fig. 4). Total transection of the rat spinal cord at the upper thoracic level did not seem to affect the SP fluorescence in the dorsal horns, while the SP-positive fibers of the ventral horns disappeared. These findings clearly indicate that SP in the first sensory neuron is biosynthesized in the spinal ganglia and migrates from there both in the central and peripheral directions, while most of the SP-positive fibers in the ventral horns arise from supraspinal cell bodies (21). Similarly, nerve fibers in the spinal trigeminal nucleus arise from the trigeminal ganglia (25,41,52).

SP is only one of several peptides present in the spinal cord and spinal ganglia. Thus, neurons containing somatostatin-, enkephalin-, neurotensin- and vasoactive intestinal peptide (VIP)-like immunoreactivity have been identified in the spinal cord (22). All these peptides, except enkephalin and neurotensin, also seem to be present in the spinal ganglia.

An important issue is the possible occurrence of two putative transmitters in the same neuron. Coexistence of 5-hydroxytryptamine (5-HT) and SP has been explored in cell bodies as well as in axons and nerve endings in the lower medulla oblongata (26). The functional significance of the coexistence in the same neurons of one inhibitory (5-HT) and one mainly excitatory (SP) compound is not clear. The storage of two putative neurotransmitters in the same neurons is, however, not unique. Thus, the presence of norepinephrine and somatostatin in peripheral neurons has been described (23) and norepinephrine and enkephalin are both present in ganglion cells (49). Although no coexistence between catecholamine and SP has histochemically been demonstrated, so far, much evidence has been given for a close interaction between these compounds (34).

Numerous studies have been devoted to the presence and action of SP in the spinal cord. Evidence is given for a release of SP during stimulation of the dorsal roots (40) and for a powerful excitatory action of SP on spinal motoneurons (19,39). These results seem to indicate that SP plays a role in the sensory transmission within the spinal cord.

Fewer studies have so far been dedicated to the function of SP in the distal terminals of the first sensory neurons. The presence of SP in cutaneous free nerve endings both around blood vessels and in the epithelium (24), as well as the recent observation of a release of SP from peripheral sensory nerves (see below), suggest that SP might be associated with both vascular and sensory mechanisms in the skin and other tissues.

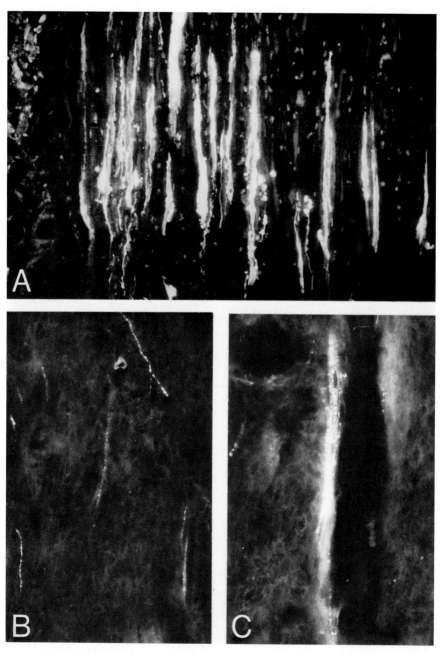

FIG. 4. Immunofluorescence micrographs of the sciatic nerve 24 hr after a ligation **(A)**, and of the dental pulp **(B,C)** after incubation with antiserum to SP. SP-like material accumulates central to the ligation **(A)**. SP immunoreactive fibers are found in the dental pulp, sometimes seemingly unrelated to blood vessels **(B)** and sometimes running close to blood vessels **(C)**. **A**, ×350 and **(B,C)**, ×300.

SP AND THE VASCULAR BED

The recent finding of SP immunoreactivity around blood vessels as well as its extreme vasodilating potency has focused our interest towards the effect and functional significance of SP in the vascular bed.

Thus in several organs, such as in the skin and the tracheobronchial tissue, SP immunoreactive nerve networks have been observed around blood vessels, particularly in the wall of the arteries (50) with a distribution pattern typical for vasomotor nerves. In addition, scattered SP-containing nerves were found in the wall of veins. In the tooth pulp of the cat SP-positive nerve fibers are frequently observed (38), some of them close to blood vessels (Fig. 4). After transection of the inferior alveolar nerve, but not of the cervical sympathetic ganglion, all SP-positive fibers disappeared.

SP is one of the most active vasodilator compounds so far known. Close arterial injections of only a few nanograms of SP significantly increases the blood flow of various vascular beds such as skin, muscle, adipose tissue, and splanchnic area (2,6,15,44). In the tooth pulp close arterial infusion of SP increases blood flow (12). This effect is evidently due to a direct action of SP on the vascular smooth muscle since it is not abolished by atropin, antihistamine, or ganglionic blocking drugs. Moreover, SP causes vasodilation also in the chronically denervated and isolated rabbit ear (27).

Intradermal injections of SP in humans induce flare, wheal, and itching (13), which are inhibited by oral pretreatment of the subjects with antihistamine or compound 48/80. These findings indicate that at least some of the effect of SP in the skin might be mediated by a release of histamine from the dermal mast cells. This conforms with the results of Johnson and Erdös (28), who found that SP was the most potent histamine liberator of a series of synthetic peptides studied.

A hypothetical mode of action of SP in the skin is shown in Fig 5. SP is supposed to stimulate the mast cells to exocytotic release of histamine, which in turn interacts with sensory nerves causing both itch sensation and antidromic vasodilation. In this model SP also serves as a mediator released from neurons involved in the vascular response. Evidences for such a release are given below. This hypothesis is based on the observations of SP immunoreactive fibers both along blood vessels and free in the skin, representing the peripheral branches of primary afferent neurons (25).

Several authors have suggested a role for SP in the regulation of local blood flow and, in particular, in the antidromic reflex vasodilation. It was originally suggested by Dale (3) that a compound, which was liberated at the distal terminals of the sensory neurons and was responsible for the vasodilation during the axon reflex, might also be the transmitter of the central terminals of the same neuron. We now know that SP is transported from the spinal ganglion to both central and peripheral terminals of the first sensory neuron, that it depolarizes the motoneurons, and that it is a potent vasodilator. In the spinal cord SP is released following stimulation of the dorsal roots (39). Similarly, a

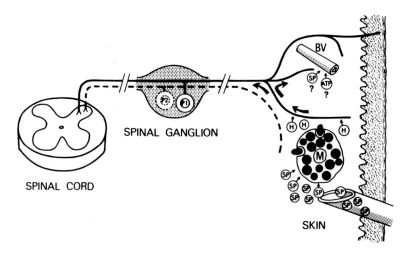

FIG. 5. Schematic drawing of the hypothetical events induced by intradermal injection of synthetic SP. SP releases histamine (H) from mastcells (M). Histamine stimulates peripheral branches of SP-containing primary sensory neurons. Antidromic activation of collaterals of the SP neurons close to blood vessels (BV) causes release of SP reducing vasodilation. ATP, adenosine triphosphate. P1 and P2 indicate two hypothetically separate populations of "pain" (P1) and "itch" (P2) nerves. From Hägermark et al., ref. 13, with permission.

series of observations have been accumulated at our institute during the last years which clearly indicate that SP is released from peripheral, probably sensory, nerve endings in connection to antidromic nerve stimulation. Thus, electric stimulation of the inferior alveolar nerve significantly elevates the concentration of SP immunoreactivity in the superfusate of the dental pulp (37) (Fig. 6). Similarly, electrical or mechanical stimulation of the trigeminal nerve is followed by a release of SP into the aqueous humor of the rabbit eye (1). It was evident that SP appearing in the eye chamber was not derived from blood plasma as a result of increased permeability of the blood-aqueous barrier.

These observations are of interest in relation to the following facts:

SP can be extracted in high amounts from certain tissue layers in the eye (4) as well as from the dental pulp of the cat, dog, and man (36).

SP in the dental pulp is connected to nerve structures, frequently found close to the blood vessels (37).

Close arterial infusion of SP increases pulp blood flow (12), while intracameral injection of SP causes miosis, protein leakage from the blood vessels, and a breakdown of the blood-aqueous barrier (1).

Antidromic stimulation of the inferior alveolar nerve increases the blood flow of the dental pulp (12). Similarly, stimulation of the sensory nerves to the eye elicits effects that are identical with those produced by SP (1).

These observations taken together speak in favor of the hypothesis that SP is involved in the vascular effects induced by sensory nerve stimulation, referred to as the "axon reflex" (32).

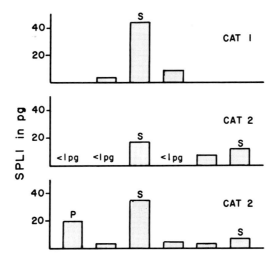

FIG. 6. SP-like immunoreactivity in superfusates of three dental pulps in adult cats. Each column represents the immunoreactivity expressed as amount of SP in picograms. S represents superfusates collected following stimulation of the inferior alveolar nerve. The superfusate indicated by P was collected immediately after preparation of the tooth. Other columns represent control periods. From Olgart et al., ref. 37, with permission.

SP has also been implicated with nociception and it has been suggested that distal nerve terminals of the first sensory neurons conveying pain release SP (18). A relationship between SP and pain was observed in 1953 when Hellauer (17) showed that local application of SP to the cornea produced a burning sensation. Similarly, intraarterial injection of SP provoked visceral pain in the lightly anesthetized dog (46). The observations by Lembeck and co-workers on the rabbit ear, isolated except for the afferent innervation, suggest that SP is released from the distal terminals of nociceptive fibers (29,31). This suggestion was supported by the findings that SP had an excitatory effect on spinal units responding specifically to noxious radiant heat applied to the skin and that it facilitates the response of these nociceptive units to the noxious stimulus (18). This evidence strongly suggests that SP is involved in the central transmission of pain. The hypothesis is further supported by the finding that the SP immunoactive nerves found in the skin are unmyelinated fibers of small diameter (25).

GASTROINTESTINAL TRACT

Another organ with a very dense SPergic innervation is the gut. Already in their original publication, Euler and Gaddum (10) presented SP as a normal constituent of extracts from intestine. Later studies have shown that SP is widely distributed in all segments and tissue layers of the mammalian gut (39). SP immunofluorescence is observed in numerous nerve fibers of the myenteric plexus both in the small intestine and in the colon. These fibers form a dense network around the cell bodies of the plexus and extend between bundles of smooth muscle. Evidence that SP in the gut is also connected to the nervous structures, notably in the Auerbach's plexus, was already given in 1952 when Ehrenpreis and Pernow (5) observed that in patients with Hirschsprung's disease (megacolon), the concentration of SP was much reduced in the inactive aganglionic segment of the rectosigmoid colon, while the proximal hyperactive part contained more SP than is normally present. Tafuri et al. (51) suggested that SP may be associated with granular vesicles seen in axon profiles from Auerbach's plexus.

Pearse and Polak (42) showed that cell bodies of both Auerbach's and Meissner's plexus react with antibodies of synthetic SP, whereas Nilsson et al. (36) were unable to identify SP immunoreactive cell bodies in the gut. More recently, strong evidence has been obtained for the existence of SP immunoreactive cell bodies in all parts of the gastrointestinal tract (48). These findings indicate that the majority of SP-positive fibers originate within the gut, but some may belong to primary sensory neurons.

SP immunoreactivity is present not only in the intrinsic nervous system of the gut but also in nerves innervating the gut. Thus extracts of the vagus nerve contain SP (10,43). Recently Lundberg et al. (35) and Gamse et al. (11) have shown by immunohistochemical technique that SP fibers account for a considerable proportion of the axons in the rat, guinea pig, and cat vagus nerve. Most of these fibers seem to be unmyelinated. Ligation of the cervical part of the vagus led to an accumulation of SP immunofluorescence central to the ligature, indicating a rapid axon transport (35). SP immunoreactive cell bodies have been observed in both the nodose and jugular ganglia (35).

In view of the presence of SP in vagal nerves, it is of special interest to note that SP is released into the central lumen of the cat stomach in response to electrical vagal stimulation (53). The same effect, which runs parallel to a release of gastrin, somatostatin, and VIP, is induced also by acetylcholine given intravenously or into the antrum. Since SP has not been observed in mucosal cells proximal to the pylorus, this finding seems to indicate a migration of SP from submucosal layers to reach the lumen. The finding of a release of several peptides in the stomach by both nervous activities and hormonal agents is of interest in the discussion of the possible significance of these peptides for the atropin-resistant vagal stimulation of secretion and motility.

Also present in the inferior mesenteric ganglion is a network of SP immunoreactive fibers, probably of a sensory nature (7). Like the spinal ganglion, the mesenteric ganglion contains several other peptide neurons besides SP. The same is true for other ganglia, particularly in the gastrointestinal tract.

Besides the nervous tissue, SP immunoreactivity has been found in endocrine cells of the intestinal mucosa. These cells occur predominantly in the proximal part of the small intestine and have a distribution which is similar to that of the enterochromaffin cells containing 5-HT (49). This view is favored by the observation of a high SP concentration in carcinoid tumor cells as well as in blood from carcinoid patients (14).

Although SP is a neurotropic compound, the site of its action on the intestinal wall seems to be exclusively on the smooth muscle. This is evident from the findings that morphine and tetrodotoxin do not affect the dose-response relationship of SP on the isolated gut (47). As was shown by Hedquist and von Euler (16), SP enhances the contraction response of the isolated guinea pig ileum to transmural nerve stimulation, while SP only weakly affected contractions induced by acetylcholine. Since the contractions induced by this type of stimulation are blocked by atropine, but not by α- or β-adrenergic blocking agents, these findings seem to suggest a prejunctional stimulating action of SP.

It has been postulated that SP plays a part in the control of the intestinal motility (9,43). These suggestions were entirely based on the presence of SP predominantly in those parts of the intestine showing the highest degree of motility and on the very high potency of SP in contracting intestinal preparations. The theory was supported by the above-mentioned findings in Hirschsprung's disease (5) and by evidence that the SP concentration of human intestinal segments was raised when motility was increased following the administration of hypertonic glucose (45). The observation of a release of SP following vagal stimulation, which is known to increase intestinal motility, is of particular interest in this respect. However, further studies are needed before the relation of SP to motility can be further clarified.

REFERENCES

1. Bill, A., Stjernschantz, J., Mandahl, A., Brodin, E., and Nilsson, G. (1979): Substance P: Release on trigeminal nerve stimulation effects in the eye. *Acta Physiol. Scand.,* 106:371–373.
2. Burcher, E., Atterhög, J. H., Pernow, B., and Rosell, S. (1977): Cardiovascular effects of substance P: Effects on the heart and regional blood flow in the dog. In: *Substance P,* edited by U. S. von Euler and B. Pernow, pp. 261–268. Raven Press, New York.
3. Dale, H. M. (1935): Pharmacology and nerve endings. *Proc. R. Soc. Med.,* 28:319–332.
4. Dunér, H., Euler, U. S. von, and Pernow, B. (1954): Catecholamines and substance P in mammalian eye. *Acta Physiol. Scand.,* 31:113–118.
5. Ehrenpreis, T., and Pernow, B. (1952/53): On the occurence of substance P in the rectosigmoid in Hirschsprung's disease. *Acta Physiol. Scand.,* 27:380–388.
6. Eklund, B., Jogestrand, T., and Pernow, B. (1976): Effect of substance P on resistance and capacitance vessels in the human forearm. In: *Substance P,* edited by U. S. von Euler and B. Pernow, pp. 275–286. Raven Press, New York.
7. Elfvin, L. G., and Dalsgaard, C. J. (1977): Retrograde axonal transport of horseradish peroxidase in afferent fibers of the inferior mesenteric ganglion of the guinea-pig. Identification of the cells of origin in dorsal root ganglia. *Brain. Res.* 126:149–153.
8. Euler, U. S. von, and Gaddum, J. H. (1931): An unidentified depressor substance in certain tissue extracts. *J. Physiol. (Lond.),* 72:74–87.
9. Euler, U. S. von (1936): Untersuchungen über Substanz P, die atropinfeste, darmerregende und gefässerweiternde Substanz aus Darm und Gehirn. *Naunyn Schmiedebergs Arch. Exp. Pathol. Pharmakol.,* 181:181–193.
10. Euler, U. S. von (1963): Substance P in subcellular particles in peripheral nerves. *Ann. NY Acad. Sci.,* 104:449–461.
11. Gamse, R., Lembeck, F., and Cuello, A. C. (1979): Substance P in the vagus nerve. Immunochemical and immunohistochemical evidence for axoplasmic transport. *Naunyn Schmiedebergs Arch. Pharmakol.,* 306:37–44.
12. Gazelius, B., Olgart, L., Edwall, L., and Trowbridge, H. O. (1977): Effect of substance P on sensory nerves and blood flow in the feline dental pulp. In: *Pain in the Trigeminal Region,* edited by Anderson and Matthews, pp. 95–101. Elsevier/North Holland, Amsterdam.

13. Hägermark, Ö., Hökfelt, T., and Pernow, B. (1978): Flare and itch induced by substance P in human skin. *J. Invest. Dermatol.,* 71:233–235.
14. Håkansson, R., Bergmark, S., Brodin, E., Ingemansson, S., Larsson, L.-I., Nilsson, G., and Sundler, F. (1977): Substance P-like immunoreactivity in intestinal carcinoid tumors. In: *Substance P,* edited by U. S. von Euler and B. Pernow, pp. 55–58. Raven Press, New York.
15. Hallberg, D., and Pernow, B. (1975): Effect of substance P on various vascular beds in the dog. *Acta Physiol. Scand.,* 93:277–285.
16. Hedquist, P., and Euler, U. S. von (1977): Effects of substance P on some autonomic neuroeffector junctions. In: *Substance P,* edited by U. S. von Euler and B. Pernow, pp. 89–95. Raven Press, New York.
17. Hellauer, H. (1953): Zur Charakterisierung der Erregungssubstanz sensibler Nerven. *Arch. Exp. Pathol. Pharmakol.,* 219:234–241.
18. Henry, J. L. (1977): Substance P and pain. A possible relation to afferent transmission. In: *Substance P,* edited by U. S. von Euler and B. Pernow, pp. 231–240. Raven Press, New York.
19. Henry, J. L., Krnjevic, K., and Morris, M. E. (1975): Substance P and spinal neurones. *Can. J. Physiol. Pharmacol.,* 53:423.
20. Hökfelt, T., Elfvin, L. G., Elde, R., Schultzberg, M., Goldstein, M., and Luft, R. (1977): Occurrence of somatostatin-like immunoreactivity in some peripheral sympathetic noradrenergic neurons. *Proc. Natl. Acad. Sci. USA,* 74:3587–3591.
21. Hökfelt, T., Johansson, O., Kellerth, J.-O., Ljungdahl, Å., Nilsson, G., Nygård, A., and Pernow, B. (1977): Immunohistochemical distribution of substance P. In: *Substance P,* edited by U. S. von Euler and B. Pernow, pp. 117–145. Raven Press, New York.
22. Hökfelt, T., Johansson, O., Ljungdahl, Å., Lundberg, J., Schultzberg, M., Fuxe, K., Pernow, B., and Goldstein, M. Peptide neurons. In: Brain Peptides: A New Endocrinology, edited by A. M. Gotto, Jr., E. J. Peck, Jr., and A. E. Boyd III, pp. 5–25. Elsevier/North Holland, Amsterdam.
23. Hökfelt. T., Kellerth. J.-O., Elde, R., Luft, R., Johansson O., Nilsson, G., Pernow, B., and Arimura, A. (1976): Immunohistochemical studies on the distribution of substance P and somatostatin in primary sensory neurons. *Sensory Functions of the Skin,* edited by Y. Zotterman, pp. 583–602. Pergamon, Oxford.
24. Hökfelt, T., Kellerth, J.-O., Nilsson, G., and Pernow B. (1975): Substance P: Localization in the central nervous system and in some primary sensory neurons. *Science,* 190:889–890.
25. Hökfelt, T., Kellerth, J.-O., Nilsson, G., and Pernow B. (1975): Experimental immunohistochemical studies on the localization and distribution of substance P in cat primary sensory neurons. *Brain Res.,* 100:235–252.
26. Hökfelt, T., Ljungdahl, Å., Steinbusch, H., Verhofstad, A., Nilsson, G., Brodin, E., Pernow, B., and Goldstein, M. (1978): Immunohistochemical evidence of substance P-like immunoreactivity in some 5-hydroxytryptamine containing neurons in the rat central nervous system. *Neuroscience,* 3:517–538.
27. Holton, F. A., and Holton, P. (1952): The vasodilator activity of spinal roots. *J. Physiol.* (Lond.), 118:310
28. Johnson, A., and Erdös, E. G. (1973): Release of histamine from mast cells by vasoactive peptides. *Proc. Soc. Exp. Biol. Med.,* 142:1252–1256.
29. Juan, H., and Lembeck, F. (1974): Action of peptides and other algesic agents on paravascular pain receptors of the isolated perfused rabbit ear. *Naunyn Schmiedebergs Arch. Pharmakol.,* 283:151–164.
30. Lembeck, F. (1953): Zur Frage der zentralen übertragung afferenten Impulse, III Mitteilung. Das Vorkommen und die Bedeutung der Substanz P in der dorsalen Wurzeln des Rüchenmarks. *Naunyn Schmiedebergs Arch. Pharmakol.,* 219:197–213.
31. Lembeck, F. (1957): Zur Frage der zentralen übertragung afferenten Impulse. *Naunyn Schmiedebergs Arch. Pharmakol.,* 230:1–9.
32. Lembeck, F., Gamse, R., and Juan, H. (1977): Substance P and sensory nerve endings. In: *Substance P,* edited by U. S. von Euler and B. Pernow, pp. 169–182. Raven Press, New York.
33. Ljungdahl, Å., Hökfelt, T., and Nilsson, G. (1978): Distribution of substance P-like immunoreactivity in the central nervous system of the rat—I. Cell bodies and nerve terminals. *Neuroscience,* 3:861–943.
34. Ljungdahl, Å., Hökfelt, T. Nilsson, G., and Goldstein, M. (1978): Distribution of substance P-like immunoreactivity in the central nervous system of the rat—II. Light microscopic localization in relation to catecholamine-containing neurons. *Neuroscience,* 3:945–976.

35. Lundberg, J. M., Hökfelt, T., Nilsson, G., Terenius, L., Rehfeld, J., Elde, R., and Said, S. (1978): Peptide neurons in the vagus splanchnic and sciatic nerves. *Acta Physiol. Scand.,* 104:499–501.

36. Nilsson, G., Larsson, L.-I., Håkansson, R., Brodin, E., Pernow, B., and Sundler, F. (1975): Localization of substance P-like immunoreactivity in the mouse gut. *Histochemistry,* 43:97–99.

37. Olgart, L., Gazelius, B., Brodin, E., and Nilsson, G. (1977): Release of substance P-like immunoreactivity from the dental pulp. *Acta Physiol. Scand.,* 101:510–512.

38. Olgart, L., Hökfelt, T., Nilsson, G., and Pernow, B. (1977): Localization of substance P-like immunoreactivity in nerves in the tooth pulp. *Pain,* 4:153–159.

39. Otsuka, M., and Konishi, S. (1976): Substance P and excitatory transmitter of primary sensory neurons. *Cold Spring Harbor Symp. Quant. Biol.,* 40:135–143.

40. Otsuka, M., and Konishi, S. (1976): Release of substance P-like immunoreactivity from isolated spinal and of newborn rat. *Nature,* 264:83.

41. Otsuka, M., Konishi, S., and Takahashi, T. (1975): Hypothalamic substance P as a candidate for transmitter of primary afferent neurons. *Fed. Proc.,* 34:1922–1928.

42. Pearse, A. G. E., and Polak, J. M. (1975): Immunocytochemical localization of substance P in mammalian intestine. *Histochemistry,* 41:373.

43. Pernow, B. (1953): Studies on substance P. Purification, occurrence and biological actions. *Acta Physiol. Scand.,* 105, (Suppl. 29): 1–90.

44. Pernow, B., and Rosell, S. (1975): Effect of substance P on blood flow in canine adipose tissue and skeletal muscle. *Acta Physiol. Scand.,* 93:139–141.

45. Pernow, B., and Wallensten, S. (1961): The relationship between substance P and the motility of the small intestine in man. International Symposium on SP, Sarajevo, edited by P. Stern. *Proc. Sci. Soc. Bosnia Herzegovina,* I:57.

46. Potter, G. D., Guzman, F., Lim, R. K. S. (1962): Visceral pain evolved by intra-arterial injection of substance P. *Nature (New Biol.)* 193:983–984.

47. Rosell, S., Björkroth, U., Chang, D., Vamaguchi, I., Wan, Y.-P., Rackur, G., Fisher, G., and Folkers, K. (1977): Effects of substance P and analogs on isolated guinea-pig ileum. In: *Substance P,* edited by U. S. von Euler and B. Pernow, pp. 83–88. Raven Press, New York.

48. Schultzberg, M., Dreyfus, C. F., Gershon, M. D., Hökfelt, T., Elde, R. P., Nilsson, G., Said, S., and Goldstein, M. (1978): VIP-, enkephalin-, substance P- and somatostatin-like immunoreactivity in neurons intrinsic to the intestine: Immunohistochemical evidence from organotypic tissue cultures. *Brain Res.,* 155:239–248.

49. Schultzberg, M., Hökfelt, T., Terenius, L., Elfvin, L. G., Lundberg, J. M., Brandt, J., Elde, R., and Goldstein, M. (1979): Enkephalin immunoreactive nerve fibers and cell bodies in synthetic ganglia of the guinea-pig and rat. *Neuroscience,* 4:249–270.

50. Sundler, F., Alumets, J., Brodin, E., Kahlberg, K., and Nilsson, G. (1977): Perivascular substance P-immunoreactive nerves in tracheobronchial tissue. In: *Substance P,* edited by U. S. von Euler and B. Pernow, pp. 271–274. Raven Press, New York.

51. Tefuru, W. A., Maria, T. A., Pittella, J. E. H., and Bogliolo, L. (1974): An electron microscope study of the Auerbach plexus and determination of substance P of the colon in Hirschsprung's disease. *Virchows Arch. (Pathol. Anat. Histol.),* 362:41–53.

52. Takahashi, T., and Otsuka, M. (1975): Regional distribution of substance P in the spinal cord and nerve roots of the cat and the effect of dorsal root section. *Brain Res.,* 87:1–11.

53. Uvnäs-Wallensten, K. (1978): Release of substance P-like immunoreactivity into the antral lumen of cats. *Acta Physiol. Scand.,* 104:464–468.

Neuropeptides and Neural Transmission,
edited by C. Ajmone Marsan and W. Z. Traczyk.
Raven Press, New York © 1980.

Binding Sites of Substance P in Brain Tissue

Norbert Mayer, Alois Saria, and Fred Lembeck

*Institute of Experimental and Clinical Pharmacology, University of Graz,
A-8010 Graz, Austria*

Substance P (SP) was found in synaptosomes by bioassay (13), radioimmunoassay (27), and immunohistochemical investigations (17). The release of SP from synaptosomes (14,27) as well as from brain or spinal cord slices (9,23) could be induced by high potassium concentrations or field stimulation. SP was visualized immunohistochemically within the nerve ending in large synaptic vesicles of a diameter of 60 to 80 nm (3,25). SP binding to phospholipids has been demonstrated and SP can be extracted from brain tissue in a phospholipid bound form (15). It was suggested that phospholipids could be involved in SP storage. An adapted lipid extraction method was used to separate synaptic vesicle bound ^{125}I-Tyr^8-SP from free tracer. Using this method to investigate binding of radiolabeled SP, high affinity binding sites were found on synaptic vesicles (20). Hydrophobic structures are assumed to be involved in binding, because SP binding sites can be extracted by unpolar solvents. Experiments were performed to investigate the chemical nature and possible function of SP binding sites in synaptic vesicles.

METHODS

Preparation of Synaptic Vesicles and Plasma Membranes

Rats (Sprague-Dawley, 200–300 g) were killed by a blow on the neck. Brains and spinal cords were removed and placed on ice. For some experiments, the brains were dissected according to Glowinski and Iversen (6). Dorsal and ventral roots of spinal cord were separated. All further handling was carried out at 4°C.

Synaptic vesicles were prepared by differential centrifugation (4). Plasma membranes were prepared from whole brains by the flotation method (11). Purity and homogeneity of synaptic vesicles and plasma membrane preparations were ascertained by electron microscopy and by estimation of the marker enzymes acetylcholinesterase, Na$^+$K$^+$-stimulated adenosinetriphosphatase, and Mg^{2+}-stimulated adenosinetriphosphatase (5,7). Protein was measured by the method of Lowry et al. (19). Phosphorus was determined according to Bartlett (2).

Binding Assay

Synaptic vesicles corresponding to 10 μg protein and plasma membranes corresponding to 80 μg protein were incubated in a final volume of 1 ml 0.03 M sodium phosphate buffer at pH 6 or in 50 mM Tris(hydroxymethyl)aminomethane-HCl at pH 7.2 (20). ^{125}I-Tyr[8]-SP (600 Ci/mmole) prepared according to Mroz et al. (21), was added to the incubates as described in Results. Substances investigated for interaction with ^{125}I-Tyr[8]-SP binding were added in solutions of identical ionic strength and pH. In the experiments investigating the influence of pH on binding, 0.1 M glycine-HCl buffer was used for incubation below pH 4. The stability of ^{125}I-Tyr[8]-SP during incubation was ascertained by gel filtration and thin layer chromatography on silica gel plates.

At the end of incubation the aqueous medium was extracted with petroleum

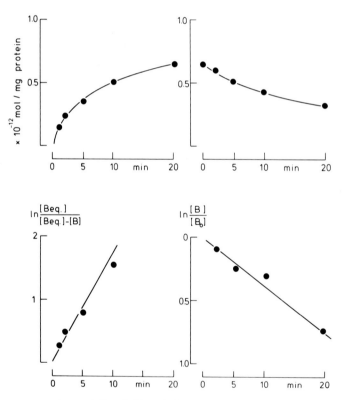

FIG. 1. Time course of association **(left)** and dissociation **(right)** of ^{125}I-Tyr[8]-SP binding to synaptic vesicles. ^{125}I-Tyr[8]-SP (0.25 nM) was incubated at 30°C, with synaptic vesicles corresponding to 12 μg protein. Binding (B) was measured at the times indicated at the *abscissa*. Dissociation was made visible by addition of 10^{-5} M unlabeled SP after reaching equilibrium in 20 min. The reactions were linearized according to a pseudo first reaction as mentioned above. Each point represents the mean of a triplicate experiment. Reproduced from Mayer et al., ref. 2, with permission of the editor.

ether-chloroform (2:1). Since in the absence of synaptic vesicles all ^{125}I-Tyr^8-SP could be recovered in the aqueous phase, radioactivity transferred to the organic solvent was assumed to be bound to synaptic vesicles.

RESULTS

Synaptic Vesicle Preparation

It was shown by electron microscopy that the synaptic vesicle preparation contained predominantly synaptic vesicles of different shape that were between 20 and 80 nm in diameter. The preparation was contaminated by a few large membrane particles. Measurements of the activity of marker enzymes showed the following results: The activity of acetylcholinesterase was 11-fold higher in plasma membranes than in the vesicle preparation; the ratio between Na$^+$K$^+$-stimulated adenosinetriphosphatase and Mg^{2+}-stimulated adenosinetriphosphatase was 22 in plasma membranes and 0.03 in synaptic vesicles.

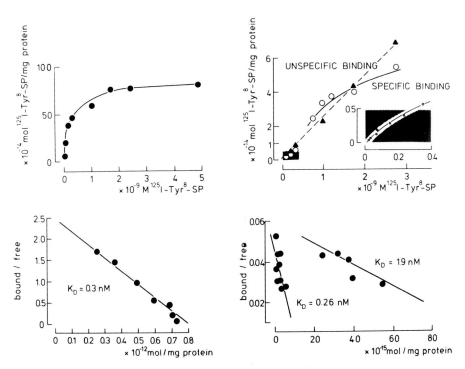

FIG. 2. Specific ^{125}I-Tyr^8-SP binding to synaptic vesicle preparations **(left)** and plasma membrane preparations **(right)**. Experiments were performed under equilibrium conditions. The binding was measured at increasing concentrations of ^{125}I-Tyr^8-SP. Synaptic vesicles (12 μg protein/ml) and plasma membranes (84 μg/ml protein were incubated at 30°C for 20 min. **Bottom:** Scatchard plot of the data. Each point represents the mean of a triplicate experiment. Reproduced partially from Mayer et al., ref. 2, with permission of the editor.

Kinetics of ^{125}I-Tyr[8]-SP Binding to Synaptic Vesicles and Plasma Membranes

The time course of ^{125}I-Tyr[8]-SP binding to synaptic vesicles was investigated. Termination of incubation after different times showed that the binding approached equilibrium after 20 min, and obeyed the kinetics of a pseudo first-order reaction (Fig. 1). Dissociation of ^{125}I-Tyr[8]-SP was demonstrated by addition of 10^{-5} M unlabeled SP after reaching equilibrium at 20 min. The rate constant of association ($k_1 = 6.6 \times 10^6$ M^{-1} sec^{-1}) and the rate constant of dissociation ($k_{-1} = 6.4 \times 10^{-4}$ sec^{-1}) resulted in a dissociation constant $K_D = k_{-1}/k_1 = 0.1$ nM (23).

For more precise determination of the K_D the incubation was performed under equilibrium conditions with increasing concentrations of ^{125}I-Tyr[8]-SP between 0.01 and 5 nM (Fig. 2). The Scatchard analysis (30) of these data gave a K_D of 0.3 nM and a number of binding sites of 800 fmoles per mg protein. Plasma membranes incubated with 0.01 to 3.7 nM ^{125}I-Tyr[8]-SP showed a K_D of 1.9 nM and 90 fmoles binding sites per mg protein (Fig. 2). Plasma membrane binding sites were therefore considered different from the binding sites found on synaptic vesicles.

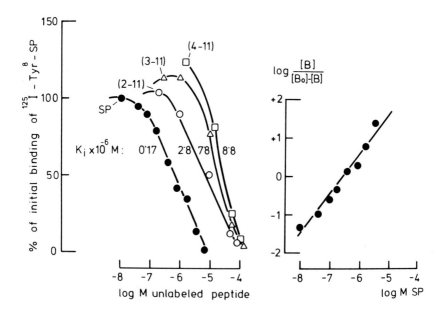

FIG. 3. Left: Incubation of the binding of 10^{-9} M ^{125}I-Tyr[8]-SP to synaptic vesicles by unlabeled SP *(closed circles)*, (2-11)-decapeptide *(open circles)*, (3-11)-nonapeptide *(triangles)*, and (4-11)-octapeptide *(squares)*. Binding *(ordinate)* is expressed as the percentage of initial binding of ^{125}I-Tyr[8]-SP in the absence of the unlabeled peptides. **Right:** Hill plot of competition for ^{125}I-Tyr[8]-SP binding sites by unlabeled SP. B is the amount of ^{125}I-Tyr[8]-SP bound. (B_0) is the measured number of binding sites. Each point is the mean of duplicate or triplicate experiments. Reproduced from Mayer et al., ref. 2, with permission of the editor.

When ^{125}I-Tyr[8]-SP was added to plasma membranes in the lowest concentrations (0.01–0.3 nM), Scatchard analysis revealed a K_D of 0.26 nM, i.e., similar to that of the synaptic vesicle preparation, but a very low number of binding sites (9 fmoles/mg protein). This apparently seems to represent a contamination of the plasma membrane preparation with some synaptic vesicles.

The specificity of ^{125}I-Tyr[8]-SP binding was investigated by addition of increasing amounts of unlabeled SP (2-11)-deca, (3-11)-nona, and (4-11)-octa SP (Fig. 3). These C-terminal SP analogs showed decreasing affinity to SP binding sites on synaptic vesicles in correspondence to the length of the chain. A Hill plot of the displacement of ^{125}I-Tyr[8]-SP by unlabeled SP showed slight cooperativity with a Hill coefficient of 1.33. Eledoisin, uperolein, and neurotensin had only weak or no affinity to the SP binding sites on synaptic vesicles.

Regional Distribution of Binding Sites in Brain Tissue

The density of synaptic vesicle binding sites within the brain and spinal cord was found to be uneven (medulla oblongata, midbrain, hypothalamus, corpus striatum, cortex, and cerebellum) (Fig. 4). This is in positive correlation with the SP content of these brain regions. A similar relationship was observed in spinal cord and in dorsal and ventral roots (Table 1).

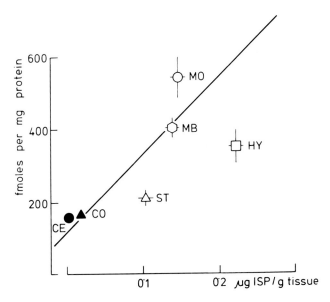

FIG. 4. Correlation between SP content of different brain regions, measured by radioimmunoassay and maximal number of binding sites, located on synaptic vesicles. CO, cortex; CE, cerebellum; ST, corpus striatum; MB, midbrain; MO, medulla oblongata; and HY, hypothalamus. *Abscissa:* Sp immunoreactivity; *ordinate:* maximum binding. The drawn straight line was calculated from linear regression without data from the hypothalamus.

TABLE 1. *Maximum binding and affinity of* ^{125}I-Tyr^8-*SP binding to synaptic vesicles of rat spinal cord, dorsal roots, and ventral roots*[a]

Regions	Max. binding (fmoles/mg prot.)	K_D (nM)
Dorsal roots	358 ± 12	0.26 ± 0.02
Ventral roots	105 ± 6	0.56 ± 0.04
Spinal cord	339 ± 14	0.43 ± 0.03

[a] $\bar{x} \pm s_{\bar{x}}$, N = 3).

Ionic Influences on the Binding

The binding of ^{125}I-Tyr^8-SP was found to be pH dependent, showing a minimum at pH 2.0 and a maximum at pH 7. Ca^{2+} and Mg^{2+} (1 mM) decreased the binding of ^{125}I-Tyr^8-SP to synaptic vesicles (Fig. 5), whereas Na^+ and K^+ decreased the binding only in concentrations higher than 10 mM (Fig. 6). Addition of 1 mM ethylenediaminetetraacetic acid (EDTA) and 1 mM ethyleneglycolbis-(aminoethyl)-*N,N,N',N'*-tetraacetic acid (EGTA) resulted in an increase of binding to synaptic vesicles (Fig. 6); it is assumed from these results that the binding is very sensitive to alterations of Ca^{2+} or Mg^{2+} concentration. The influence of Ca^{2+} and Mg^{2+} was noncompetitive as seen by Scatchard analysis (Fig. 7); the affinity of binding sites remained unchanged.

Biochemical Characteristics of the Binding

Some experiments were performed to investigate the biochemical nature of the binding site. Preincubation of synaptic vesicles with 0.5 mM *N*-ethyl maleim-

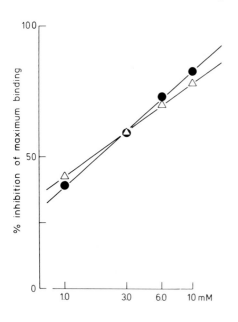

FIG. 5. Influence of Ca^{2+} and Mg^{2+} on specific ^{125}I-Tyr^8-SP binding to synaptic vesicles. *Abscissa:* concentration of both divalent cations. *Ordinate:* diminution of 100% maximal binding. *Circles,* Ca^{2+}; *Triangles,* Mg^{2+}. Each point represents the mean of five experiments.

pmol / mg protein

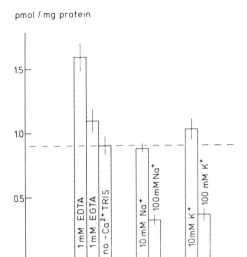

FIG. 6. Influence of EGTA, EDTA, Na+, and K+ in indicated concentrations on maximum binding of ^{125}I-Tyr^8-SP to synaptic vesicles from whole rat brain. Each bar represents the mean ± SEM of five experiments.

ide and 5 mM monoiodoacetic acid had no influence on the binding of SP to synaptic vesicles, indicating that SH-groups were not involved in the binding (Fig. 8). Preincubation of synaptic vesicles with phospholipases A$_2$, C, and D and with trypsin led to a total loss of binding activity (Fig. 8).

DISCUSSION

The presence of a specific binding of SP within the synaptic region was investigated. Such binding sites may be considered as receptor or as storage sites,

B / F

[mg protein / l] × 10^{-3}

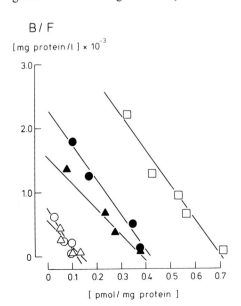

[pmol / mg protein]

FIG. 7. Scatchard plots of specific ^{125}I-Tyr^8-SP binding to synaptic vesicles in the presence of 1 mM *(closed circles)* and 10 mM *(open circles)* Ca$^{2\pm}$, and 1 mM *(closed triangles)* and 10 mM *(open triangles)* Mg$^{2\pm}$; controls *(squares)*. Each point represents the mean of triplicate experiments.

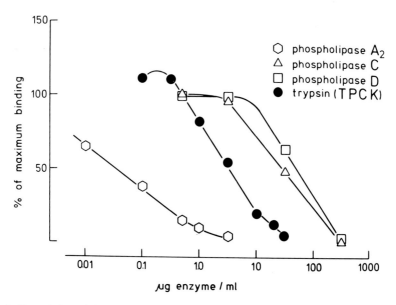

FIG. 8. Degradation of the binding sites for specific ^{125}I-Tyr^8-SP binding to synaptic vesicles by preincubation with different enzymes: Trypsin (TPCK treated 3.5 U/mg), phospholipase A_2 (800 U/mg), phospholipase C (54 U/mg), and phospholipase D (20 U/mg). In the case of phospholipase D, 5 mM EDTA was added after preincubation to inactivate the added essential Ca^{2+} (5 mM).

depending on their binding characteristics and subcellular distribution. Since binding of SP to phospholipids in brain lipid extracts was observed earlier (15), an involvement of phospholipids in the specific binding to synaptic vesicles and plasma membranes seemed likely. Other biologically active substances, like serotonin (10), opiates (18), and acetylcholine (28), were also shown to be bound to phospholipids or proteolipids. A lipid extraction method (see introductory remarks) was applied to remove bound SP from the incubate.

Nakata et al. (22) reported a specific binding of SP on crude synaptic membranes with a K_D of 2.74 nM. Our experiments show a high affinity site (K_D = 0.3 nM) on synaptic vesicles, which may be regarded as a storage site, and a low affinity site (K_D = 1.9 nM) in plasma membranes, which might possibly represent a receptor site. The view of a storage site on synaptic vesicles is supported by the positive correlation between SP concentrations and the number of high affinity binding sites in different regions of the central nervous system. The presence of a small number of high affinity binding sites in plasma membrane preparations might be explained by a contamination of plasma membranes with synaptic vesicles.

The rate constants of association and dissociation for ^{125}I-Tyr^8-SP binding to synaptic vesicles ($k_1 = 6.6 \times 10^6$ moles^{-1} sec^{-1} and $k_{-1} = 6.4 \times 10^{-4}$ sec^{-1}) were comparable to those found by Kitabgi et al. (12) in the specific neurotensin binding to plasma membranes. Since the SP concentration of about 3 ng/mg protein in synaptic vesicles (3) is even higher than the K_D value (0.3 nM), a high occupancy of these binding sites can be expected *in vivo*. The binding capacity of nearly 1 pmole/mg protein is high enough to bind the most part of endogenous SP. These facts favor the assumption of a storage function of binding sites located on synaptic vesicles.

Information on the biochemical nature of the binding site was obtained by preincubation of synaptic vesicles with different hydrolytic enzymes. Trypsin was able to destroy the binding ability, indicating a protein involved in binding, which is in agreement with the specificity inferred from the displacement data. Preincubation with N-ethyl-maleimide (NEM) (0.5 mM) and monoiodoacetic acid (5 mM) exclude involvement of SH groups in binding. In contrast, opiate binding sites were inhibited by SH group blockers (24). Since all phospholipases used were able to destroy the binding ability, phospholipids as constituents of the binding site or the importance of the phospholipid environment can be assumed. The SP binding to phospholipids is sensitive to alterations of pH and ionic environment indicating ionic interactions (16). A similar sensitivity was found in the binding of ^{125}I-Tyr^8-SP to synaptic vesicles. It is not unlikely that cations interact at a phospholipid part of the binding site.

The alterations of binding characteristics by Ca^{2+} and Mg^{2+} may be seen in connection with the SP release from this assumed storage site. Some speculations on this release can be added. The K^+-induced release of SP from slices or synaptosomes was shown to be Ca^{2+} dependent (9,14,23,27). Concentrations less than 1 mM Ca^{2+} or Mg^{2+} already decreased the binding of SP to synaptic vesicles. These concentrations are expected within the nerve ending [10 μM ionized Ca^{2+} (1)]. Complete removal of Ca^{2+} or Mg^{2+} from synaptic vesicles increased the binding. The capacity of synaptic vesicles to bind SP is therefore highly dependent on minute changes of the cation concentrations in their environment. Recently, Ca^{2+} binding sites which might regulate transmitter release were found on synaptic vesicles (9). The K_D of these binding sites (2 mM) is comparable with the IC_{50} value for the inhibition of ^{125}I-Tyr^8-SP binding to synaptic vesicles by Ca^{2+}.

SP binding sites on synaptic vesicles are therefore assumed to be involved in storage and release mechanism which could be modulated by alteration of the concentration of Ca^{2+} and Mg^{2+}. The definition of binding sites on plasma membranes remains uncertain at present and requires further experiments.

ACKNOWLEDGMENTS

This study was supported by the Austrian Scientific Research Funds Grant No. 3.400 and by the Austrian National Bank Funds Grant No 1.293. For electron microscopy we thank Dr. M. Pabst from the Institute of Histology and Embryology, University of Graz, Austria.

REFERENCES

1. Baker, P. F. (1972): Transport and metabolism of calcium ions in nerve. *Progr. Mol. Biophys. Biol.,* 24:177–223.
2. Bartlett, G. R. (1958): Phosphorous assay in column chromatography. *J. Biol. Chem.,* 234:466–468.
3. Cuello, A. C., Jessell, T. M., Kanazawa, I., and Iversen, L. L. (1977): Substance P: Localization in synaptic vesicles in rat central nervous system. *J. Neurochem.,* 29:747–781.
4. De Robertis, E., Rodriguez de Lores Arneiz, G., Salganicoff, L., Pellegrino de Iraldi, A., and Zieher, L. M. (1963): Isolation of synaptic vesicles and structural organization of the acetylcholine system within brain nerve endings. *J. Neurochem.,* 10:225–235.
5. Ellman, G. L., Courtney, K. D., Andres, V., Jr., and Featherstone, R. M. (1961): A new and rapid colorimetric determination of acetylcholinesterase activity. *Biochem. Pharmacol.,* 7:88–95.
6. Glowinski, J., and Iversen, L. L. (1966): Regional studies of catecholamines in the rat brain. 1. The disposition of 3H-norepinephrine, 3H-dopamine and 3H-DOPA in various regions of the brain. *J. Neurochem.,* 13:655–669.
7. Hosie, R. J. A. (1965): The localization of adenosine triphosphatases in morphologically characterized subcellular fractions of guinea-pig brain. *Biochem. J.,* 96:404–412.
8. Hoss, W., Okumura, K., Formaniak, M., and Tanaka, R. (1979): Relation of cation binding sites on synaptic vesicles to opiate action. *Life Sci.,* 24:1003–1010.
9. Iversen, L. L., Jessel, J., and Kanazawa, J. (1976): Release and metabolism of substance P in rat hypothalamus. *Nature,* 264:81.
10. Johnson, D. A., Cho, T. M., and Loh, H. H. (1977): Identification of 5-hydroxytryptamine binding substances from rat brain stem. *J. Neurochem.,* 29:1105–1109.
11. Jones, D. H., Matus, A. J. (1974): Isolation of synaptic plasma membranes from brain by combined flotation-sedimentation density gradient centrifugation. *Biochim. Biophys. Acta,* 356:276–287.
12. Kitabgi, P., Carraway, R., Van Rietschoten, J., Granier, C., Morgat, J. L., Menez, A., Leeman, S. E., and Freychet, P. (1977): Neurotensin: Specific binding to synaptic membranes from rat brain. *Proc. Natl. Acad. Sci. USA,* 74:1846–1850.
13. Lembeck, F., and Holasek, A. (1960): Die intracelluläre Lokalisation der Substanz P. *Naunyn Schmiedebergs Arch. Exp. Pathol. Pharmakol.,* 238:542–545.
14. Lembeck, F., Mayer, N., and Schindler, G. (1977): Substance P in rat brain synaptosomes. *Naunyn Schmiedebergs Arch. Pharmacol.,* 301:17–22.
15. Lembeck, F., Mayer, N., and Schindler, G. (1978): Substance P: Binding to lipids in the brain. *Naunyn Schmiedebergs Arch. Pharmacol.,* 303:79–86.
16. Lembeck, F., Saria, A., and Mayer, N. (1979): Substance P: Model studies of its binding to phospholipids. *Naunyn Schmiedebergs Arch. Pharmacol.,* 306:189–194.
17. Ljungdahl, A., Hökfelt, T., and Nilsson, G. (1978): Distribution of substance P-like immunoreactivity in the central nervous system of the rat. I. Cell bodies and nerve terminals. *Neuroscience,* 3:861–943.
18. Loh, H., Law, D. Y., Ostwald, T., Cho, T. M., and Way, E. L. (1978): Possible involvement of cerebroside sulfate in opiate receptor binding. *Fed. Proc.,* 37:147–152.
19. Lowry, O. H., Rosebrough, N. J., Farr, A. L., and Randall, R. J. (1951): Protein measurement with the folin phenol reagent. *J. Biol. Chem.,* 193:265–275.
20. Mayer, N., Lembeck, F., Saria, A., and Gamse, R. (1979): Substance P: Characteristics of binding to synaptic vesicles of rat brain. *Naunyn Schmiedebergs Arch. Pharmacol.,* 306:45–51.
21. Mroz, E. A., Brownstein, M. J., and Leeman, S. E. (1977): Distribution of immunoassayable substance P in the rat brain. Evidence for the existing of substance P-containing tracts. In: *Substance P,* edited by U. S. von Euler and B. Pernow. Raven Press, New York.
22. Nakata, Y., Kusaka, Y., Segawa, T., Yajima, H., and Kitagawa, K. (1978): Substance P: Regional distribution and specific binding to synaptic membranes in rat central nervous system. *Life Sci.,* 22:259–268.
23. Otsuka, M., and Konishi, S. (1976): Release of substance P-like immunoreactivity from isolated spinal cord of newborn rat. *Nature,* 264:83–84.
24. Pasternak, G. W., Wilson, H. A., and Snyder, S. H. (1975): Differential effects of protein modifying reagents on receptor binding of opiate agonists and antagonists. *Mol. Pharmacol.,* 11:340–359.

25. Pickel, V. M., Reis, D. J., and Leeman, S. E. (1977): Ultrastructural localization of substance P in neurones of rat spinal cord. *Brain Res.,* 122:534–540.
26. Scatchard, G. (1949): The attraction of proteins for small molecules and ions. *Ann. NY Acad. Sci.,* 51:660–670.
27. Schenker, C., Mroz, E. A., and Leeman, S. E. (1976): Release of substance P from isolated nerve endings. *Nature,* 264:790–792.
28. Taylor, R. F. (1978): Isolation and purification of cholinergic receptor proteolipids from rat gastrocnemius tissue. *J. Neurochem.,* 31:1183–1189.

Neuropeptides and Neural Transmission,
edited by C. Ajmone Marsan and W. Z. Traczyk.
Raven Press, New York © 1980.

Action of Substance P on Trigeminal Nucleus Caudalis Neurones in Capsaicin-treated Rats

R. G. Hill, M. L. Hoddinott, and P. M. Keen

*Department of Pharmacology, University of Bristol Medical School,
Bristol BS8 1TD, United Kingdom*

Large amounts of substance P (SP) are present in the trigeminal nucleus caudalis (19) where the peptide is localised within nerve fibres in the substantia gelatinosa and in the reticular formation adjacent to the main nucleus (8). There is now evidence from immuno-peroxidase studies that SP is associated with synaptic vesicles contained within unmyelinated fibre terminals (16) and that it is released from central nervous tissue in a calcium-dependent manner (7,19). There is some controversy in the literature, however, over the action of SP when applied by microiontophoresis to single sensory neurones in the dorsal horn of the spinal cord and in the trigeminal nucleus caudalis. Some groups find that SP preferentially excites those neurones that are also excited by noxious stimuli, and therefore presumably by the transmitter released from small diameter afferents (2,11,12). Other workers find that neurones responding to a wide variety of sensory input are excited by SP (21,27), and indeed, neurones with an exclusively low threshold input in the cuneate nucleus are readily excited by it (22). An approach to this problem is to examine the change in sensitivity to SP produced by denervation of the experimental area, and one such study using dorsal rhizotomy has been performed (26). A gross lesion such as rhizotomy, however, does not remove only the small diameter afferents believed to utilize SP, but also the large myelinated fibres. The picture is further complicated by the recent finding that some small afferents enter the spinal cord by way of the ventral roots (6) and hence would *not* be sectioned. A more selective lesion can be produced using capsaicin, the active constituent of red pepper (24), which first stimulates and then blocks those nerve fibres responsible for chemical and thermal nociception (16), and believed on electrophysiological grounds to be exclusively unmyelinated C fibres (4). Some time ago it was demonstrated that capsaicin reduces the fluoride-resistant acid phosphatase activity in the substantia gelatinosa of the dorsal horn of the rat spinal cord (17), and this has subsequently been shown to be associated with depletion of the SP content of the substantia gelatinosa (20). We have therefore examined the neuronal activity of the rat trigeminal nucleus caudalis in control rats and in rats previously injected with capsaicin, applying SP and other relevant substances by microiontophoresis to monitor changes in neuronal sensitivity.

METHODS

Capsaicin Pretreatment

Animals were sorted into control and capsaicin groups on the second day of life; the capsaicin group was injected with 70 μl sc of a 10 mg/ml solution of capsaicin (Sigma) in 10% ethanol, 10% Tween 80, and 80% normal saline, this being equivalent to a dose of 87.5 mg/kg. The controls received injections of vehicle only. The two groups were housed in the same room and treated identically thereafter. Between 8 and 10 months of age, pairs of control and capsaicin-treated animals were examined for their sensitivity to noxious stimuli and then used for acute electrophysiological testing of neuronal sensitivity on consecutive days.

Acute Preparation

Anaesthesia was induced with halothane (2–3%) and maintained with urethane (0.5 ml of 25% wt/vol solution per 100-gm rat ip). Animals were mounted in a stereotaxic frame and prepared for recording from the trigeminal nucleus caudalis as previously described (3). Multibarrelled micropipettes for extracellular recording and microiontophoretic application of drugs were inserted perpendicular to the surface of the lateral dorsal medulla using a motor driven hydraulic micromanipulator. Trigeminal neurones were identified by their responses to natural and electrical stimulation of ipsilateral oro-facial structure (3). Following each experiment the anatomical location of the neurones studied was confirmed when electrode tracks were traced in formalin fixed transverse sections of caudal medulla, the location of the track being aided by dye spots produced by the iontophoretic deposition of pontamine sky blue (10).

Micropipette Preparation

Micropipettes were conventional five- or six-barrelled pipettes constructed from fibre-filled glass tubing as previously described (13). SP (synthetic) was obtained from Peninsula Labs, San Diego, and a 2.5-mM solution was prepared. Aliquots (200μl) were freeze-dried and reconstituted on the day of each experiment by the addition of 150 mM NaCl solution, the solutions being kept on ice until the micropipettes were filled a few minutes later. Solutions of eledoisin-related peptide (ERP, 5 mM in 150 mM NaCl, Sigma) were made fresh on the day of the experiment. Other drug solutions used were glutamic acid (Sigma), 0.5 M, pH 8.5; acetylcholine (Sigma), 0.5 M, pH 3.5; aspartic acid (Sigma), 0.2 M, pH 8.5; and pontamine sky blue (Gurr), 2% in acetate buffer. Recording barrels of all pipettes contained 4 M NaCl and one barrel was filled with 1 M NaCl for current balancing and to provide a return path for the iontophoresis currents.

Tail Flick Latency Measurement

Various tests are available for the determination of nociception threshold in rats, but most workers accept the hot water-tail immersion test (18,25) as a valid measure of the animal's sensitivity to noxious heat. Control and capsaicin-treated rats were tested for their tail flick latency before being used in acute electrophysiological experiments. Each capsaicin-treated animal was compared with a control animal of the same age. The animals were placed in open-ended restraining tubes, the head ends of which were clamped against a grill to prevent the animal from leaving the tube during the test. The rats were allowed to settle in their new environment for 10 min; their tails were then dipped in water at 60°C and the time period for withdrawal was recorded. The test was repeated at 15-min intervals until a total of five measurements was obtained for each rat. The first two readings showed considerable variation, probably because the rats were still unsettled in their unfamiliar environments, and these readings were therefore discarded and mean values calculated from the last three readings for each animal.

Recordings from Trigeminal Neurones

Neurones were located at depths from 200 to 2,500 μ below the surface of the medulla and initially classified as spontaneous or non-spontaneous on the basis of their responses to microiontophoretic application of glutamate (20–50 nA) which was used as a search stimulus. Those neurones which had fired no action potentials 2 min after removal of the glutamate current, but which could be repeatedly excited by glutamate, were classed as non-spontaneous. Neurones showing stable responses were selected for further study involving repeated testing over periods of 30 to 60 min. An extensive study of the responses of neurones in capsaicin-treated animals to various natural stimuli has been made, in comparison with our earlier study on control animals (3), but since the results of this study are too complex to elaborate on in this chapter, they will therefore be the subject of a separate publication. However, it is relevant to this study to be able to classify the type of response shown by some of the neurons to noxious and non-noxious natural stimuli (3). Use has therefore been made of the convention of Iggo (14) which describes those neurones responding exclusively to low intensity stimulation as type 1, those responding to both low intensity and noxious stimuli (i.e., polymodal) as type 2, and lastly, those with exclusively high-threshold responses as type 3. As this classification was made after full pharmacological testing, some neurones were lost before this could be completed.

RESULTS

Rats treated with capsaicin showed the characteristic appearance described by previous workers (17,24) with patchy thin fur, very pink skin, and self-inflicted abrasions probably caused by excessive grooming. These animals were otherwise healthy, however, and tolerated the anaesthesia and surgical procedures as well as the controls.

Tail Flick Latencies

The results for five pairs of rats are illustrated in histogram form in Fig. 1. Although there was considerable variation in the responses of control animals, probably explicable in terms of diurnal variation in tail flick latency (9), in every pair tested the reaction time of the capsaicin-treated animal was longer, and in each case the result was statistically significant. This result taken together with the gross appearance of the rats, indicates that the animals subsequently used for electrophysiological experiments were affected in a characteristic manner by the capsaicin.

Responses of Trigeminal Neurones

Stable recordings were obtained from 35 neurones in control animals and from 39 in capsaicin-treated animals. Some of these neurones were further classi-

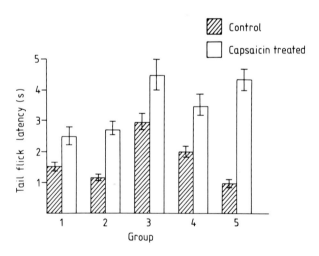

FIG. 1. Histograms showing the variation in tail flick latency between control animals *(hatched bars)* and capsaicin pre-treated rats *(open bars)* for five pairs of rats tested on different days. The error bars show the mean ± SEM for three successive measurements of latency (see text). In each case the latency of the control animals' response was significantly less than that of the capsaicin-treated animal tested on the same occasion. (paired *t*-test, *p* > 0.01)

TABLE 1. *Comparison of the relative percentage of neurones spontaneously active and excited by either SP or ERP in control and capsaicin-treated animals*

	Spontaneously active	Excited by SP	Excited by ERP
Controls n = 35	31%	54%	54%
Capsaicin treated n = 39	77%	84%	93%

The percentages in the columns referring to SP and ERP are expressed as a percentage of the number of neurones tested with each substance and includes those neurones excited by combined application of peptide and glutamate.

fied on the basis of their responses to natural stimuli (see Methods). Responses obtained to iontophoretic application of synthetic SP were indistinguishable from those obtained following application of ERP, and results with the two substances have therefore been considered together (Table 1).

Neuronal Responses in Control Animals

Only 7 of the 35 neurones (18%) tested were directly excited by SP or ERP when applied with currents between 80 and 160 nA and, as noted by other workers (21), those neurones that were firing spontaneously when encountered (31% of the total) were more likely to be excited by the peptides. These responses were entirely characteristic (21,27) with a latency of up to 40 sec before excitation started and often showing a peak firing rate increase after the application of peptide had been discontinued. Responses continued for 1 min or more after the end of the drug application. All neurones were readily excited by application of glutamate (10–100 nA) or aspartate (20–100 nA) and some neurones that failed to be excited by peptide application alone readily showed enhancement of their responses to glutamate (12 of the 35). Together with those neurones that were directly excited by the peptides, this gave a total of 19 of the 35 neurones (54%) that showed an excitatory response to either SP or ERP (Table 1). A proportion of neurones were excited by application of acetylcholine (20–100 nA), but there was no obvious correlation between sensitivity to acetylcholine and sensitivity to the peptides.

Seventeen neurones were classified according to their responses to natural stimulation (3,11,14); it was found that five out of nine type 1 low-threshold neurones were excited by the peptides, four out of five type 2 polymodal neurones were excited, and one out of three type 3 high-threshold neurones was excited. No support was therefore gained for the hypothesis that substance P exclusively excites nociceptive neurones (2,11,12).

Neuronal Responses in Capsaicin-Treated Animals

The first difference noted between neurones in capsaicin-treated animals and those in the controls was the much higher incidence of spontaneous activity [77% as compared with 31% (Table 1)]. A far higher proportion of neurones was sensitive to the peptides, with 23 of the 39 neurones studied (60%) directly excited. When neurones were included that were initially insensitive, but showed enhancement of the glutamate response during concurrent application of SP or ERP, then 84% (21 of 25) of those neurones tested with SP were excited as were 95% (13 of 14) of those tested with ERP.

The responses, which were in no way abnormal, resembled those seen in control animals and those described in the literature by other workers (2,11, 21,22,27). A photographic record of the firing of a neurone in a capsaicin-treated rat is shown in Fig. 2. The neurone was firing spontaneously with an irregular pattern before application of SP 60 nA and after a considerable latency showed a marked increase in firing rate in response to application of the peptide. The increased firing rate was maintained for some time after discontinuing the SP application. After recovery from the application of SP had been obtained, subsequent application of glutamate 30 nA produced a characteristic rapid onset–rapid offset response. Analogue rate meter traces of the firing of the same neurone are shown in Fig. 3, and clearly show the difference in time course of the effects of SP and glutamate when both were applied with a current of 60 nA,

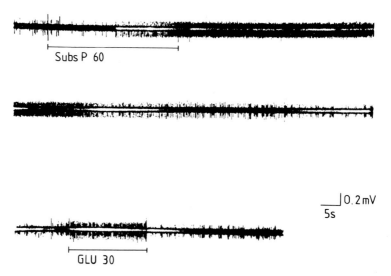

FIG. 2. Photographic records of the firing of a trigeminal nucleus caudalis neurone in a capsaicin-treated rat. The application of SP *(first horizontal bar)* with a current of 60 nA caused excitation of the neurone after a long latency and the evoked firing continued well after the end of the SP application. The application of glutamate *(second horizontal bar)* 30 nA caused a short latency, rapidly decaying excitation of the neurone.

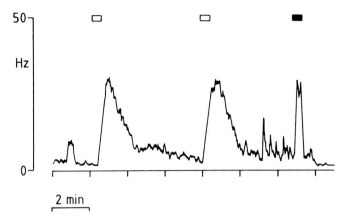

FIG. 3. Analogue rate meter records of the firing of the neurone also illustrated in Fig. 2. *Open bars* indicate the application of SP 60 nA and *filled bars* the application of gluta-mate 60 nA. Note the difference in time course of the responses to the two excitant sub-stances.

even though both substances caused the cell to achieve approximately the same peak firing rate.

Responses of a neurone that was not directly excited by SP but which showed enhancement of the effects of glutamate are illustrated in Fig. 4. In the left-hand panel of the figure responses to repeated pulses of glutamate 30 nA are shown; in the right-hand panel, however, it can be seen that pulses of glutamate 10 nA were ineffective until SP 80 nA was also applied to the neurone, at

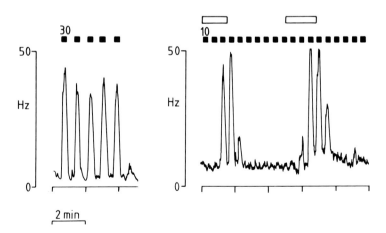

FIG. 4. Analogue rate meter records of the firing of a second trigeminal neurone in a capsaicin-treated rat. The **left panel** illustrates excitation of the neurone by repeated application of glutamate *(filled bars)* 30 nA. The **right panel** shows the initial lack of response to glutamate *(filled bars)* 10 nA, which turns into a powerful excitation when SP *(open bars)* 80 nA is applied concurrently.

which point each glutamate pulse caused a sharp increase in firing rate. As with the direct excitant effect of the peptide, this type of response showed a long latency and persisted after the termination of the SP application.

Fifteen neurones were classified according to their responses to natural stimulation (3,11,14) and it was found that all seven type 1 low-threshold neurones were excited as were all nine type 2 polymodal neurones tested. It was interesting to note that no type 3 high-threshold neurones were identified in these animals.

It was important to decide if the differences between normal and capsaicin-treated animals were explicable solely by the increased proportion of spontaneously active neurones seen in the capsaicin-treated sample, for it seemed in the control animals that spontaneously firing neurones were more readily excited by the peptides. A detailed comparison of the currents needed to produce an adequate excitatory effect was therefore made and the results of this are illustrated in Table 2. The first column of the table shows the mean current of SP or ERP applied to all neurones in the study regardless of whether they responded or not. This shows that in the controls, where likelihood of finding neurones that responded to the peptides was lower, higher currents were used, thus validating the broad conclusion that neurones in capsaicin-treated animals were more likely to be sensitive. In the second column of the table the currents needed to directly excite neurones in control and capsaicin-treated animals are compared. This shows quite clearly that, in control animals, only those neurones where higher than average peptide applying currents were used were excited, whereas in capsaicin-treated animals much lower currents than this were needed. This strongly suggests that, in addition to there being a greater number of responding neurones in these experiments, these neurones were abnormally sensitive to the peptides.

The last column of the table compares currents needed for excitation produced by a combination of peptide and glutamate, and here too neurones in the capsaicin-treated animals required markedly lower currents.

Thus, lesioning of the SP-containing fibres produced a large increase in the

TABLE 2. *Comparison of the effective currents (nA) needed to produce excitation in control and in capsaicin-treated rats*

	Mean current all tests	Excited by SP/ERP	Excited by SP/ERP + GLU
Controls	91.8 ± 6.9 (33)	124.3 ± 13.6 (7)	75.0 ± 9.8 (12)
Capsaicin treated	**44.1 ± 2.8 (39)	**48.9 ± 2.7 (23)	*32.3 ± 5.2 (11)

(n) for each group
Significantly differs from control (*t*-test)
** $p < 0.001$; * $p < 0.01 > 0.001$

proportion of neurones sensitive to SP and its analogue, ERP, and also increased the sensitivity of neurones to these peptides. In this context it is noteworthy that no changes in sensitivity to glutamate were detected between control and capsaicin-lesioned animals.

DISCUSSION

It is tempting to interpret the results of this investigation as evidence for denervation super-sensitivity (5), but such a conclusion may be unwarranted. In control animals it was found that some type 1 low-threshold neurones were excited by SP or ERP, and that in capsaicin-treated animals a larger number of type 1 neurones showed an increased sensitivity to the peptides. As these neurones appear to receive their synaptic input exclusively from A β-fibres (3,14), such a result is not consistent with an increase in sensitivity of those neurones that are effectively denervated by the capsaicin lesioning of SP-containing fibres. Indeed, as this investigation failed to find any type 3 high-threshold neurones in capsaicin-treated animals, perhaps some of those neurones that lost their synaptic connection with SP-containing fibres had become unresponsive, although a larger sample of neurones would have to be taken in order to be certain of this conclusion.

Unlike animals in which complete trigeminal rhizotomy has been made (1,23), there was no obvious abnormality in the capsaicin-treated animals with respect to the behaviour of neurones in trigeminal nucleus caudalis, other than the increase in the proportion of spontaneous activity and sensitivity to SP and ERP. No neurones corresponding to the "hyperactive" classification made by Anderson and his colleagues (1) were seen and sensitivity to applied amino acids was normal with none of the hyposensitive neurones described by Macon (23). Treatment with capsaicin therefore appears to produce a relatively specific lesion, producing changes in sensitivity only to SP and analogues.

It is not apparent at the present time just how the increase in sensitivity to SP and ERP occurs, particularly as it is not restricted to neurones receiving synaptic contact with C fibres, but appears to occur on all neurones having SP receptors. It is possible that enzymic removal processes for SP in the trigeminal nucleus caudalis degenerate when terminals fail to release the peptide over long periods of time, but the results obtained in this study could be equally well explained by an increase in receptor sensitivity. Only detailed neurochemical investigation will elucidate this problem.

The undoubted change in sensitivity of neurones in the trigeminal nucleus caudalis to SP following the specific lesion of the fibres containing this substance supports the contention that the peptide may have a physiological role in this area. The fact that neurones responding to a variety of sensory modalities changed their SP sensitivity suggests that the importance of SP as a sensory transmitter may extend beyond its possible role in nociception.

ACKNOWLEDGMENT

This work was supported by grants from the Wellcome Trust and the Royal Society. We are grateful to S. Stoter and A. Duncan for skilled technical assistance.

REFERENCES

1. Anderson, L. S., Black, R. G., Abraham, J., and Ward, A. A. (1971): Neuronal hyperactivity in experimental trigeminal deafferentation. *J. Neurosurg.*, 35:444–452.
2. Andersen, R. K., Lund, J. P., and Puil, E. (1977): The effects of iontophoretic applications of morphine and putative neurotransmitters on neurons of the trigeminal nuclei oralis and caudalis. In: *Pain in the Trigeminal Region,* edited by D. Anderson and B. Matthews, pp. 271–284. Elsevier/North-Holland, Amsterdam.
3. Ayliffe, S. J., and Hill, R. G. (1979): Responses of cells in the trigeminal subnucleus caudalis of the rat to noxious stimuli. *J. Physiol. (Lond.)* 287:18–19P.
4. Burgess, P. R., and Perl, E. R. (1973): Cutaneous mechanoreceptors and nociceptors. In: *Handbook of Sensory Physiology, Vol. II,* edited by A. Iggo, pp. 29–78. Springer-Verlag, Berlin.
5. Cannon, W. B. (1939): A law of denervation. *Am. J. Med. Sci.,* 198:737–750.
6. Coggeshall, R. E., Applebaum, M. L., Frazer, M. L., Stubbs, M., and Sykes, M. T. (1975): Unmyelinated axons in human ventral roots, a possible explanation for the failure of dorsal rhizotomy to relieve pain. *Brain,* 98:157–166.
7. Cuello, A. C., Jessell, T. M., Kanazawa, I., and Iversen, L. L. (1977): Substance P: Localization in synaptic vesicles in rat central nervous system. *J. Neurochem.,* 29:747–751.
8. Cuello, A. C., and Kanazawa, I. (1978): The distribution of substance P immunoreactive fibers in the rat central nervous system. *J. Comp. Neurol.,* 178:129–156.
9. Frederickson, R. C. S., and Norris, F. H. (1977): Enkephalins as inhibitory neurotransmitters modulating nociception. In: *Iontophoresis and Transmitter Mechanisms in the Mammalian Central Nervous System,* edited by R. W. Ryall and J. S. Kelly, pp. 320–322. North Holland, Amsterdam.
10. Hellon, R. F. (1971): The marking of electrode tip positions in nervous tissue. *J. Physiol. (Lond.),* 214:12P.
11. Henry, J. L. (1976): Effects of substance P on functionally identified units in cat spinal cord. *Brain Res.,* 114:439–451.
12. Henry, J. L., Hu, J. W., Lucier, G. E., and Sessle, B. J. (1977): Responses of units in the trigeminal sensory nuclei to oral-facial stimuli and to substance P. In: *Pain in the Trigeminal Region,* edited by D. Anderson and B. Matthews, pp. 295–306. Elsevier/North-Holland, Amsterdam.
13. Hill, R. G., and Pepper, C. M. (1978): Selective effects of morphine on the nociceptive responses of thalamic neurones in the rat. *Br. J. Pharmacol.,* 64:137–143.
14. Iggo, A. (1974): Activation of cutaneous nociceptors and their actions on dorsal horn neurons. *Adv. Neurol.,* 4:1–9.
15. Iversen, L. L., Jessell, T., and Kanazawa, I. (1976): Release and metabolism of substance P in rat hypothalamus. *Nature,* 264:81–83.
16. Jansco, G., Jansco-Gabor, A., and Szolcsanyi, J. (1967): Direct evidence for neurogenic inflammation and its prevention by denervation and by pretreatment with capsaicin. *Br. J. Pharmacol.,* 31:138–151.
17. Jansco, G., and Knyihar, E. (1975): Functional link between nociception and fluoride resistant acid phosphatase activity in the Rolando substance. *Neurobiology,* 5:42–43.
18. Janssen, P. A. J., Niemegeers, C. J. E., and Dony, J. G. H. (1963): The inhibitory effect of fentanyl and other morphine-like analgesics on the warm water induced tail withdrawal reflex in rats. *Arzneim. Forsch.,* 13:502–507.
19. Jessell, T. M., and Iversen, L. L. (1977): Opiate analgesics inhibit substance P release in rat trigeminal nucleus. *Nature,* 268:549–551.
20. Jessell, T. M., Iversen, L. L., and Cuello, A. C. (1978): Capsaicin-induced depletion of substance P from primary sensory neurones. *Brain Res.,* 152:183–188.

21. Krnjevic, K. (1977): Effects of substance P on central neurons in cats. In: *Substance P,* edited by U. S. von Euler and B. Pernow, pp. 217–230. Raven Press, New York.
22. Krnjevic, K., and Morris, M. E. (1974): An excitatory action of substance P on cuneate neurones. *Can. J. Physiol. Pharmacol.,* 52:736–744.
23. Macon, J. B. (1978): Neuronal responses to amino acid iontophoresis in the deafferent spinal trigeminal nucleus. *Exp. Neurol.,* 60:522–540.
24. Szolcsanyi, J., Jansco-Gabor, A., and Joo, F. (1975): Functional and fine structural characteristics of the sensory neurone blocking effect of capsaicin. *Naunyn. Schmeidebergs Arch. Pharmacol.,* 287:157–169.
25. Woolf, C. J., Barrett, G. D., Mitchell, D., and Myers, R. A. (1977): Naloxone-reversible peripheral electroanalgesia in intact and spinal rats. *Eur. J. Pharmacol.,* 45:311–314.
26. Wright, D. M., and Roberts, M. H. T. (1978): Supersensitivity to a substance P analogue following dorsal root section. *Life Sci.,* 22:19–24.
27. Zieglgänsberger, W., and Tulloch, I. F. (1979): Effects of substance P on neurones in the dorsal horn of the spinal cord of the cat. *Brain Res.,* 166:273–282.

Neuropeptides and Neural Transmission,
edited by C. Ajmone Marsan and W. Z. Traczyk.
Raven Press, New York © 1980.

Effects of Substance P and Capsaicin on Isolated Spinal Cord of Newborn Rat

M. Yanagisawa, S. Konishi, T. Suzue, and M. Otsuka

Department of Pharmacology, Faculty of Medicine, Tokyo Medical and Dental University, Bunkyo-ku, Tokyo 113, Japan

Substance P (SP) exerts a powerful excitatory action on spinal neurons (4,7,8,11). The mechanisms of SP action, however, are still not entirely clear, and in order to clarify the functional role of SP in synaptic transmission in the spinal cord, we need further detailed information about the action of the peptide. In the present study, therefore, we have examined the effects of SP on spinal motoneurons in the isolated rat spinal cord by intra- and extracellular recordings. Furthermore, some additional experiments were made on the effects of capsaicin that seem to cause SP release from primary afferent neurons.

METHODS

Spinal cord below Th5 was isolated from 0- to 4-day-old Wistar rats (10). The hemisected spinal cord was placed in a bath of about 0.2 ml in volume, and was perfused with artificial cerebrospinal fluid (CSF) gassed with 95% O_2 and 5% CO_2. The composition of the artificial CSF was as follows (mM): NaCl, 138.6; KCl, 3.35; $CaCl_2$, 1.26; $MgCl_2$, 1.15; $NaHCO_3$, 20.9; NaH_2PO_4, 0.58; and glucose 10 (cf. 3). The temperature of the bath was kept at 27°C and the perfusion rate was 2 to 7 ml/min. Intracellular recordings were made from motoneurons of L3-L5 segments using a 2M-potassium acetate-filled microelectrode of 30 to 50 MΩ resistance. For measuring the membrane resistance, hyperpolarizing current pulses were injected into the motoneurons through the recording microelectrode by the use of bridge circuit. Potential changes were also recorded extracellularly from a ventral or dorsal root (L3-L5) using a suction electrode as described previously (10).

In order to measure the release of SP from spinal cord, the hemisected cord was placed in a test tube containing 1 ml incubation solution. Dithiothreitol (6 μM) was added to the solution which was bubbled with 95% O_2 and 5% CO_2. After incubation for 30 min the cord was removed. Samples were lyophilized and submitted to radioimmunoassay for SP (15,16).

RESULTS AND DISCUSSION

Intracellular Recordings of SP Effects on Spinal Motoneurons

When a microelectrode was inserted into a lumbar motoneuron, a negative resting potential of 50 to 90 mV was recorded. Antidromic stimulation of the corresponding ventral root produced an overshooting action potential. Perfusion with artificial CSF containing SP (2×10^{-6} M) induced a depolarization of 10 to 20 mV (Fig. 1A). The depolarization was accompanied by a definite increase in membrane conductance (9,12). Addition of tetrodotoxin (TTX) in a concentration of 1.3×10^{-7} M completely blocked the spinal reflexes as well as the antidromic action potentials of motoneurons. In the presence of TTX, SP still produced the depolarization of motoneurons, although its amplitude was markedly depressed and the time course was much slower than in the absence of TTX (Fig. 1B).

Effects of Calcium and TTX on SP-Induced Depolarization

The above results obtained with intracellular recordings suggest that the SP-induced depolarization of motoneurons is due to both transsynaptic and direct actions on the motoneurons. In order to further examine this notion, the effect of SP as well as of L-glutamate was studied in varied Ca concentrations while the Mg concentration was kept constant at 2 mM. When Ca concentration

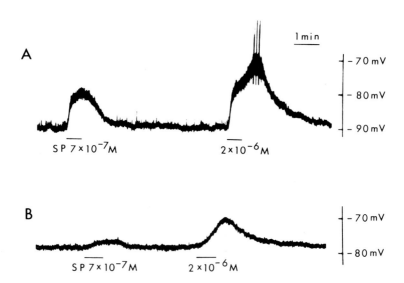

FIG. 1. Intracellular recordings from a lumbar motoneuron of isolated rat spinal cord showing the effects of bath-applied SP. **A:** In normal artificial CSF; **B:** after the addition of TTX (1.3×10^{-7} M). SP solutions were perfused through the bath during the periods indicated by the *horizontal bars* under records.

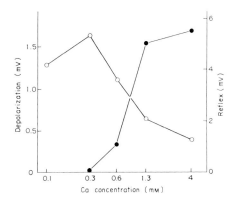

FIG. 2. Effects of Ca concentration on the size of monosynaptic reflex *(closed circles)* and the amplitude of the SP-induced depolarization *(open circles)*. Extracellular recordings from L4 ventral root. Spinal reflexes were evoked by a single supramaximal stimulation of L4 dorsal root with intervals of 11 sec. Mg concentration was kept constant at 2 mM. SP (10^{-7} M) was applied during the periods of 30 sec. (From Otsuka and Yanagisawa, ref. 13, with permission.)

was reduced below 0.3 mM, the spinal reflexes induced by single dorsal root stimulation and recorded from the corresponding ventral root were completely abolished. By contrast, the depolarization induced by SP (10^{-7} M) or by L-glutamate (2×10^{-4} M) was larger in the 0.1-mM Ca medium than in the normal Ca (1.26 mM) medium (Fig. 2). Addition of TTX (1.3×10^{-7} M) to the 0.1-mM Ca medium, however, markedly depressed the depolarizations produced by both SP and glutamate (13). Although further studies are needed to clarify the mechanisms of the action of TTX, a possible explanation is that a TTX-sensitive Na conductance of the motoneuron membrane is involved in the SP-induced depolarization. Another explanation is that the block of synaptic transmission in the spinal cord is incomplete in the 0.1-mM Ca medium, but is complete only after the addition of TTX.

Time Course of SP-Induced Depolarization

Studies of SP action with electrophoretic application showed that the SP-induced excitation of spinal neurons began after a delay of 15 to 30 sec and persisted for 1 to 2 min after the application of SP was stopped (4). However, the slow time course of SP action observed in these experiments might be accounted for by a delayed release and/or a slow diffusion of SP from the micropipette to the site of action. We have therefore examined the time course of the depolarization of spinal motoneurons produced by bath application of SP. In the experiment illustrated in Fig. 3, potentials were recorded extracellularly from a ventral root. To facilitate the penetration of drugs, pia mater was carefully removed under collagenase treatment (0.05 mg/ml). When normal artificial CSF-containing SP (8×10^{-5} M) was introduced into the bath, the depolarization began after a delay of 1.1 ± 0.1 sec (mean $\pm$ SEM). Similarly, the application of L-glutamate (10^{-3} M) induced the depolarization after a delay of 0.4 ± 0.1 sec. When a lower concentration of SP (10^{-6} M) was applied, the delay was about 3 sec, the rise time and the half-decline were 9 to 14 sec in both normal and low Ca mediums (Fig. 3B). It is likely that a large part of the delay time

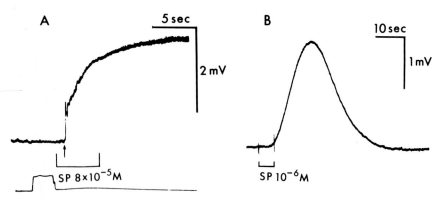

FIG. 3. Time course of the depolarization produced by bath application of SP. **A:** Extracellular recording from L4 ventral root *(upper trace)*. Isolated spinal cord of 1-day-old rat was perfused with normal artificial CSF, and SP (8×10^{-5} M) was bath-applied during the period indicated under the record. The end of the square pulse in *lower trace* marks the moment when the SP solution entered the bath. *Arrow* indicates the beginning of the depolarization. **B:** Depolarization induced by SP (10^{-6} M) in artificial CSF containing 0.1 mM Ca and 3.5 mM Mg. Extracellular recording from L4 ventral root. During the period marked under the record, SP solution was perfused through the bath.

of SP-induced depolarization is due to the diffusion of the peptide through the tissue (13).

Capsaicin-Induced Release of SP from Primary Afferent Fibers

Jessell et al. (6) have shown that the repeated injections of capsaicin into the rat produce a depletion of SP from the primary afferent terminals in substantia gelatinosa of the spinal cord. In the experiment illustrated in Fig. 4A, the application of capsaicin (5×10^{-7} M) to the isolated spinal cord produced a depolarizing response of primary afferent fibers that could be recorded extracellularly from a dorsal root. The response was potentiated in the medium containing 0.1 mM Ca and 2 mM Mg. When the potentials were recorded from a ventral root, the application of capsaicin produced a depolarizing response of faster time course (Fig. 4B). In the medium containing 0.1 mM Ca and 2 mM Mg, or in the presence of baclofen (2.3×10^{-6} M), the depolarizing response of motoneurons produced by capsaicin was markedly reduced or completely abolished (Figs. 4B and 5). Baclofen has previously been shown to antagonize the depolarizing action of SP on rat motoneurons (11,14).

These results, together with those of Jessell et al. (6), suggest that capsaicin acts on the nerve terminals of certain primary afferent fibers to produce the depolarization and the release of SP therefrom in a Ca-dependent manner. This notion was further supported by the direct measurements of SP release from isolated spinal cords. The results are summarized in Table 1. Addition of capsaicin (10^{-6} M) to normal artificial CSF increased the SP release by about fivefold.

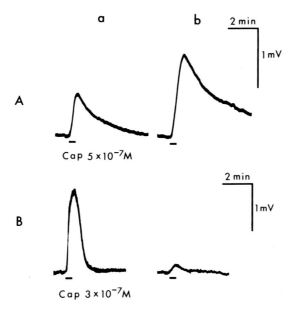

FIG. 4. Capsaicin-induced potential changes recorded from dorsal and ventral roots, and the effects of Ca concentration. Extracellular recordings from **(A)** L5 dorsal root and **(B)** L4 ventral root. Capsaicin was applied by perfusion during the periods of 20 sec, as marked by *horizontal bars* under records, in **(a)** normal artificial CSF and **(b)** the medium containing 0.1 mM Ca and 2 mM Mg. Depolarization upwards. Cap, capsaicin.

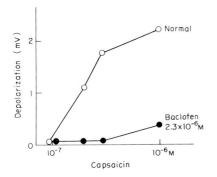

FIG. 5. Effect of baclofen on the capsaicin-induced depolarization recorded from L4 ventral root. *Ordinate:* Extracellularly recorded potential change produced by bath application of capsaicin for 20 sec. *Abscissa:* Concentration of capsaicin on a logarithmic scale.

By contrast, in the medium containing 0.1 mM Ca and 2 mM Mg, the same concentration of capsaicin did not cause any significant change in SP release (15).

CONCLUSIONS

SP in quite a low concentration produced a depolarization of rat spinal motoneurons in the medium containing 0.1 mM Ca or TTX (1.3×10^{-7} M), suggesting

TABLE 1. *Capsaicin-evoked release of SP from newborn rat spinal cord*

Incubating solution	SP released during 30-min period (fmoles)
Artificial CSF	56.5 ± 29.6
Artificial CSF $+10^{-6}$ M capsaicin	287.3 ± 33.9 [a]
Artificial CSF containing: 0.1 mM Ca 2.0 mM Mg $+10^{-6}$ M Capsaicin	60.8 ± 24.2 [b]

[a] $p < 0.01$ when compared with the value in normal artificial CSF.

[b] $p < 0.01$ when compared with the value in normal artificial CSF plus capsaicin.

Each value is the mean $\pm$ SEM from three separate experiments.

Data from Theriault et al., ref. 15.

that SP has a direct action on motoneurons in addition to its transsynaptic action. This notion is consistent with the immunohistochemical findings that SP-containing nerve terminals occur around cell soma and dendrites of spinal motoneurons (1,2,5).

The depolarization of the motoneurons produced by bath-applied SP began after a delay of about 1 sec. It is likely that the real delay time at the site of action is less than a few hundred milliseconds, which is consistent with the role of SP as a neurotransmitter (cf. Vincent and Barker, *this volume*).

Capsaicin is a powerful pain-inducing substance and the present study suggests that the capsaicin-induced pain may be mediated by the release of SP from primary afferent terminals. Furthermore, capsaicin is likely to serve as a useful tool for elucidating the physiological role of SP in central nervous system.

REFERENCES

1. Barber, R. P., Vaughn, J. E., Slemmon, J. R., Salvaterra, P. M., Roberts, E., and Leeman, S. E. (1979): The origin, distribution and synaptic relationships of substance P axons in rat spinal cord. *J. Comp. Neurol.*, 184:331–352.
2. Cuello, A. C., Polak, J. M., and Pearse, A. G. E. (1976): Substance P: A naturally occurring transmitter in human spinal cord. *Lancet*, 2:1054–1056.
3. Feldberg, W., and Fleischhauer, K. (1960): Penetration of bromophenol blue from the perfused cerebral ventricles into the brain tissue. *J. Physiol. (Lond.)*, 150:451–462.
4. Henry, J. L., Krnjević, K., and Morris, M. E. (1975): Substance P and spinal neurones. *Can. J. Physiol. Pharmacol.*, 53:423–432.
5. Hökfelt, T., Kellerth, J.-O., Nilsson, G., and Pernow, B. (1975): Experimental immunohistochemical studies on the localization and distribution of substance P in cat primary sensory neurons. *Brain Res.*, 100:235–252.
6. Jessell, T. M., Iversen, L. L., and Cuello, A. C. (1978): Capsaicin-induced depletion of substance P from primary sensory neurons. *Brain Res.*, 152:183–188.

7. Konishi, S., and Otsuka, M. (1974): Excitatory action of hypothalamic substance P on spinal motoneurones of newborn rats. *Nature,* 252:734–735.
8. Konishi, S., and Otsuka, M. (1974): The effects of substance P and other peptides on spinal neurons of the frog. *Brain Res.,* 65:397–410.
9. Nicoll. R. A. (1978): The action of thyrotropin-releasing hormone, substance P and related peptides on frog spinal motoneurons. *J. Pharmacol. Exp. Ther.,* 207:817–824.
10. Otsuka, M., and Konishi, S. (1974): Electrophysiology of mammalian spinal cord in vitro. *Nature,* 252:733–734.
11. Otsuka, M., and Konishi, S. (1976): Substance P and excitatory transmitter of primary sensory neurons. *Cold Spring Harbor Symp. Quant. Biol.,* 40:135–143.
12. Otsuka, M., and Konishi, S. (1977): Electrophysiological and neurochemical evidence for substance P as a transmitter of primary sensory neurons. In: *Substance P,* edited by U. S. von Euler and B. Pernow, pp. 207–214. Raven Press, New York.
13. Otsuka, M., and Yanagisawa, M. (1978): The action of substance P on motoneurons of the isolated rat spinal cord. In: *Advances in Pharmacology and Therapeutics, Vol. 2: Neurotransmitters,* edited by P. Simon, pp. 181–190. Pergamon, Oxford.
14. Saito, K., Konishi, S., and Otsuka, M. (1975): Antagonism between Lioresal and substance P in rat spinal cord. *Brain Res.,* 97:177–180.
15. Theriault, E., Otsuka, M., and Jessell, T. (1979): Capsaicin-evoked release of substance P from primary sensory neurons. *Brain Res.,* 170:209–213.
16. Yanaihara, C., Sato, H., Hirohashi, M., Sakagami, M., Yamamoto, K., Hashimoto, T., Yanaihara, N., Abe, K., and Kaneko, T. (1976): Substance P radioimmunoassay using N^2-tyrosyl-substance P and demonstration of the presence of substance P-like immunoreactivities in human blood and porcine tissue extracts. *Endocrinol. Jap.* 23:457–463.

Neuropeptides and Neural Transmission,
edited by C. Ajmone Marsan and W. Z. Traczyk.
Raven Press, New York © 1980.

Substance P and Chemosensitive Neurones

F. Lembeck, R. Gamse, P. Holzer, and A. Molnar

*Institut für Experimentelle und Klinische Pharmakologie der Universität
Graz, A-8010 Graz, Austria*

The Bell-Magendie law, stating that the anterior fibres are purely efferent and that the fibres of the posterior roots are purely afferent, was apparently contradicted by Stricker's (65) and Gaertner's (15) findings of vasodilator fibres that leave the spinal cord through the dorsal roots. Stricker's method was very simple: he stimulated the peripheral portion of the transsected dorsal roots and observed the vasodilation in the paw by visual inspection and by the rise of temperature seen on a mercury thermometer placed between two toes. He ruled out the possibility that the vasodilator fibres were spinal efferent nerves and he also excluded any implication of the sympathetic nervous system in this "antidromic vasodilation."

The first and almost neglected pharmacological experiments on these vasodilator fibres were made by Bruce (3) in Vienna. He showed that mustard oil locally applied onto the eye did not cause any vasodilation and plasma exudation after chronic denervation of the trigeminal branch going to the eye. Therefore, he concluded that the skin irritant mustard oil produces vasodilation and plasma exudation obviously by an action on sensory nerves. Comprehensive work by Bayliss (2), Langley (41), Lewis and Marvin (51), Kibjakow (37), and others (for a review, see ref. 7) extended these early observations and unanimously resulted in the conclusion that a "histamine-like" agent is released at the peripheral endings of sensory neurones which produces vasodilation and plasma extravasation. These studies also supported the concept that "neurogenic inflammatory responses" are based on "axon reflexes" taking place at the bifurcating end branchings of sensory nerves. Also, the flare of arteriolar vasodilation following a minor injury of the skin is most likely brought about by activation of axon reflexes in sensory nerve fibres (51).

In trying to characterize the nature of these vasodilator fibres, Hinsey and Gasser (25) showed that cutaneous vasodilation upon antidromic stimulation of sensory nerves occurred only if the stimulus was intense enough to evoke a C wave in the neurogram. Later, Celander and Folkow (5) clearly demonstrated that only pain fibres are provided with an axon reflex arrangement. The brilliant work of Jancsó et al. (32) amounted to convincing evidence (a) that plasma extravasation elicited by antidromic stimulation is brought about by the release of a neuromediator from chemosensitive small diameter afferent fibres which carry impulses of pain, and (b) that pretreatment of adult rats with a large dose of capsaicin causes a long-lasting morphological (67) and functional impairment of afferent C_2 fibres without any influence on other neurones (66). Neonatal capsaicin pretreatment was shown to result in a selective and irreversible degeneration of these chemosensitive fibres and in an irreversible impairment of neurogenic plasma extravasation (33). Beginning with Otto Loewi's discovery of the humoral transmission of nerve impulses in 1921, pharmacologists were busy and successful in investigating the transmitter amines of efferent nerves. From that time, there exists only the suggestion by Dale (11) that antidromic vasodilation might be produced by release of the same substance that mediates the centripetal transmission from sensory neurones. This idea was taken up by Hellauer and Umrath (23) who investigated the biological effects of extracts from ventral and dorsal roots. The discovery that there is 10 times more substance P (SP) in dorsal than in ventral roots (42), and the first results on a very selective distribution of SP within the CNS (39), resulted in the rather premature consideration of this peptide as a neurotransmitter of sensory afferents. This early suggestion obtained increasing support from the immunohistochemical localization of SP to a distinct population of unmyelinated primary sensory neurones (27) and from the work of Otsuka's group (for a review, see ref. 58). The isolation and synthesis of SP by Leeman's group (for a review, see ref. 54) enabled us to resume investigations by more adequate methods concerning the following questions:

1. Is SP released from peripheral endings of certain sensory fibres?
2. Is SP released from their central endings in the spinal cord?
3. Does SP fulfill the requirements for a neurotransmitter?

METHODS

Capsaicin Pretreatment

Rats were injected subcutaneously with a single dose of 50 mg/kg capsaicin on the 2nd, 10th, 15th, or 20th day of life. Control rats received solvent only (10% ethanol, 10% Tween 80 in saline). Adult rats were pretreated with 50 mg/kg subcutaneous capsaicin on 2 consecutive days; control rats received solvent only (16).

Intraarterial Infusion into the Hind Leg

Rats were anaesthetized with pentobarbital (50 mg/kg i.p.). Drugs, dissolved in isotonic phosphate buffer pH 7.4, were infused into the femoral artery via the superficial epigastric artery.

Assessment of Plasma Extravasation in the Hind Paw

Rats were anaesthetized with pentobarbital. Plasma extravasation following intraarterial infusion of drugs into the hind leg, antidromic electrical stimulation of the cut saphenous nerve or cutaneous application of mustard oil (5% in liquid paraffin) was assessed by the Evans blue test (32). Extravasated Evans blue in the dorsal skin paw was extracted with formamide for 24 hr at 60°C for colorimetric determination at 620 nm. The amount of Evans blue exceeding that of the control paw, or that produced by solvent only in case of intraarterial infusion of drugs, was used to quantify plasma extravasation (16).

Assessment of Vasodilation in the Hind Paw

The day before the experiments, rats were pretreated with 20 mg/kg subcutaneous guanethidine. Rats were anaesthetized with pentobarbital. Vasodilation in the hind paw following antidromic electrical stimulation of the cut saphenous nerve or intraarterial infusion of drugs was determined by measuring the outflow from the femoral vein with a drop recorder. Systemic blood pressure, measured in the carotid artery, was kept constant by infusion of rat blood into the jugular vein (46).

Tail Flick Test

The reaction time of the tail flick response to heat from a lamp focussed on the tip of the tail was measured (30).

Hot Plate Test

Rats were placed on a 56°C hot metal plate and the reaction time of the response (paw licking or jumping) was measured (30).

Chronic Denervation of Paw Skin

The saphenous nerve on one side was cut in the thigh under pentobarbital anaesthesia. Eight days later, the skin area innervated by the saphenous nerve was removed from the denervated and the control paw. The skin of 5 rats was pooled and used for determination of SP (16).

Determination of SP

SP was extracted from various brain regions dissected according to Glowinski and Iversen (21); dorsal and ventral half of the spinal cord, dorsal roots, vagus and saphenous nerve with hydrochloric acid as described (16). SP in the skin and intestine was extracted with acetone-HCl (6) after pulverization in liquid nitrogen. SP was measured with a sensitive radioimmunoassay (18), the minimum detection limit being 25 pg SP per sample. The antibody used showed less than 0.01% cross-reactivity for any of the known neuropeptides.

Release of SP

Hypothalamus, substantia nigra, or spinal cord were chopped to slices less than 0.3 mm in size. Tissue weighing about 90 mg (hypothalamus), 20 mg (substantia nigra), or 150 mg (spinal cord) was transferred to a superfusion chamber and superfused with Krebs-bicarbonate solution at room temperature. The composition of the Krebs solution was: NaCl 118 mM, KCl 4.6 mM, MgSO$_4$ 1.17 mM, CaCl$_2$ 2.5 mM, KH$_2$PO$_4$ 1.17 mM, NaHCO$_3$ 25 mM, glucose 10 mM, with 0.1% bovine serum albumin and bacitracin 20 μM added. After an initial wash period of 12 min, 2-min fractions were collected into glacial acetic acid (final concentration: 2M). At the end of each experiment, SP remaining in the slices was extracted with hydrochloric acid (18). After lyophylization, samples were redissolved and SP was determined by radioimmunoassay (18). The amount of SP released is expressed as the efflux rate constant, i.e.:

$$\frac{\text{pg SP per 2-min fraction}}{\text{pg SP in the slices at time of release}} \times 50\%$$

The total evoked release was calculated as the sum of the efflux rate constants minus mean efflux rate of the three fractions preceding a pulse (19).

Binding Studies

Binding of ^{125}I-Tyr[8]-SP to synaptic vesicle preparations from various regions of the rat CNS and from dorsal and ventral roots was assayed as described by Mayer et al. (53).

Binding of ^{3}H-diprenorphine to homogenates of the whole spinal cord of the rat or to the upper dorsal horn of the spinal cord was assayed as described by Gamse et al. (17).

RESULTS

Observations on the Peripheral Endings of Chemosensitive Fibres

SP Content After Capsaicin Pretreatment

Capsaicin pretreatment (50 mg/kg s.c.) of rats on the 2nd day of life caused a reduction of the SP content, measured at the age of 3 months, in the paw skin, saphenous and vagus nerve, dorsal roots, dorsal half of the spinal cord, and medulla oblongata, but not in any other part of the CNS (Table 1) (16)

TABLE 1. *Percentage decrease of SP 3 months after capsaicin pretreatment at the indicated age*

	Capsaicin pretreatment on day of life[a]		
Structure	2nd	10th	20th
Hind paw skin	*68*	*45*	4
Saphenous nerve	*65*	*36*	8
Vagus nerve	*62*	*44*	0
Dorsal roots	*69*	*48*	*30*
Dorsal spinal cord	*52*	*42*	*31*
Ventral spinal cord	7	0	0
Medulla oblongata	*16*	*17*	*9*
Midbrain	5	0	10
Hypothalamus	0	0	0
Striatum	15	6	6
Cortex	0	0	0
Cerebellum	22	0	3

[a] Values in italics represent statistically significant changes ($p < 0.05$).
Data from Gamse et al., ref. 16.

or in any part of the gastrointestinal tract (29). The decrease of the SP content was similar when capsaicin pretreatment was performed on the 10th day of life, but almost absent when made on the 20th day of life (Table 1). Since SP in the skin was decreased by 58% 4 days after capsaicin pretreatment on the 20th day of life (16), but not 3 months later, it is evident that capsaicin pretreatment up to the 10th day of life results in an irreversible SP decrease, and pretreatment on the 20th day of life and later results in a reversible decrease.

The results show that neonatal capsaicin pretreatment causes a decrease of SP only in areas of the nervous system where primary afferent fibres are located, but not in any other part of the CNS or in the gastrointestinal tract. This can be well explained by the fact that neonatal capsaicin pretreatment causes selective degeneration of chemosensitive primary sensory neurones (33). The decrease of the SP content never exceeded 70%; at present, it cannot be said whether the remaining amount is located in other capsaicin-insensitive primary afferents and/or whether the capsaicin-sensitive afferents did not undergo complete degeneration.

Antidromic Vasodilation

Antidromic vasodilation, exclusively mediated by chemosensitive pain fibres (5,25,32), was measured in the rat hind paw 4 months after capsaicin pretreatment on the 2nd day of life. As antidromic stimulation of the saphenous nerve caused severe vasoconstriction in pretreated as well as in control rats, but was absent after guanethidine and, therefore, was of sympathetic origin, all animals were routinely pretreated with guanethidine (20 mg/kg s.c.). Antidromic vasodilation was almost completely abolished in capsaicin pretreated rats (Fig. 1)

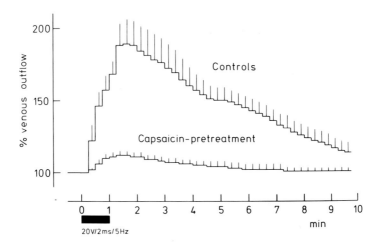

FIG. 1. Hind paw vasodilation induced by antidromic stimulation of the cut saphenous nerve 4 months after pretreatment on the 2nd day of life. Vasodilation was determined by measuring the outflow from the femoral vein. Rats were injected with guanethidine (20 mg/kg s.c.) the day before the experiment. Means ± SEM, $N = 5$ (From Lembeck and Holzer, ref. 46, with permission.)

(46). Thus, antidromic vasodilation is mediated by a distinct population of capsaicin-sensitive primary afferents. Furthermore, there is a striking parallelism between the decreased SP content of sensory nerves (see Table 1) and the absence of antidromic vasodilation.

Intraarterial infusion of SP caused vasodilation in a dose-dependent manner (Figs. 2 and 3) with a threshold dose of 0.5 pmoles/min, thus mimicking antidromic vasodilation. These doses were too low to exert any effect on systemic blood pressure (Fig. 2). During a 3-min intraarterial infusion of SP, venous outflow reached its peak increase within 1 min and then slowly declined (Fig. 2). This might be explained by rapidly developing desensitization. Antidromic vasodilation was unaffected by pretreatment with indomethacin, methysergide, cimetidine, and atropine, but was markedly reduced under the combination of cimetidine and mepyramine and under compound 48/80 (46) (Fig. 4).

Further experiments should clarify whether the vasodilator effect of intraarterial infused SP is a direct effect or is mediated via release of histamine from mast cells. Such a release has been shown by Johnson and Erdös (36) and by Hägermark et al. (22). As shown in Fig. 4, vasodilation induced by antidromic nerve stimulation as well as by intraarterial infusion of SP was diminished after pretreatment with compound 48/80 or with a combination of an H_1-antagonist and an H_2-antagonist, but not with indomethacin.

So it is very likely that the vasodilator effect of intraarterially infused SP is brought about, at least partially, by release of histamine from mast cells, similarly to antidromic vasodilation associated with degranulation of skin mast cells (38). On the other hand, it was not possible to clearly demonstrate a vasodilator

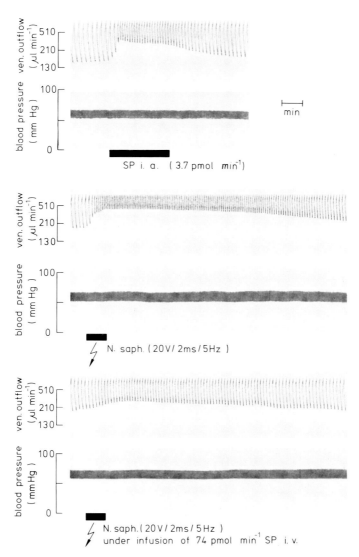

FIG. 2. Hind paw vasodilation induced by infusion of SP into the femoral artery *(upper tracing)*, by antidromic stimulation of the cut saphenous nerve *(middle tracing)*, and by antidromic stimulation of the cut saphenous nerve under continuous i.v. infusion of SP (started 5 min prior, *lower tracing*). Systemic blood pressure was recorded from a carotid artery. Rats were injected with guanethidine (20 mg/kg s.c.) the day before the experiment (From Lembeck and Holzer, ref. 46, with permission.)

effect of intraarterially infused histamine, since doses higher than 9 nmoles/min also caused a marked fall of systemic blood pressure (46), which decreased peripheral circulation. The implication of serotonin, also localized in mast cells, can be ruled out, since intraarterial infusion of doses higher than 0.6 nmoles/

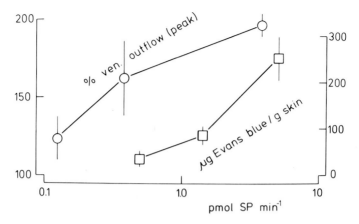

FIG. 3. Dose-dependent vasodilation (measured by the outflow from the femoral vein) and plasma extravasation (measured by Evans blue exudation) induced by infusion of SP into the rat femoral artery. Means ± SEM, *N* = 5 (From Lembeck and Holzer, ref. 46, with permission.)

min produces severe vasoconstriction. Due to the ineffectiveness of indomethacin, an implication of prostaglandins in antidromic vasodilation and vasodilation induced by SP is also excluded.

The experiments concerning the vasodilator effects of SP show that SP acts

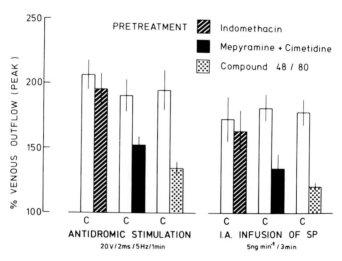

FIG. 4. Hind paw vasodilation induced by antidromic stimulation of the cut saphenous nerve (20 V, 2 msec, 5 Hz; duration: 1 min) or by infusion of SP into the femoral artery (3.7 pmoles/min; duration: 3 min). Effect of pretreatment with indomethacin 10 mg/kg i.p., 1 hr prior), cimetidine (10 mg/kg i.p., 15 min prior) and mepyramine (10 mg/kg i.p., 15 min prior), and compound 48/80 (5 mg/kg s.c., on 2 preceding days). C, controls. All rats were injected with guanethidine (20 mg/kg s.c.) the day before the experiment. Means ± SEM, *N* = 4–10 (From Lembeck and Holzer, ref. 46, with permission.)

in physiologically relevant doses, i.e., in amounts likely to be provided by release from peripheral nerve endings. To further confirm this, the effect of desensitization against SP on antidromic vasodilation was investigated. An intravenous infusion of 74 pmoles/min SP was started 5 min prior to the stimulation of the saphenous nerve. This intravenous infusion initially led to a transient fall in systemic blood pressure, which, however, soon returned to its previous level. Antidromic vasodilation was reduced by 66% under SP infusion (46) (Fig. 2).

Neurogenic Plasma Extravasation

Rats were pretreated with 50 mg/kg subcutaneous capsaicin on the 2nd, 10th, 15th, and 20th day of life and used for experiments 3 months later. Upon local application of mustard oil, plasma extravasation was reduced by 84 and 92% in rats pretreated on the 2nd and 10th day of life, respectively (Fig. 5A). Rats pretreated on the 15th or 20th day of life did not show a reduction of plasma extravasation 3 months after pretreatment (Fig. 5A). However, there was a significant impairment of neurogenic plasma extravasation 4 and 11 days after pretreatment on the 20th day of life (Fig. 5B).

This shows that the impairment of neurogenic plasma extravasation is irreversible after capsaicin pretreatment up to the 15th day of life, i.e., while the nervous

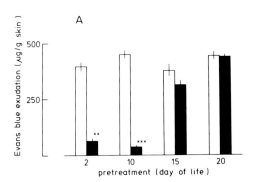

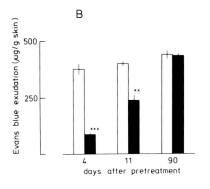

FIG. 5. **A:** Neurogenic plasma extravasation induced by mustard oil 3 months after pretreatment at the indicated age. *Open bars,* controls; *closed bars,* capsaicin. Means ± SEM, N = 6, $^{xx}p <$ 0.01, $^{xxx}p < 0.001$. **B:** Neurogenic plasma extravasation induced by mustard oil at the indicated time after pretreatment on the 20th day of life. *Open bars,* controls; *closed bars,* capsaicin. Means ± SEM, N = 6, $^{xx}p < 0.01$, $^{xxx}p < 0.001$ (From Gamse et al., ref. 16, with permission.)

system of the rat is still undergoing substantial development (12). Furthermore, there is a close parallelism between impaired neurogenic plasma extravasation and impaired antidromic vasodilation, on the one hand, and a decreased SP content in the saphenous nerve and the skin area innervated by it, on the other hand.

Chronic denervation of the skin innervated by the saphenous nerve resulted in a marked decrease of the SP content of the skin and impairment of neurogenic plasma extravasation (Fig. 6), similar to that after neonatal capsaicin pretreatment. This is a further indication that SP could mediate neurogenic plasma extravasation upon its release from peripheral nerve endings (16).

The time courses of the development of plasma extravasation following stimulation of the saphenous nerve and intraarterial infusion of SP were almost identical (Fig. 7). The somewhat slower onset after intraarterial infusion of SP may result from a delayed access of SP to the smooth muscle via the endothelium compared with the release from nerve endings which are located closely to the vascular smooth muscle.

Plasma extravasation is generally slower in onset than vasodilation (compare Figs. 1 and 2 with Fig. 7), and furthermore requires higher doses of SP (Fig. 3). So it is to be expected that plasma extravasation follows the initial vasodilation.

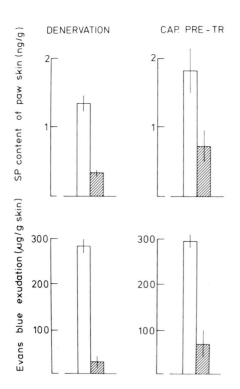

FIG. 6. Neurogenic plasma extravasation (induced by mustard oil) and SP content of the paw skin after chronic denervation (8 days after cutting the saphenous nerve) or capsaicin treatment of adult rats (50 mg/kg s.c. on 2 consecutive days, SP determination 4 days later). Means ± SEM, N = 4–6 (From Gamse et al., ref. 16; and Lembeck et al., ref. 44, with permission.)

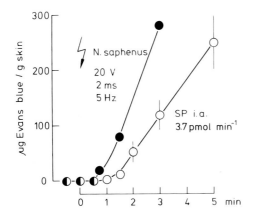

FIG. 7. Time course of plasma extravasation induced by antidromic stimulation of the cut saphenous nerve or by infusion of SP into the femoral artery. Means ± SEM, $N = 4$–6 (From Lembeck and Holzer, ref. 46, with permission.)

To prove the specificity of the vascular permeability increasing action of SP, the effect of SP was compared with the effect of neuropeptides known so far to be present in peripheral neurones. These neuropeptides—including vasoactive intestinal polypeptide, somatostatin, FK 33-824 (Sandoz, Basle) as a Met-enkephalin analogue, and caerulein as a CCK and gastrin analogue—were ineffective in doses 100-fold higher than those of SP which produced plasma extravasation (16). Physalaemin, another tachykinin, was about three times more potent than SP; it does not, however, occur in mammals. Bradykinin was shown to have only about 1/30th of the potency of SP (44). Plasma extravasation upon intraarterial infusion of SP was not altered after chronic denervation of the paw skin

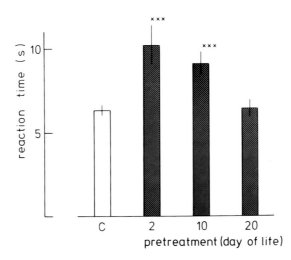

FIG. 8. Hot plate test (56°C), performed 3–4 months after capsaicin pretreatment at the indicated age. C, controls. Means ± SEM of at least 10 animals. [xxx]$p < 0.001$ (From Holzer et al., ref. 30, with permission.)

(44) or in rats pretreated with capsaicin on the 2nd day of life (16), thus excluding a neural mediation of the action of SP (16).

Pain Threshold

Pain threshold, measured as the reaction time in the tail flick and hot plate tests, was assessed 3 to 4 months after capsaicin pretreatment (30). The reaction time of the tail flick response was significantly prolonged in rats pretreated on the 2nd day of life (6.7 ± 0.5 sec versus 12.8 ± 1.2 sec, $p < 0.001$, $N = 15$). Capsaicin pretreatment on the 2nd and 10th day of life also resulted in a prolonged reaction time in the hot plate test (Fig. 8), whereas later pretreatment failed to change reaction time. Thus, the increase of pain threshold corresponds to the impairment of neurogenic plasma extravasation (Fig. 5A), and this shows again that neonatal capsaicin pretreatment causes functional impairment of pain fibres.

Observations on the Central Endings of Chemosensitive Fibres

SP Release by Capsaicin

Exposure of slices from hypothalamus, substantia nigra, or spinal cord to a superfusion medium containing 47 mM K^+ resulted in an increased efflux of SP (Fig. 9). In contrast to elevated K^+, capsaicin increased the SP efflux only from the spinal cord, but not from the hypothalamus or from the substantia nigra (Fig. 9). Thus, the SP-releasing action of capsaicin seems to be confined

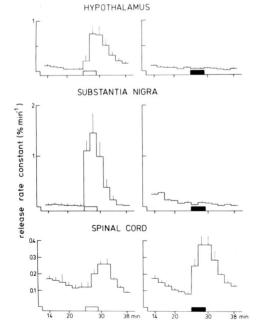

FIG. 9. Effect of 47 mM K *(open rectangles)* or 3.3×10^{-5} capsaicin *(closed rectangles)* on SP release from slices of hypothalamus, substantia nigra, and spinal cord. Means $\pm$ SEM, $N = 3-6$ (From Gamse et al., ref. 19, with permission.)

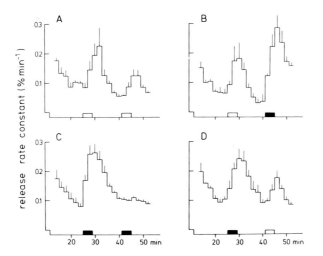

FIG. 10. SP release from spinal cord slices. Pulses of 47 mM K *(open rectangles)* or 3.3 × 10⁻⁶ M capsaicin *(closed rectangles)* were applied in the sequences indicated. Means ± SEM, *N* = 4 (From Gamse et al., ref. 19, with permission.)

to chemosensitive afferent fibres, and this again underlines the specificity of the action of capsaicin.

The release by capsaicin of SP from spinal cord slices was found to be dose-dependent and Ca²⁺-dependent. Capsaicin-induced SP exhibited rapid and specific tachyphylaxis since a second pulse of capsaicin did not increase SP efflux (Fig. 10C), whereas a second pulse of 47 mM K⁺ did (Fig. 10D). However, capsaicin was still able to increase SP efflux after K⁺ (Fig. 10A,B) (19). It is important to note that exposure of spinal cord slices to capsaicin for 18 min caused only an initial SP release which subsequently declined despite the continuous presence of capsaicin; the time course of an 18-min pulse of capsaicin did not differ from that of a 4-min pulse (19). Thus, the SP-depleting action of capsaicin cannot simply be explained by an exhaustion of the releasable pool of SP.

SP Binding Sites on Synaptic Vesicles

Neonatal capsaicin pretreatment as well as pretreatment of adult rats led to a decrease of SP binding sites in synaptic vesicle preparations from dorsal roots and dorsal spinal cord (52) (Fig. 11). Since these SP binding sites on synaptic vesicle membranes are considered as SP storage sites rather than as recognition sites of an SP receptor (53), it can be inferred that capsaicin interferes with the storage of SP in chemosensitive primary sensory neurones.

Opiate Receptors on Chemosensitive Neurones

La Motte et al. (40) presented evidence that opiate receptors are located presynaptically on primary afferent neurones terminating in the substantia gelati-

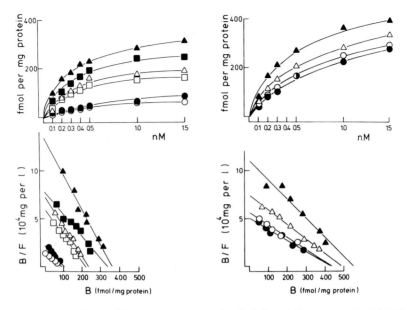

FIG. 11. Influence of capsaicin pretreatment on the 2nd day of life on specific ^{125}I-Tyr[8]-SP binding to synaptic vesicles from various regions. *Closed symbols* refer to control rats; *open symbols* to capsaicin pretreated rats. **Left:** *triangles,* dorsal roots; *circles,* ventral roots; *squares,* spinal cord. **Right:** *triangles,* midbrain; *circles,* hypothalamus. The corresponding Scatchard plots are shown below. Each point represents the mean of four determinations on two different synaptic vesicle preparations, each obtained from 4 rats (From Mayer et al., ref. 52, with permission.)

nosa of the spinal cord. Therefore, it was investigated whether neonatal capsaicin pretreatment leading to degeneration of chemosensitive afferents (33) is associated with a decrease of opiate receptors in the upper dorsal horn of the spinal cord. The number of ^{3}H-diprenorphine binding sites was reduced by 37% in the upper dorsal horn of the spinal cord without any change in their affinity (17) (Fig. 12). The difference of 37% was significantly different: $p < 0.01$ (Student's t-test). This suggests that a considerable number of opiate receptors are located presynaptically on chemosensitive primary sensory neurones. It also shows that these opiate receptors may be located on primary SP-containing afferents, confirming earlier results of Jessell and Iversen (34) and Mudge et al. (55).

DISCUSSION

Release of SP from the Peripheral Endings of Chemosensitive Afferent Neurones

Neonatal capsaicin pretreatment up to the 10th day of life was shown to result in an irreversible decrease of SP in the skin and in areas of the nervous

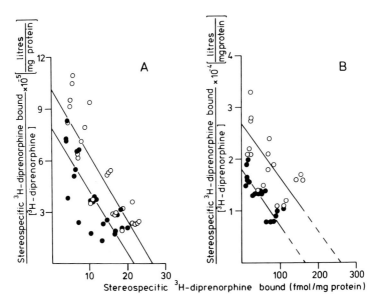

FIG. 12. Scatchard plots of ³H-diprenorphine binding to homogenates of rat whole spinal cord **(A)** or of upper dorsal horn of rat spinal cord **(B)**. Rats were pretreated with capsaicin (50 mg/kg s.c.) on the second day of life *(closed circles)* or solvent only *(open circles)*. Points are single values, obtained from at least 5 capsaicin and 5 control rats (From Gamse et al., ref. 17, with permission.)

system known to contain primary sensory neurones (16). In other areas of the central nervous system and in the gastrointestinal tract no change of the SP content following capsaicin pretreatment was detected (16,29). Since neurogenic plasma extravasation and antidromic vasodilation were almost abolished concomitantly, it is suggested that these phenomena are mediated by peripheral release of SP from a distinct population of capsaicin-sensitive pain fibres.

Capsaicin pretreatment from the 15th day of life on led only to a reversible functional impairment of the fibres subserving neurogenic plasma extravasation (16) and to a decrease of SP in the skin which was reversible within 3 months (16). In the more central portions of the capsaicin-sensitive fibres, i.e., the dorsal roots, the restoration of the SP content seemed to take place much slower there since the SP content was still decreased 5 months after pretreatment (16). Capsaicin pretreatment of adult rats or chronic denervation of the paw skin led to a similar decrease of SP in the skin and to a similar impairment of neurogenic plasma extravasation (16). As far as SP neurones are concerned, capsaicin has obviously a selective action on primary sensory SP neurones.

In every case, a decreased SP content of skin and sensory nerves was accompanied by functional impairment of chemosensitive sensory neurones (16,30,46) which are known to subserve antidromic vasodilation and neurogenic plasma extravasation (32) and to conduct impulses from polymodal nociceptors (66). Neurogenic plasma extravasation (16) and antidromic vasodilation (46) were almost absent and pain threshold was markedly increased as assessed by the tail flick and hot plate tests (30). These effects were irreversible after capsaicin pretreatment up to the 10th day of life and can well be explained by selective degeneration of capsaicin-sensitive afferent neurones (33).

Taken together, these findings have two major implications: (a) A major part of afferent SP neurones are chemosensitive primary sensory neurones pharmacologically characterized by their sensitivity to capsaicin. (b) SP is the most likely transmitter candidate which, upon its peripheral release, mediates both antidromic vasodilation and neurogenic plasma extravasation.

In agreement with the second statement, SP is able to mimic the effects of antidromic stimulation of sensory nerves. Intraarterial infusion of physiologically relevant doses (about 1 pmole/min) causes vasodilation and plasma extravasation (16,46). Furthermore, antidromic vasodilation is greatly reduced under intravenous infusion of SP (46). Since the vascular effects of SP exhibit desensitization, and desensitization to SP can be used for the identification of SP (14,50), the reduction of antidromic vasodilation after infusion of SP is a strong indication for SP being the mediator of this phenomenon. Among the neuropeptides so far demonstrated in peripheral neurones, SP was the only one able to mimic neurogenic plasma extravasation (16). Prostaglandins were also found to be very potent in producing plasma extravasation (44); however, neurogenic plasma extravasation is not affected by indomethacin (46).

In contrast to the findings of Jancsó et al. (32), antidromic vasodilation was found to be associated with degranulation of mast cells, and both antidromic vasodilation and neurogenic plasma extravasation seem to involve release of vasoactive constituents from mast cells, especially histamine (22,38,46). Both antidromic vasodilation and vasodilation induced by SP are significantly reduced after pretreatment with mepyramine or compound 48/80 (46). Thus, a further requirement for SP being a mediator of antidromic vasodilation is fulfilled: SP apparently has the same mode of action as antidromic stimulation of sensory nerves. This also confirms earlier results that SP releases histamine from mast cells (22,36). There is also good evidence that plasma extravasation induced by SP is not mediated by a neural action of SP since chronic denervation of the paw skin (44) or neonatal capsaicin pretreatment (16) does not alter the effect of SP.

In view of the low SP content in the skin, no attempt was made to directly estimate SP released from the peripheral endings of sensory neurones. The amount of released SP is by all means far too low to be measureable even by the most sensitive methods. In spite of this, the parallelism between the decreased SP content of chemosensitive pain fibres and the functional impairment of these fibres after neonatal capsaicin pretreatment provides indirect evidence that (a) SP is a transmitter of chemosensitive primary sensory neurones and that (b) release of SP at their peripheral branchings accounts for the signs of the axon reflex, i.e., cutaneous vasodilation and plasma extravasation.

Release of SP from the Central Endings of Chemosensitive Afferent Neurones

The SP content of the dorsal roots and the dorsal half of the spinal cord was decreased by 50 to 70% after neonatal capsaicin pretreatment (16). A similar but less pronounced fall of SP in the dorsal spinal cord was seen after pretreatment of adult rats (20,35). This decrease is also reflected in a reduction of SP binding sites in synaptic vesicle preparations from dorsal roots and spinal cord (52). This reduction was seen not only after neonatal capsaicin pretreatment, but also after pretreatment of adult rats. It is worth noting here that capsaicin pretreatment of adult rats leads only to functional impairment of chemosensitive pain fibres and a decrease of microvesicles therein (67), but not to axonal degeneration.

Since plasma extravasation induced by cutaneous application of capsaicin is thought to be mediated by release of a factor from chemosensitive sensory neurones (32), it should be possible that capsaicin releases this substance also from the central terminals of these neurones in the spinal cord. It was shown that capsaicin releases SP from spinal cord slices and it was concluded that the SP-releasing action of capsaicin is confined to primary afferent SP neurones (19). This capsaicin-induced release of SP from spinal cord slices was Ca^{2+}-dependent and, in contrast to K^+-induced SP release, underwent rapid and specific tachyphylaxis. Thus, the SP-depleting action of capsaicin in adult rats cannot be solely attributed to a protracted SP release; but there are other possibilities to be considered such as interference with synthesis, storage, axonal transport, and metabolism of SP. An interference with the storage of SP is possibly reflected by the decreased number of SP binding sites in synaptic vesicle preparations from dorsal roots and spinal cord of capsaicin-treated rats (52).

The 37% fall in the number of opiate receptors in the upper dorsal horn after neonatal capsaicin pretreatment suggests a presynaptic location of opiate receptors on chemosensitive sensory neurones (17). These findings confirm the hypothesis that part of the analgesic action of opiates takes place already at the level of the substantia gelatinosa Rolandi by inhibiting the transmitter release from pain fibres. Since SP is considered to be this transmitter (16,42,59), opiates would suppress the release of SP, and this indeed was found by Jessell and Iversen (34) and Mudge et al. (55).

SP and Requirements for a Neurotransmitter

For identification of new neurotransmitters several criteria have to be fulfilled:

1. Presence of the transmitter candidate in the considered population of neurones, together with the following:
2. Presence of an enzyme system for its synthesis and metabolism.
3. Evidence for (a) axoplasmic transport and (b)
4. Storage in synaptic vesicles.

5. Demonstration of a Ca^{2+}-dependent release from nerve endings.

6. Definition and characterization of postsynaptic receptors.

7. Knowledge of the manner in which synaptic transmission is terminated.

8. Ability to mimic the synaptic effects for which the candidate is considered to be responsible.

9. Pharmacological characterization, i.e., pharmacological modulation of synthesis, transport, storage, release, and action of the transmitter on receptors, and termination of synaptic transmission.

Concerning SP as primary sensory transmitter, a number of these criteria are already fulfilled. In the following, short references are made to each of the headings.

1. SP was immunohistochemically demonstrated in a population of unmyelinated primary sensory neurones terminating in the skin and substantia gelatinosa of the spinal cord (8,10,27). The recent findings using capsaicin have shown that these neurones include a major part of chemosensitive sensory neurones (16,35).

2. Although information about the synthesis steps of SP is still not available, there is indirect evidence that SP is synthesized in spinal ganglion cells (1,27,68) as well as in trigeminal ganglion cells (8) and in nodose ganglion cells (18).

3. Axoplasmic transport of SP in the bifurcating sensory neurones was demonstrated both towards the central endings (1,8,18,27,68) and towards the periphery (8,18,26,28,68).

4. Like all known putative neurotransmitters, SP was found to be present in synaptosomes (31,45,48,63) and more specifically in synaptic vesicles (9,26,61). Synaptic vesicles from rat brain and spinal cord (52,53) possess high affinity binding sites for SP which could be considered as storage sites for SP.

5. In the spinal cord SP is released upon electrical stimulation of the dorsal roots (60). SP was also shown to be released by antidromic stimulation from the peripheral endings of sensory nerves in the tooth pulp (57). Furthermore, a Ca^{2+}-dependent stimulus-evoked release of SP from synaptosomes (48,63) and from trigeminal sensory nucleus slices (34) and spinal cord slices (19) was described. Jessell et al. *(personal communication)* showed by intrathecal perfusion of the cat spinal cord that SP is released by stimulation of the sciatic nerve only if the stimulus is intense enough to excite C fibres.

6. The existence of SP receptors is postulated because the actions of SP cannot be antagonized by antagonists of any other putative neurotransmitter (for reviews, see refs. 49,50). Recent biochemical studies have revealed high affinity binding of SP to crude synaptic membranes (56) and purified plasma membranes (N. Mayer et al., *this volume*) which possibly could represent an interaction with synaptic receptors for SP.

7. No information on the manner in which "SPergic" transmission is terminated is presently available. The demonstration of a reuptake system for SP has not succeeded (64). In peripheral vascular beds where the axon reflex takes

place, a highly effective inactivating system for SP was demonstrated (47).

8. Antidromic vasodilation and neurogenic plasma extravasation, which are likely to be mediated by peripheral release of SP, can be mimicked by intraarterial infusion of SP (46). In the spinal cord, SP selectively excites units that are also activated by noxious stimulation of the skin (24,62). Thus, SP can mimic "transmission of pain" in the spinal cord.

9. Pharmacological characterization of SPergic transmission exists only to a very limited extent. Neonatal capsaicin pretreatment leads to degeneration of SP-containing sensory neurones; pretreatment of adult rats causes only depletion of SP (16). The mode of action of capsaicin is still unknown, but it seems to interfere with the storage of SP (52). Furthermore, capsaicin releases SP from primary sensory neurones in a Ca^{2+}-dependent manner (19); however, in view of rapidly developing tachyphylaxis the SP-depleting action of capsaicin cannot be simply explained by the SP-releasing action of capsaicin. Whether capsaicin acts specifically on SP neurones remains to be clarified. Release of SP from sensory neurones is suppressed by opiates (34,55) acting on presynaptic opiate receptors (17,40). No competitive antagonist of SP is presently known; in the spinal cord baclofen is considered as an antagonist of SP (M. Otsuka, *this volume*). On smooth muscle, the action of SP can specifically be depressed by previous administration of SP (see ref. 50). Antidromic vasodilation is also greatly reduced under intravenous infusion of SP (46). The highly effective inactivating system found for SP in peripheral vascular beds can be inhibited by the protease inhibitor bacitracin (47).

Open Questions

Despite accumulating evidence that SP is a neurotransmitter of primary sensory neurones, several questions are still unsolved and areas remain that require comprehensive work:

1. If SP is regarded as the transmitter of chemosensitive small diameter fibres, what are the transmitters of all the other afferent fibres?

2. Antidromic vasodilation, now known for more than 100 years, can be explained by peripheral release of SP from chemosensitive sensory fibres. What is the physiological significance of this vasodilation and the following plasma extravasation?

3. Afferent fibres of the vagus nerve contain SP. In contrast to the detailed knowledge of the cholinergic efferent part, no information about the afferent SP-containing part is known.

4. Apart from the consideration of SP as transmitter of chemosensitive pain fibres in the spinal cord, SP does not stimulate pain receptors in the periphery (43). This is reminiscent of the concept of "alternative transmission" formulated by Feldberg and Vogt (13) that central neurones are not excited by the transmitter that they themselves release at their endings.

ACKNOWLEDGMENTS

This work was supported by Grant Nos. 3400 and 3506 of the Austrian Scientific Research Funds and by Grant No. 1293 of the Jubiläumsfonds der Österreichischen Nationalbank. The SP antibody used in these studies was generously provided by Dr. S. E. Leeman. The expert technical assistance of Mr. J. Donnerer, Mrs. U. Hetzendorf, and Mr. W. Schluet is gratefully acknowledged.

REFERENCES

1. Barber, R. P., Vaughn, J. E., Slemmon, J. R., Salvaterra, P. M., Roberts, E., and Leeman, S. E. (1979): The origin, distribution and synaptic relationships of substance P axons in rat spinal cord. *J. Comp. Neurol.,* 184:331–351.
2. Bayliss, W. M. (1901): On the origin from the spinal cord of the vasodilator fibres of the hind limb, and on the nature of these fibres. *J. Physiol. (Lond.),* 26:173–209.
3. Bruce, A. N. (1910): Über die Beziehung der sensiblen Nervenendigungen zum Entzündungsvorgang. *Arch. Exp. Pathol. Pharmakol.,* 63:424–433.
4. Bury, R. W., and Mashford, M. L. (1977): A pharmacological investigation of synthetic substance P on the isolated guinea-pig ileum. *Clin. Exp. Pharmacol. Physiol.,* 4:453–461.
5. Celander, O., and Folkow, B. (1953): The nature and distribution of afferent fibres provided with the axon reflex arrangement. *Acta Physiol. Scand.,* 29:359–370.
6. Chang, M. M., and Leeman, S. E. (1970): Isolation of a sialogogic peptide from bovine hypothalamic tissue and its characterization as substance P. *J. Biol. Chem.,* 245:4784–4790.
7. Chapman, L. F., and Goodell, H. (1964): The participation of the nervous system in the inflammatory reaction. *Ann. NY Acad. Sci.,* 116:990–1017.
8. Cuello, A. C., del Fiacco, M., and Paxinos, G. (1978): The central and peripheral ends of the substance P-containing sensory neurones in the rat trigeminal system. *Brain Res.,* 152:499–509.
9. Cuello, A. C., Emson, P., del Fiacco, M., Gale, J., Iversen, L. L., Jessell, T. M., Kanazawa, J., Paxinos, G., and Quik, M. (1978): Distribution and release of substance P in the central nervous system. In: *Centrally Acting Peptides,* edited by J. Hughes, pp. 135–155. Macmillan, London.
10. Cuello, A. C., Polak, J. M., and Pearse, A. G. E. (1976): Substance P: A naturally occurring transmitter in human spinal cord. *Lancet,* 2:1054–1056.
11. Dale, H. H. (1935): Pharmacology and nerve endings. *Proc. Roy. Soc. Lond. (Biol.),* 28:319–332.
12. Dobbing, J. (1968): The development of the blood brain barrier. *Prog. Brain Res.,* 29:417–427.
13. Feldberg, W., and Vogt, M. (1948): Acetylcholine synthesis in different regions of the central nervous system. *J. Physiol. (Lond.),* 107:372–381.
14. Gaddum, J. H. (1953): Tryptamine receptors. *J. Physiol. (Lond.),* 119:363–368.
15. Gaertner, G. (1889): Über den Verlauf der Vasodilatoren. *Wien. Klin. Wochenschr.,* 51:980–981.
16. Gamse, R., Holzer, P., and Lembeck, F. (1979): Decrease of substance P in primary afferent neurones and impairment of neurogenic plasma extravasation by capsaicin. *Br. J. Pharmacol.,* 68:207–21.
17. Gamse, R., Holzer, P., and Lembeck, F. (1979): Indirect evidence for presynaptic localization of opiate receptors on chemosensitive primary sensory neurones. *Naunyn Schmiedebergs Arch. Pharmacol.,* 308:281–285.
18. Gamse, R., Lembeck, F., and Cuello, A. C. (1979): Substance P in the vagus nerve: Immunochemical and immunohistochemical evidence for axoplasmic transport. *Naunyn Schmiedebergs Arch. Pharmacol.,* 306:37–44.
19. Gamse, R., Molnar, A., and Lembeck, F. (1979): Substance P release from spinal cord slices by capsaicin. *Life Sci.,* 25:629–636.
20. Gasparović, J., Hadzović, S., Huković, S., and Stern, P. (1964): Contribution to the theory that substance P has a transmitter role in sensitive pathways. *Med. Exp.,* 10:303–306.

21. Glowinski, J., and Iversen, L. L. (1966): Regional studies of catecholamines in the rat brain. I. The disposition of ^{3}H-norepinephrine, ^{3}H-dopamine and ^{3}H-DOPA in various regions of the brain. J. Neurochem., 13:655–669.
22. Hägermark, Ö., Hökfelt, T., and Pernow, B. (1978): Flare and itch induced by substance P in human skin. J. Invest. Dermatol., 71:233–235.
23. Hellauer, H., and Umrath, K. (1947): The transmitter substance of sensory nerve fibres. J. Physiol. (Lond.), 106:20.
24. Henry, J. L. (1976): Effects of substance P on functionally identified units in cat spinal cord. Brain Res., 114:439–452.
25. Hinsey, J. C., and Gasser, H. S. (1930): The component of the dorsal root mediating vasodilatation and the Sherrington contraction. Am. J. Physiol., 92:679–689.
26. Hökfelt, T., Johansson, O., Kellerth, J.-O., Ljungdahl, A., Nilsson, G., Nygards, A., and Pernow, B. (1977): Immunohistochemical distribution of substance P. In: Substance P, edited by U. S. von Euler and B. Pernow, pp. 177–145. Raven Press, New York.
27. Hökfelt, T., Kellerth, J.-O., Nilsson, G., and Pernow, B. (1975): Experimental immunohistochemical studies on the localization and distribution of substance P in cat primary sensory neurons. Brain Res., 100:235–252.
28. Holton, P. (1960): Substance P concentration in degenerating nerve. In: Polypeptides Which Affect Smooth Muscles and Blood Vessels, edited by M. Schachter, pp. 192–194. Pergamon, Oxford.
29. Holzer, P., Gamse, R., and Lembeck, F. (1979): Distribution of substance P in the rat gastrointestinal tract—lack of effect of capsaicin pretreatment. Eur. J. Pharmacol., 61:303–307.
30. Holzer, P., Jurna, I., Gamse, R., and Lembeck, F. (1979): Nociceptive threshold after neonatal capsaicin pretreatment. Eur. J. Pharmacol., 58:511–514.
31. Inouye, A., Kataoka, K. (1962): Subcellular distribution of substance P in the nervous tissues. Nature, 193:585.
32. Jancsó, N., Jancsó-Gábor, A., and Szolcsányi, J. (1967): Direct evidence for neurogenic inflammation and its prevention by denervation and by pretreatment with capsaicin. Br. J. Pharmacol., 31:138–151.
33. Jancsó, G., Kiraly, E., and Jancsó-Gábor, A. (1977): Pharmacologically induced selective degeneration of chemosensitive primary sensory neurones. Nature, 270:741–743.
34. Jessell, T. M., and Iversen, L. L. (1977): Opiate analgesics inhibit substance P release in rat trigeminal nucleus. Nature, 268:549–551.
35. Jessell, T. M., Iversen, L. L., and Cuello, A. C. (1978): Capsaicin-induced depletion of substance P from primary sensory neurones. Brain Res., 152:183–188.
36. Johnson, A. R., and Erdös, E. G. (1973): Release of histamine from mast cells by vasoactive peptides. Proc. Soc. Exp. Biol. Med., 142:1253–1256.
37. Kibjakow, A. W. (1931): Zur Frage des Vasodilatations—mechanismus bei der Reizung antidromer Nerven. Pfluegers Arch. Ges. Physiol., 228:30–39.
38. Kiernan, J. A. (1975): A pharmacological and histological investigation of the involvement of mast cells in cutaneous axon reflex vasodilatation. Quart. J. Exp. Physiol., 60:123–130.
39. Kopera, H., and Lazarini, W. (1953): Zur Frage der zentralen Übertragung afferenter Impulse. IV. Mitteilung. Die Verteilung von Substanz P im Zentralnervensystem. Arch. Exp. Pathol. Pharmakol., 219:214–222.
40. La Motte, C., Pert, C. B., and Snyder, S. H. (1976): Opiate receptor binding in primate spinal cord: Distribution and changes after dorsal root section. Brain Res., 112:407–412.
41. Langley, J. N. (1923): Antidromic action. J. Physiol. (Lond.), 57:428–446.
42. Lembeck, F. (1953): Zur Frage der zentralen Übertragung afferenter Impulse. III. Mitteilung. Das Vorkommen und die Bedeutung der Substanz P in den dorsalen Wurzeln des Rückenmarks. Arch. Exp. Pathol. Pharmakol., 219:197–213.
43. Lembeck, F., and Gamse, R. (1977): Lack of algesic effect of substance P on paravascular pain receptors. Naunyn Schmiedebergs Arch. Pharmacol., 299:295–303.
44. Lembeck, F., Gamse, R., and Juan, H. (1977): Substance P and sensory nerve endings. In: Substance P, edited by U. S. von Euler and B. Pernow, pp. 169–181. Raven Press, New York.
45. Lembeck, F., and Holasek, A. (1960): Die intracelluläre Lokalisation der Substanz P. Arch. Exp. Pathol. Pharmakol., 238:542–545.
46. Lembeck, F., and Holzer, P. (1979): Substance P as a mediator of antidromic vasodilation and neurogenic plasma extravasation. Naunyn Schmiedebergs Arch. Pharmacol., 310:175–183.
47. Lembeck, F., Holzer, P., Schweditsch, M., and Gamse, R. (1978): Elimination of substance P

from the circulation of the rat and its inhibition by bacitracin. *Naunyn Schmiedebergs Arch. Pharmacol.*, 305:9–16.

48. Lembeck, F., Mayer, N., and Schindler, G. (1977): Substance P in rat brain synaptosomes. *Naunyn Schmiedebergs Arch. Pharmacol.*, 301:17–22.

49. Lembeck, F., and Zetler, G. (1962): Substance P: A polypeptide of possible physiological significance, especially within the nervous system. *Int. Rev. Neurobiol.*, 4:159–215.

50. Lembeck, F., and Zetler, G. (1971): Substance P. *Int. Encycl. Pharmacol. Ther., Sect. 72*, 1:29–71.

51. Lewis, T., and Marvin, H. M. (1927): Observations relating to vasodilatation arising from antidromic impulses, to herpes zoster and trophic effects. *Heart*, 14:27–46.

52. Mayer, N., Gamse, R., and Lembeck, F. (1980): Effect of capsaicin-pretreatment on substance P binding sites on synaptic vesicles. *J. Neurochem. (in press)*.

53. Mayer, N., Lembeck, F., Saria, A., and Gamse, R. (1979): Substance P: Characteristics of binding to synaptic vesicles of rat brain. *Naunyn Schmiedebergs Arch. Pharmacol.*, 306:45–51.

54. Mroz, E. A., and Leeman, S. E. (1977): Substance P. *Vitam. Horm.*, 35:209–281.

55. Mudge, A. W., Leeman, S. E., and Fischbach, G. D., (1979): Enkephalin inhibits release of substance P from sensory neurons in culture and decreases action potential duration. *Proc. Natl. Acad. Sci. USA*, 76:526–530.

56. Nakata, Y., Kusaka, Y., Segawa, T., Yajima, H., and Kitagawa, K. (1978): Substance P: Regional distribution and specific binding to synaptic membranes in rabbit central nervous system. *Life Sci.*, 22:259–268.

57. Olgart, L., Gazelius, B., Brodin, E., and Nilsson, G. (1977): Release of substance P-like immunoreactivity from the dental pulp. *Acta Physiol. Scand.*, 101:510–512.

58. Otsuka, M. (1977): Substance P and sensory transmitter. *Adv. Neurochem.*, 2:193–211.

59. Otsuka, M., and Konishi, S. (1976): Substance P and excitatory transmitter of primary sensory neurons. *Cold Spring Harbor Symp. Quant. Biol.*, 40:135–143.

60. Otsuka, M., and Konishi, S. (1976): Release of substance P-like immunoreactivity from isolated spinal cord of newborn rat. *Nature*, 264:83–84.

61. Pickel, V. M., Reis, D. J., Leeman, S. E. (1977): Ultrastructural localization of substance P in neurons in rat spinal cord. *Brain Res.*, 122:534–540.

62. Randić, M., and Miletić, V. (1977): Effect of substance P in cat dorsal horn neurones activated by noxious stimuli. *Brain Res.*, 128:164–169.

63. Schenker, C., Mroz, E. A., and Leeman, S. E. (1976): Release of substance P from isolated nerve endings. *Nature*, 264:790–792.

64. Segawa, T., Nakata, Y., Yajima, H., Kitagawa, K. (1977): Further observation on the lack of active uptake system for substance P in the central nervous system. *Jap. J. Pharmacol.*, 27:573–580.

65. Stricker, S. (1876): Untersuchungen über die Gefässwurzeln des Ischiadicus. *Stitz.-Ber. Kaiserl. Akad. Wiss. (Wien)*, 3:173–185.

66. Szolcsányi, J. (1977): A pharmacological approach to elucidation of the role of different nerve fibres and receptor endings in mediation of pain. *J. Physiol. (Paris)*, 73:251–259.

67. Szolcsányi, J., Jancsó-Gábor, A., and Joó, F. (1975): Functional and fine structural characteristics of the sensory neurone blocking effect of capsaicin. *Naunyn Schmiedebergs Arch. Pharmacol.*, 287:157–168.

68. Takahashi, T., and Otsuka, M. (1975): Regional distribution of substance P in the spinal cord and nerve roots of the cat and the effects of dorsal root section. *Brain Res.*, 87:1–11.

Neuropeptides and Neural Transmission,
edited by C. Ajmone Marsan and W. Z. Traczyk.
Raven Press, New York © 1980.

Substance P as a Modulator of Physiological and Pathological Processes

P. Oehme, *K. Hecht, L. Piesche, H. Hilse, **E. Morgenstern, and *M. Poppei

*Academy of Sciences of GDR, Institute of Drug Research, 1136 Berlin; *Department of Psychiatry and Neurology, Charité, 104 Berlin; and **Pharmacological Research Institute of the Pharmaceutical Industry, 1136 Berlin, German Democratic Republic*

Substance P (SP) has long been known for its marked effects on the central nervous system. It has been thought to be a neurotransmitter in sensory pathways ever since its concentrations were found to be high in the dorsal roots and columns of the spinal cord (6). Strong depolarising action of SP on spinal neurons in frogs and rats was reported by Otsuka and co-workers (11). SP has been found to produce potent, long-lasting analgesic activity in mice in more recent studies in which the hot plate technique was used (3,17).

In 1978, SP was found to be a long-lasting analgesic also in the tail flick test of rats to which it had been intracerebrally administered (9). Oehme et al. (10), on the other hand, had proposed that SP produces hyperalgesia. Frederickson et al. (3) tried to explain those conflicting data and postulated dual action of SP on nociperception.

Only preliminary results have been presented so far regarding the action of SP on behaviour. Starr et al. (15) found that peripheral administration of synthetic SP, according to Stern et al.'s earlier results (16), induced behavioral depressant properties in mice. SP, endorphins, and other brain peptides were recently discussed by Barchas et al. (1) who proposed that those peptides acted as neuromodulators. This would mean that they were not responsible for the direct transfer of nerve signals from presynaptic to postsynaptic elements, but rather altered neuronal activities in other ways, for instance, by affecting transmitter synthesis, release, uptake, receptor interaction, and metabolism. Some results by Magnusson et al. (8), Starr et al. (15), Reubi et al. (13) and the authors' own group (10,12) showed that such postulated interaction could really exist between SP and the mono-aminergic neurons.

The experiments reported in this chapter were conducted with the view of obtaining more information about the action of SP on nociperception, behaviour, and mono-aminergic neurons.

METHODS AND RESULTS

Action of SP on Nociperception

The experiments described in this chapter are likely to suggest that the dual property of SP to produce analgesia or hyperalgesia depends, last but not least, on the given condition of the individual animal—that is, on individual control response latency before SP testing. SP was tested by the authors for its action on nociperception by means of the hot plate procedure.

ICR standard mice were used in the studies, body weights being between 18 and 22 g. Hot plate testing was based on an apparatus with a thermostatically heated metal plate (57°C). A Plexiglass cylinder, 10.0 cm in height and 20.5 cm in inner diameter, and with open top, was used to confine the mice to a certain area of the plate surface. SP administration was intraperitoneal and intravenous. Control mice received isotonic saline.

The time, in seconds, which elapsed from first contact with the plate to first hind-paw licking was recorded as response latency. Control latencies were estimated one day before testing and 15 min before SP treatment. The resulting value before SP treatment gave the mean control latency. Experiments published earlier had shown that in hot plate testing, response latencies were reduced by SP (hyperalgesia) (10): the mice used in the experiments reported herein had received intraperitoneal SP injections, the dose being 500 µg/kg. The authors, when conducting these experiments, were under the impression that the action of SP differed in mice with shorter or longer control response latencies. Therefore, a selection procedure was applied to the mice.

Estimation of control response latencies in the manner described was followed by selection of mice and their grouping: group I included mice with control response latencies below 15 sec, group II included mice with latencies between 15 and 29 sec, and group III included those with values between 30 and 44 sec. The response latencies of the three groups were measured again 30, 60, 90, and 120 min after injection of SP. The latencies recorded 60 min after SP treatment are given in Fig. 1. The response latencies of the three groups were altered in different ways by SP treatment. For group I, with short control response latencies, SP proved to cause analgesic activity, the latency between first contact and first hind-paw licking being prolonged. For group III, with the longest control response latencies, the response latency was reduced by SP, a sign of hyperalgesia. For group II, with control response latencies between groups I and III, response latencies were also depressed by SP treatment, albeit slightly. These results would suggest that the action of SP on nociperception depends on the given condition of the individual mouse. One and the same dose of SP, consequently, would be capable of producing different effects, analgesia or hyperalgesia, depending on different conditions in each of the mice involved (Fig. 2).

The next step taken by the authors was to compare the above three groups,

	n	Increase(+) or decrease(−) in latency [seconds]	Significance [p]
① Latency < 15 sec.			
Control	40	− 0.9 ± 5.9	n. s.
SP-treatment	74	+ 5.0 ± 20.1	< 0.05
② Latency 15 − 29 sec.			
Control	40	− 0.7 ± 21.5	n. s.
SP-treatment	75	− 6.7 ± 14.1	< 0.001
③ Latency ≦ 30 sec.			
Control	20	− 7.2 ± 32.3	n. s.
SP-treatment	50	−16.6 ± 19.1	< 0.001

FIG. 1. Changes in mean response latency of mice with different control values before SP treatment (hot plate procedure, 57°C); response latency being the time from first contact with the plate to first hind-paw licking.

under the same experimental conditions, for the absolute values of response latency, 60 min after SP treatment. The result was surprising for the mean values of all three groups were almost identical. This suggests that SP was capable of producing "standardisation" of responsiveness to pain.

    The authors then investigated dose-dependence of SP action on nociperception

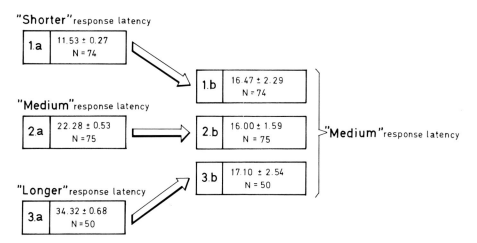

FIG. 2. Mean response latencies of mice before and after SP treatment (same test procedure as in Fig. 1). **1a–3a:** Mean response latency (sec) ± SEM before SP treatment. **1b–3b:** Mean response latency (sec) ± SEM 60 min after SP treatment (500 μg/kg i.v.).

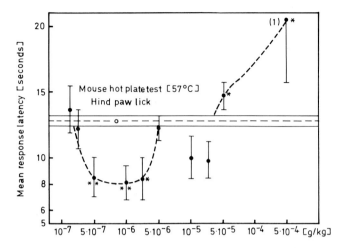

FIG. 3. Dose-response curve for SP action on nociperception (same test procedure as in Fig. 1). *Filled circles* give the mean latency (± SE) at 60 min after SP treatment (i.p.). (1): i.v. application. *Open circles:* saline-treated mice. *N:* 10 mice per treatment. **$p < 0.005$, *$p < 0.05$.

(Fig. 3), and the intraperitoneal administration of SP was found to produce dose-related effects. The mice used in this test had control response latencies below 15 sec. Small but significant analgesic activity, i.e., increase in latency, was recordable from the same mice, following application of 500 μg/kg (5×10^{-4} g/kg). Lower doses switched this analgesic action to hyperalgesia, with the latter's maximum being close to 10^{-6} g/kg. Another but insignificant maximum was recordable in response to something close to 10^{-5} g/kg.

The above findings would suggest that SP had a dual action also on mice with defined short control response latencies. This particular kind of dual action was dose-dependent: higher doses of SP produced analgesia and lower doses produced hyperalgesia.

In summary the point can be made that SP exerts different effects upon nociperception, since it is capable of causing both analgesia and hyperalgesia. High responsiveness to thermic stimuli can be reduced, and low responsiveness can be increased. Such effect will, in any case, result in "normalisation" or "standardisation" of individual responsiveness to pain.

Action of SP on Behaviour

In this field, too, the authors supported the hypothesis that SP action might depend on the given condition of the individual animal. For this reason intact rats and stressed rats with disorders in behaviour were used in the experiments. An avoidance response test was used to investigate the action of SP on behaviour. This method was published in detail by Hecht et al. (5). The working principle was as follows: An electric foot shock was applied to the paws of the rat. The

Procedure for daily noise application:

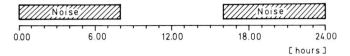

FIG. 4. Diagram of noise application.

task of the animal was to cover a distance of 40 cm to press down a lever that cut off the electric current. The rats then were trained to avoid the unconditioned stimulus (US) in response to a conditioned stimulus (CS), a tone of 3,000 Hz over 5 sec. The procedure for acquisition training included 15 CS per session and per day on the first 2 days and 20 on each of the following days. A conditioned reflex was considered to be established if avoidance response was produced by the rats to 90% of the CS applied. The conditioned avoidance response (CAR) was the ratio between correctly performed avoidance reactions, on the one hand, and the number of possible CS, on the other.

In intact adult rats, aged 14 weeks, no change was found in acquisition of this avoidance response, following SP treatment (250 and 500 μg/kg i.v.) (5). The situation was quite different in stressed rats; i.e., rats exposed to noise stress. The procedure of noise application is shown in Fig. 4. Avoidance acquisition by the rats was impaired after 5 weeks (Fig. 5). The effect of SP treatment on noise-induced disorders in avoidance behaviour was investigated in experiments which followed. During 4 days of acquisition SP was always applied 1 hr before the learning experiments were started (Fig. 6). SP treatment led to complete normalisation of avoidance acquisition in stressed rats. A smaller dose of SP (25 μg/kg i.v.) had the same effect. The effect was not obtained in response to 2.5 μg/kg intravenous SP.

The avoidance-normalising effect of SP was associated with state-dependent learning in response to the higher dose (250 μg/kg), but not following the smaller dose (25 μg/kg). Such normalising effect of SP in noise-stressed rats

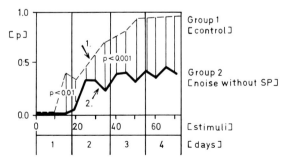

FIG. 5. Effect of noise (30 days) on CAR *(p)* learning of female rats. $N = 10$ rats per group, controls received 10 μl aqua dest. per rat i.p.

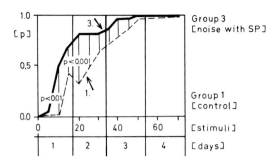

FIG. 6. Effect of noise and of noise together with SP application (250 μg/kg i.p.) on CAR (p) learning of female rats. N = 10 rats per group, controls received 10 μl aqua dest. per rat i.p.

was found not only in the context of avoidance learning, for noise application over 5 weeks also induced in the same rats persistent increase in blood pressure and other changes in vegetative functions. Elevated blood pressure and other changes in vegetative functions were in the same way completely normalised by SP pretreatment (Fig. 7).

The normalising effect of SP on avoidance learning was studied also in rats stressed by immobilisation in a plastic tube. Disorders in avoidance learning and blood pressure were also recordable from such rats. The stress-induced disorders in avoidance learning and increased blood pressure were restored to normal by the same SP dose (4). This part of the authors' work reaffirmed the conclusion that the action of SP depends on the given situation of the individual animal. SP is inactive in intact rats, but in stressed rats it can normalise disorders in avoidance learning and changes in vegetative functions.

Action of SP on Mono-Aminergic Neurons

It has become known that certain stresses, such as exposure to averse stimuli, seem to alter the re-uptake mechanism for norepinephrine (1). The authors established earlier from intact rats that SP, *in vitro* and *in vivo,* could cause slight

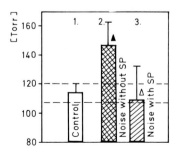

FIG. 7. Effect of noise (30 days) and of noise together with SP application (250 μg/kg i.p.) on blood pressure of female rats. N = 10 rats per group, controls received 10 μl aqua dest. per rat i.p. Significance: 2 vs 1, $p < 0.001$ *(filled triangles);* 3 vs 2, $p < 0.001$ *(open triangles).*

but significant inhibition of norepinephrine uptake in hypothalamic synaptosomes (10,12). Now, some more information can be offered on the problem.

SP was injected in intact rats and, after killing the animals, synaptosomes were prepared from the hypothalamus, according to the technique of Whittaker et al. (18). Isolated synaptosomes, P_2, were treated according to Whittaker et al. by incubation in McIlwain buffer for 10 min with different concentrations of D,L-^{3}H-norepinephrine. The uptake of ^{3}H-norepinephrine by synaptosomes of rat hypothalamus can be described as a two-stage process with two uptake constants: K_m (I) = 0.9 μM, and K_m (II) = 0.06 μM. The existence of a dual uptake system in the norepinephrine concentrations studied may be correlated with the heterogeneous nature of the synaptosomal fraction which has different storage sites, mostly presynaptic but also postsynaptic terminals.

Two- to fourfold increase of K_m (I) was observed under the influence of SP. Injection of SP was more effective than addition of SP to the incubation medium. The change of K_m (I) seems to reflect a competitive type of inhibition. On the other hand, in the high-affinity uptake II a non-competitive type of inhibition (decrease of V_{max} by 60%) was observed after injection of SP, but not after incubation. This shows that in hypothalamic synaptosomes of rat SP can inhibit norepinephrine uptake in two different ways, competitive and non-competitive (Table 1).

Opposite results were recorded from SP treatment by incubation of hypothalamus slices. SP was again administered intravenously. The rats were killed 15 min after injection and the brains were removed immediately. Hypothalamic tissue was dissected in slices and incubated in McIlwain buffer with D,L-^{3}H-norepinephrine. Ten minutes were allowed for incubation before the hypothalamus slices were re-centrifuged, according to Whittaker's procedure. Norepinephrine uptake was found to have been markedly stimulated under such conditions.

These results are only of a preliminary nature and need completion. Nevertheless, it is again shown that SP seems to exercise dual action on norepinephrine uptake (Fig. 8).

DISCUSSION

Frederickson et al. (3) showed that SP produced analgesia in mice on administration of very small doses, which effect was blocked by naloxone. With higher doses that analgesic activity was lost, but hyperalgesia did occur when such higher doses were given in combination with naloxone. The conclusion drawn from those data by Frederickson et al. (3) was that very small doses of SP probably released endorphin, while higher doses caused direct excitation of neuronal activity in nociperceptive pathways.

The present authors also found the property of SP to produce analgesia or hyperalgesia to be dose-dependent. Yet, their results were contrary to those of Frederickson et al. (3), who used the hot plate procedure and found that higher SP doses entailed analgesia and lower doses entailed hyperalgesia. A possible

TABLE 1. Influence of SP, in vitro or in vivo, on uptake of ^{3}H-norepinephrine by synaptosomes of hypothalamus of rat (V_{max} in n moles g^{-1} proteins, 10 min^{-1}; K_m in μmoles)

	High affinity uptake I			High affinity uptake II		
	K_m	V_{max}	n	K_m	V_{max}	n
Controls	0.94 ∓ 0.05 (5)	51.4 ∓ 5.7 (5)		0.061 ∓ 0.026 (5)	5.6 ∓ 1.7 (5)	
Injection [15 min. before killing, 500 μg/kg]	3.77 ∓ 2.04 (3) ▲	87.7 ∓ 76.4 (3)		0.038 ∓ 0.007 (3)	1.7 ∓ 0.1 (3) ▲▲	
Incubation [10^{-5} M]	1.81 ∓ 0.60 (4) ▲	82.5 ∓ 38.0 (4)		0.103 ∓ 0.050 (4)	5.1 ∓ 1.2 (4)	

Significance (versus controls): ▲ $p < 0.02$ ▲▲ $p < 0.01$

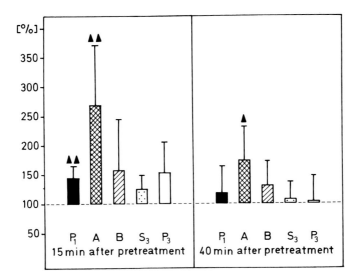

FIG. 8. Influence of SP (500/μg/kg i.v.), *in vivo*, on uptake of ³H-norepinephrine by slices of hypothalamus of rat. The values are means ± SEM (% controls). ▲ $p < 0.01$ vs controls; ▲▲ $p < 0.05$ vs controls. $N = 4$. P_1, nuclei and cell debris; A, synaptosomes (light fraction); B, synaptosomes (heavy fraction); P_3 microsomes and ribosomes; B_3, final supernatant.

explanation for this discrepancy may be found in the differences between the control response latencies in the mice used by Frederickson et al. and those used by the authors: The authors used mice with control response latencies below 15 sec and Frederickson et al. used mice with an average value of 23 sec. It is possible that this difference may be a result of an existing relationship between the given condition of the individual animal, i.e., the individual response latency before SP treatment, and the direction of SP action.

Madden et al. (7) investigated stress-induced parallel changes to central opioid levels and pain responsiveness of rat and suggested that the level of endogenous opioids in the brain played a role in responsiveness to pain. For SP it was postulated that analgesia was due to the release of endorphin. Applied to the authors' own experiments, such postulation would mean that SP was capable of releasing endorphin only in mice with short control response latencies. For mice with longer control response latencies SP would produce hyperalgesia through direct excitation of neuronal activity in nociperceptive pathways. In view of the capability of SP to cause two opposite effects, depending on the condition of the individual animal and on dosage, the authors suggest that the physiological effect of SP might be "normalisation" or "adaptation."

The same normalising effect was found in stressed rats with disorders in avoidance learning and vegetative functions. To the authors' knowledge this is the first evidence, so far, of such a normalising action of SP on disturbed behavior in rats. It is known from Rodgers (14) that the endogenous opiate system may be involved in mood regulation and can modify an animal's responsiveness to averse stimulation.

It might be possible that the release of endorphin is involved in SP action on behaviour. This assumption appears to be supported by the authors' findings to the effect that higher SP doses could induce state-dependent learning, just as morphine could. Yet, lower concentrations did not reveal any relationship between the normalising effect of SP on avoidance acquisition and state-dependent learning. Therefore, it might be a good guess that normalisation was a direct effect of SP.

There is compelling evidence that behavioral events alter neurochemical functions and that altered neurochemical functions can change behaviour. Yet, interpretation of biochemical data on neurotransmitters is extremely difficult. This is also true for the authors' opposite effects of SP on norepinephrine uptake by hypothalamic synaptosomes or hypothalamus slices. One explanation might be the following: In the authors' experiments with slices, the whole nervous cells were in the incubation system. In the authors' incubation system with synaptosomes of hypothalamus, there were only cell terminals, most of them presynaptic. It is suggested that SP can act in different ways on different parts of the cell. Inhibition of uptake may result from change in the synaptic area, while stimulation of uptake may be caused by change outside that area. The receptors in the synaptic area can be identical with the postulated presynaptic inhibitory opiate receptors (7). Some evidence to the possible existence of such

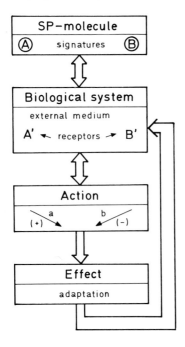

FIG. 9. Working model of mechanism of *regulatory peptides* ("regulides"), e.g., SP.

different SP receptors has been provided by Bergmann et al. (2) in particular, who investigated SP action on smooth muscle preparations.

CONCLUSIONS

If SP has the potential of dual action, its molecule can be the carrier of different signatures. This suggestion was made by Oehme et al. at the Nobel Symposium on Substance P in Stockholm, 1976 (10). In terms of the information theory, such phenomenon, with several signatures in one molecule determining different functions for one and the same molecule, is referred to as principle of ambiguity or indetermination of effect. This principle can be important to molecules with flexible structures, such as the linear flexible SP undecapeptide, for which different conformational situations are possible. Which of the properties of the signature-carrying molecule is decisive for the actual effect will depend, as well, on the second component of the reaction (e.g., receptors) and the surrounding medium (e.g., ions).

The last two points are of importance for the responsiveness of the individual animal. These were the considerations which led the authors to the working model of SP action which is shown in Fig. 9. According to the hypothesis proposed in this figure *regula*tory pept*ides* (or "regulides") might be a good name for such peptides.

REFERENCES

1. Barchas, J. D., Akil, H., Elliott, G. R., Holman, R. B., and Watson, S. J. (1978): Behavioral neurochemistry: Neuroregulators and behavioral states. *Science,* 200:964–973.
2. Bergmann, J., Oehme, P., and Bienert, M. *(in preparation).*
3. Frederickson, R. C. A., Burgis, V., Harrell, C. E., and Edwards, J. D. (1978): Dual actions of substance P on nociception: Possible role of endogenous opioids. *Science,* 199:1359–1362.
4. Hecht, K., Oehme, P., and Poppei, M. (1979): A substance P analogue—its effects upon learning and memorising processes, behavioral patterns, and blood pressure in neurotic hypertensive rats. *Pharmazie,* 34:653–657.
5. Hecht, K., Oehme, P., Poppei, M., and Hecht, T. (1979): Conditioned-reflex learning of normal juvenile and adult rats exposed to action of substance P and of an SP analogue. *Pharmazie,* 34:419–423.
6. Lembeck, F. (1972): Substance P. *Int. Encycl. Pharmacol. Ther.,* 1:29–71.
7. Madden, J., Akil, H., Patrick, R. L., and Barchas, J. D. (1977): Stress-induced parallel changes in central opioid levels and pain responsiveness in the rat. *Nature (New Biol.),* 265:358–360.
8. Magnusson, T., Carlsson, A., Fisher, G. H., Chang, D., and Folkers, K. (1976): Effect of synthetic substance P on monoaminergic mechanisms in brain. *J. Neural Transmission,* 38:89–93.
9. Malick, J. B., and Goldstein, J. M. (1978): Analgesic activity of substance P following intracerebral administration in rats. *Life Sci.,* 23:835–844.
10. Oehme, P., Bergmann, J., Bienert, M., Hilse, H., Piesche, L., Minh Thu, P., and Scheer, E. (1977): Biological action of Substance P—Its differentiation by affinity and intrinsic efficacy. In: *Substance P,* edited by U. S. von Euler and B. Pernow, pp. 327–335. Raven Press, New York.
11. Otsuka, M., Konishi, S., and Takahashi, T. (1975): Hypothalamic substance P as a candidate for transmitter of primary afferent neurons. *Fed. Proc.,* 34:1922–1928.
12. Piesche, L., Hilse, H., Scheer, E., Bienert, M., and Oehme, P. (1977): Über die Hemmung

der ^{3}H-Noradrenalin-Aufnahme in Synaptosomen durch Substanz P. *Acta Biol. Med. Germ.,* 36:1351–1354.

13. Reubi, J. C., Emson, P. C., Jessell, T. M., and Iversen, L. L. (1978): Effects of GABA, dopamine, and substance P on the release of newly synthesized ^{3}H-5-hydroxytryptamine from rat substantia nigra in vitro. *Naunyn Schmiedebergs Arch. Pharmacol.,* 304:271–275.

14. Rodgers, R. J. (1978): Opioid peptides, brain and behaviour: A brief review. *Irish J. Med. Sci.,* 147(Suppl. 1):57–62.

15. Starr, M. S., James, T. A., and Gaytten, D. (1978): Behavioural depressant and antinociceptive properties of substance P in the mouse: Possible implication of brain monoamines. *Eur. J. Pharmacol.,* 48:203–212.

16. Stern, P., Hukovic, S., and Radivojevic, M. (1976): Hemmung von Morphin-Effekten durch synthetische Substanz P. *Experientia,* 32:1326–1327.

17. Stewart, J. M., Getto, C. J., Nesdner, K., Reeve, E. B., Krivoy, W. A., and Zimmermann, E. (1976): Substance P and analgesia. *Nature,* 262:784–785.

18. Whittaker, V. P., Michaelson, I. A., and Kirkland, R. J. A. (1964): The separation of synaptic vesicles from nerve-ending particles ('Synaptosomes'). *Biochem. J.,* 90:293.

Neuropeptides and Neural Transmission,
edited by C. Ajmone Marsan and W. Z. Traczyk.
Raven Press, New York © 1980.

Substance P as a Synaptic Modulator

*William A. Krivoy, **James R. Couch, †John M. Stewart, and
††Emery Zimmermann

*NIDA Addiction Research Center, Lexington, Kentucky 40583; **Department of
Medicine, Southern Illinois University, College of Medicine, Springfield, Illinois 62708;
†Department of Biochemistry, University of Colorado, School of Medicine, Denver, Colorado
80262; and ††Department of Anatomy and Brain Research Institute, University of
California, School of Medicine, Los Angeles, California 90024

The term "synaptic modulation" was introduced to describe actions of bradykinin, substance P (SP), and β-melanocyte-stimulating hormone (β-MSH) (8,12,13) because their actions appeared different from those of other putative neurohumors. SP and β-MSH each had potent facilitatory actions on evoked reflexes, but did not cause spontaneous discharge of motoneurons, convulsions, or overt changes in behavior of intact animals commensurate with their capacity to alter reflex activity. Bradykinin depressed evoked spinal reflex activity, but did not produce behavioral changes in intact animals commensurate with its potent action on spinal cord. The neurotropic actions of these three peptides became manifest gradually and lasted sometimes for hours. The obvious differences between the neurotropic actions of these peptides and those of the then accepted putative transmitters led the authors to recognize that an updated nomenclature was needed. They utilized the term "synaptic modulator" and suggested this to be a normal physiological role of certain substances including these peptides.

Within this communication we use *synaptic modulation* to describe altered excitability of synapses by a substance that does not ordinarily produce a propagated spike potential at the synapse in question. *Synaptic transmission* is used in its traditional sense, i.e., as the process of conveying information across a synaptic cleft. We use *neurotransmitter* in its conventional sense to describe a substance that can produce a postsynaptic spike potential, and *detonation* is used to indicate a propagated spike potential. One might criticize these definitions as being artificial; for example, in low doses neurotransmitters can produce modulation, as can a number of pathological, physical, or chemical changes in environment. These considerations will be addressed later. For the present it should be emphasized that in using these definitions we are referring to the physiological role and capacity of a given substance at a given synapse. Further, as pointed out in our opening sentence, although various substances may be physiological modulators of synaptic transmission, and this may be their physiological role, we shall confine our comments in this chapter to actions of SP.

SOME OBSERVATIONS SUGGESTING THAT A PHYSIOLOGICAL ROLE OF SP IS TO MODULATE SYNAPTIC EXCITABILITY

Evolution of the Concept

Early conclusions (8,12,13) that SP may be a neurohumor were derived from recognition that, in general, it fulfilled the criteria prescribed by Chang and Gaddum (1) before acetylcholine could be considered a neurohumor. Although some of these criteria had to be modified because of differences between actions of acetylcholine and SP, they included demonstration of an enzyme capable of degrading the putative neurohumor, and that substances inhibiting this enzyme *in vitro* will potentiate actions of the neurohumor *in vivo*. Both the enzyme which inactivates SP (5) and its inhibition by LSD (7) have been described. LSD was subsequently found to potentiate actions of SP on cat spinal cord (9). However, unexpected of a detonator substance, the potentiation included frequency-dependent augmentation both of potentials associated with supernormality during the recovery process and of the monosynaptic segmental reflex (8,9,12,13). These effects of SP were long-lasting and not associated with convulsive activity or spontaneous discharge. Although these actions clearly differed from those produced by more generally accepted putative transmitter substances, they did allow the conclusion that SP is a putative neurohumor. However, failure of SP to produce detonation, or alter conduction, while producing slow and sustained alteration of evoked reflexes and recovery processes led to the conclusion that one physiological role of SP is to modulate synaptic excitability (8,12,13).

Subsequent studies with synthetic SP showed that it produces detonation when applied to *certain* neurons of frog (18) or cat (6) spinal cord. However, three additional observations were again noted. First, the actions of SP appeared only after a relatively long latent period, and second, they outlasted the period of application, leading to the conclusion that SP was not acting as a fast-acting transmitter, but as a modulator of synaptic activity (6,15). The third observation was confirmation that administration of SP did not result in discharge of cat motoneurons (6,14). Because of this third observation, and as SP altered transmission through monosynaptic pathways without causing their detonation (8,9, 12,13), α-motoneurons of the monosynaptic pathway of cat spinal cord seemed a particularly attractive model for studying modulation. Further, since actions of SP on this pathway were known to be frequency-dependent and to be partly associated with altered postdetonation recovery processes (9), we attempted to test the modulatory role of SP by studying its influence on the recovery cycle of α-motoneurons.

Influence of SP on Postdetonation Recovery

This was studied using single lumbar α-motoneurons (of decerebrate, low spinal cats) impaled with single-barrel micropipettes so that their intracellular potentials could be recorded (11). The units chosen were those of monosynaptic reflex pathways, identified by both ortho- and antidromic invasion. They were activated via their dorsal roots, stimuli being applied in pairs. The first stimulus of each pair was a conditioning stimulus, the second a test stimulus. Each stimulus of the pair was supramaximal when applied alone, but because the test stimulus was presented during the relative refractory period following the conditioning stimulus, only a fraction of the test stimuli evoked a postsynaptic spike potential during the control period. After intravenous SP, 5 ng/kg, each of the test stimuli evoked a postsynaptic spike potential. There was no evidence of SP-induced spontaneous discharge. This increased responsivity to orthodromic invasion was slow in onset, long in duration, and frequency-dependent. Similar observations were made by Krnjević (14) who pointed out that whereas SP fails to discharge motoneurons, it facilitated orthodromic synaptic transmission. Using the isolated hemisected spinal cord of the frog, Nicoll (16) also found that SP facilitated synaptic transmission, but did not cause spontaneous discharge. Thus, these various laboratories appear to agree on the fact that SP may facilitate synaptic transmission without per se causing detonation of spinal motoneurons. There is some disagreement on the possible mechanisms in that Krivoy et al. (11) found no change in membrane potential or excitatory postsynaptic potential (EPSP) after SP, whereas Krnjević (14) observed partial depolarization of membrane potential and increased size of EPSP. Nicoll (16) also observed membrane depolarization. Thus, the evidence would suggest that SP acts postsynaptically to facilitate synaptic transmission, although there may also be a presynaptic component (16,19).

Modulation of Monosynaptic Reflexes by Iontophoretically Applied SP

To gain more information on the role of SP in synaptic modulation and at the same time reduce artifacts due to intravenous administration, we decided to investigate this peptide's influence on synaptic excitability of single units by recording extracellularly while administering SP by iontophoresis. Decerebrate low-spinal cats were paralyzed with succinylcholine and artificially respired. A seven-barrel micropipette was lowered into the lumbar spinal cord until it approximated the α-motoneuron of a monosynaptic reflex. The only neurons used were those that responded to suprathreshold orthodromic stimulation with a single spike potential. The unit was then stimulated using just threshold stimuli applied to its dorsal root such that the unit responded with a spike potential to approximately 50% of the stimuli. The ratio of responses to number of stimuli is reported as percentage of response. Once the percentage response had stabilized (at a value less than 70) SP was applied to the neuron. The percentage response of the unit before, during, and after the period of SP application was plotted as a continuous time histogram. Iontophoresis currents of 80, 40, 20, 10, or 5 nA were used to eject SP; a current of 5 nA was employed to retain SP. When ejection currents of 20 to 80 nA were employed there was no evidence of spontaneous discharge, but the percentage response increased (Fig. 1A). Application of SP using currents of 40 or 80 nA caused a clear increase in percentage response in 3 of 3 and 13 of 17 experiments, respectively. When 20 nA was used it was also followed by an increased percentage response in 13 of 16 experiments, although in 5 of these experiments the response was biphasic (i.e., excitation preceded or followed by inhibition) (Fig. 1B). In 10 of 13 experiments utilizing an ejection current of 10 nA the percentage response decreased (Fig. 1C), and in 2 it changed in a biphasic manner. Five nA produced no statistically significant change in percentage response (no change in 4 experiments, a decrease in 1, and an increase in another). Thus, the modulating influ-

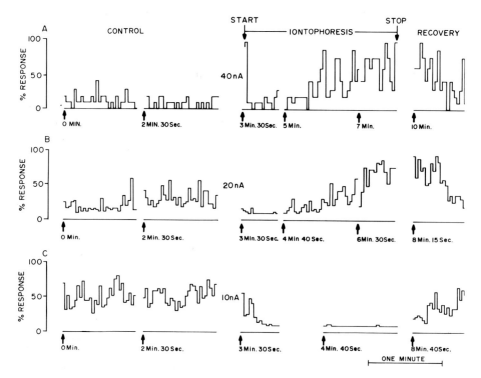

Fig. 1. Actions of SP on synaptic transmission assayed by facilitation or inhibition of detonation of single α-motoneurons of cat spinal cord during stimulation of dorsal roots at a repetition rate of 0.5 Hz. Time under each panel is from beginning of illustrated control. Histograms in **A, B,** and **C** (each being a separate experiment) represent percentage of stimuli that detonated the neuron. After the control period SP was applied by iontophoresis using currents of 80, 40, 20, or 10 nA during the period indicated. Note that the high dose produced facilitation **(A),** the intermediate dose **(B)** both inhibition and facilitation, whereas the lowest effective dose (10 nA) was followed by inhibition **(C).** No change was produced when the ejection current was 5 nA.

ence of SP appears to be biphasic and dose-dependent. Further, as may be seen from the histograms in Fig. 1 the effect of SP on response to stimulation appeared after a relatively long delay and significantly outlasted the period of administration.

There was no evidence in any of our experiments that iontophoretic application of SP caused discharge of these motoneurons unrelated to orthodromic stimulation. Auditory and visual monitoring of the evoked response evidenced only the fact that more stimuli caused a postsynaptic spike potential. Further, the percentage response never exceeded 100 during or after SP administration.

As in the experiments related in the preceding section which demonstrate an influence of SP on recovery processes, we have no hard data to explain its influence on synaptic excitability. In fact, it is doubtful that these two phenomena can be rigidly differentiated within the design of our experiments. The problem of mechanism of modulation is compounded in the present experiments by the fact that iontophoretic application of SP resulted in biphasic modulation. Although biphasic actions of SP on neural excitability have been reported by others (17,19), except for the observations of Frederickson et al. (4) it has been difficult to determine whether or not they are dose-related. In our own experiments, low doses were inhibitory and higher doses caused excitation, a result opposite to that obtained with transmitter substances and at variance with generally accepted concepts of synaptic transmission. Thus, although these may both be a result of direct postsynaptic actions of SP, it seems appropriate to examine and recognize the possibility that the biphasic action is a result of interaction with one receptor at two sites, or with two different receptors. These might be on the neuron whose activity is being recorded, or a slight distance away, but sufficiently close to allow SP to migrate to them. Considering the inhibitory component from the point of view that it may be the consequence of an indirect action, migration to neighboring Renshaw cells might excite them (2), thereby causing postsynaptic inhibition. Similarly, SP could migrate presynaptically to cause inhibition of release of transmitter in a manner analogous to its action at the neuromuscular junction (19).

Possible mechanisms by which SP produces facilitation have already been considered. It may be due to a direct action of SP on motoneurons causing partial depolarization (14,16), or facilitation of the EPSP as described by Krnjević (14). Or it may be a presynaptic influence as described by Nicoll (16) and by Steinaker (19). Finally, SP has been shown to reduce actions of acetylcholine on Renshaw cells (2), an action that could be manifest as facilitation of synaptic transmission.

DISCUSSION

Although there has been considerable recent use and abuse both of the word "modulation" as applied to physiology, pharmacology, and behavior, and of the term "synaptic modulation," we have chosen to use the latter in its original context, i.e., to describe actions of a group of putative neurohumors which do not produce detonation, but which alter excitability of a synapse (8,12,13). A number of criteria might be used to test the hypothesis that one physiological role of a substance may be to function as a synaptic modulator. These criteria could obviously include those used by Chang and Gaddum (1) to evaluate the hypothesis that acetylcholine is a neurohumor, but necessarily modified as dictated by such differences as duration of action (compared to acetylcholine). More importantly, compared to the criteria used to accept acetylcholine, the suspected synaptic modulator must cause altered excitability without producing detonation. In the experiments of Henry et al. (6), Krivoy (9), and Krnjević (14) SP was not found to detonate cat spinal α-motoneurons. In the most recent experiments, described herein, even the highest concentration of SP used failed to cause cells to fire more than once per stimulus or to fire spontaneously. Thus, the burden of evidence would indicate that SP does not per se produce detonation of these motoneurons.

Whereas SP-induced detonation was not observed during these experiments, the data presented in Fig. 1 clearly illustrate an altered postsynaptic response to presynaptic stimuli in the presence of SP. At higher doses (20 nA or more) these alterations were manifest as facilitation of synaptic transmission, whereas at lower doses (10 nA) they were manifest as inhibition. It would seem, therefore, that SP is capable of modulating synaptic excitability biphasically, with low doses modulating in an inhibitory direction and higher doses in an excitatory direction.

Many heretofore confusing data on *in vivo* effects of SP can now be understood in light of these results. First, they may explain the observations of von Euler and Pernow (3) that SP produces a mixture of behavioral excitation and depression in the cat, and those of Frederickson et al. (4) that SP has a biphasic influence on response to painful stimuli, with lower doses causing analgesia and higher ones hyperalgesia. Thus, if the analgesic properties of morphine are due to its ability to inhibit or gate synaptic transmission (10), then by analogy low concentrations of SP would be expected to be analgesic. Conversely, high doses (which facilitate synaptic transmission) would be hyperalgesic. A second point is that the presence of a purely modulating system provides the brain with an analog as well as a digital system for integration including coding, storage, and retrieval of information. The importance of having two such systems is demonstrated in the field of analgesia by the fact that morphine reduces pain perception without interfering with other neural functions such as voluntary movement. A third area of importance is that a modulator, incapable of causing detonation, would tend to reduce the possibility of errors in transmission as discussed below.

Commentary on Use of the Word "Modulation"

There have been two major criticisms of our use and conceptualization of synaptic modulation. The first of these has been concerned with the question of whether or not such physical agents as temperature and pH should be classified as modulators. The second criticism is that the dissociation of detonation and modulation is artificial and useless. In the first instance we propose that SP, and a variety of other substances, are specific physiological modulators as opposed to modifiers of physiology. Such things as artificially altered temperature of a synapse *in vitro* or of a patient undergoing surgery using hypothermia to help produce anesthesia obviously modify a number of physiological functions, but are not themselves physiological modulators. The second criticism is that our definition, distinguishing transmitters and modulators, is artificial because low doses of transmitter substances modulate without producing detonation. This is indeed the case. However, SP, which has been reported to produce detonation at a number of synapses, seems not to detonate α-motoneurons of monosynaptic reflex pathways, but only modulates excitability of these pathways. Thus, as in other forms of information transfer, it would appear that two forms of specificity are involved with actions of SP. One is dependent on those physico-chemical characteristics of SP which influence its ability to gain access to a receptor and to combine therewith. The second form of specificity is dependent on the configuration of a receptor, the nature of its coupling with the effector tissue, and the function of the effector tissue. Thus, SP may be a transmitter at one synapse where its combination with the receptor produces a propagated response. However, its combination with other receptors, or the same species of receptor but at a different site (or effector tissue) may culminate only in modulation.

There are two closing points to be made regarding modulation and detonation. The first of these concerns our earlier statement that the presence of separate modulator and detonator systems would reduce the probability of biochemical accidents in neural integration (including storage and retrieval of information, movement, conditioned behavior, etc.). If physiological detonator-transmitters were the only available facilitatory modulators, even minor changes in their release or of the end result of their combination with receptors might result in confusion of digital and analog-based integration. Thus, modulation would allow a broader range of inputs to affect the process of synaptic transmission and would also reduce the possibility of producing synaptic misfiring.

The second and final point is the question of the general applicability of this principle (of separate types of synaptic transfer of information) to other synapses. This needs much more investigation. We have already pointed out above that a substance acting as a modulator at one type of synapse may act as a transmitter at another. This classification and separation of synaptic functions should prove to be an important basis for further investigation.

REFERENCES

1. Chang, H. C., and Gaddum, J. H. (1933): Choline esters in tissue extracts. *J. Physiol. (Lond.),* 79:255–285.

2. Davies, J., and Dray, A. (1977): Substance P and opiate receptors. *Nature,* 268:351–352.
3. Euler, U. S. von, and Pernow, B. (1956): Neurotropic effects of substance P. *Acta Physiol. Scand.,* 36:265–275.
4. Frederickson, R. C. A., Burgis, V., Harrell, C. E., and Edwards, J. D. (1978): Dual actions of substance P on nociception: A possible role of endogenous opioids. *Science,* 199:1355–1362.
5. Gullbring, B. (1943): Inactivation of substance P by tissue extracts. *Acta Physiol. Scand.,* 6:246–255.
6. Henry, J. L., Krnjević, K., and Morris, M. E. (1975): Substance P and spinal neurons. *Can. J. Physiol. Pharmacol.,* 53:423–432.
7. Krivoy, W. (1957): The preservation of substance P by lysergic acid diethylamide. *Br. J. Pharmacol.,* 12:361–364.
8. Krivoy, W. (1961): A comparison of the actions of substance P and other naturally occurring polypeptides on spinal cord. *Proceedings of the Scientific Society of Bosnia and Herzegovina-Jugoslavia, Vol. I,* pp. 131–137.
9. Krivoy, W. (1961): Potentiation of substance P by lysergic acid diethylamide *in vivo. Br. J. Pharmacol.,* 16:253–256.
10. Krivoy, W., and Huggins, R. (1961): The action of morphine, methadone, meperidine and nalorphine on dorsal root potentials of cat spinal cord. *J. Pharmacol. Exp. Ther.,* 134:210–213.
11. Krivoy, W., Kroeger, D., and Zimmermann, E. (1977): Additional evidence for a role of Substance P in modulation of synaptic transmission. In: *Substance P,* edited by U. S. von Euler and B. Pernow, pp. 187–193. Raven Press, New York.
12. Krivoy, W., Lane, M., and Kroeger, D. (1963): The actions of certain polypeptides on synaptic transmission. *Ann. NY Acad. Sci.,* 104:312–325.
13. Krivoy, W., and Zimmermann, E. (1973): A possible role of polypeptides in synaptic transmission. In: *Chemical Modulation of Brain Function,* edited by H. Sabelli, pp. 111–121. Raven Press, New York.
14. Krnjević, K. (1977): Effects of substance P on central neurons in cats. In: *Substance P,* edited by U. S. von Euler and B. Pernow, pp. 217–230. Raven Press, New York.
15. Krnjević, K., and Morris, M. E. (1974): An excitatory action of substance P on cuneate neurons. *Can. J. Physiol. Pharmacol.,* 52:736–744.
16. Nicoll, R. A. (1978): The action of thyrotropin-releasing hormone, substance P and related peptides on frog spinal motoneurons. *J. Pharmacol. Exp. Ther.,* 207:817–824.
17. Otsuka, M., and Konishi, S. (1974): Excitatory action of hypothalamic substance P on spinal motoneurons of newborn rats. *Nature,* 252:734–735.
18. Otsuka, M., Konishi, S., and Takahashi, T. (1975): Hypothalamic substance P as a candidate for transmitter at primary afferent neurons. *Fed. Proc.,* 34:1922–1928.
19. Steinacker, A. (1977): Calcium dependent presynaptic action of substance P at the frog neuromuscular junction. *Nature,* 267:268–270.

Neuropeptides and Neural Transmission,
edited by C. Ajmone Marsan and W. Z. Traczyk.
Raven Press, New York © 1980.

Substance P Pharmacology of Cultured Mouse Spinal Neurons

Jeffery L. Barker, *Jean-Didier Vincent, and **John F. MacDonald

Laboratory of Neurophysiology, National Institute of Neurological and Communicative Disorders and Stroke, National Institutes of Health, Bethesda, Maryland 20205

There is now good evidence that the undecapeptide "substance P" (SP) is synthesized in sensory ganglia for bidirectional transport out to the periphery and into the spinal cord (see ref. 8). It appears to be released from sensory nerve endings upon noxious chemical and mechanical stimulation and to act in a neurohormonal manner to initiate reflex vasodilatation and local plasmaphoresis (see Lembeck et al., *this volume*). It is also released from primary afferents in the spinal cord (22), where it has been shown to have excitatory effects on spinal neurons (11–14,16,21). The relatively slow time course of the excitatory response has led some investigators to conclude that the peptide may not be a good candidate for a neurotransmitter mediating fast excitatory synaptic input at the first synapse into the central nervous system (CNS) (15,16,21). However, the peptide has never been applied pharmacologically in a way that would mimic the physiological release of SP at intraspinal synapses. Most of the observations have been made *in vivo* or *in situ* with the peptide being applied either by iontophoresis or in the bathing medium. The complexity of the intact spinal cord does not permit precise placement of the iontophoretic pipette with respect to the neuron being recorded. Bath application is a rather imprecise method of applying the peptide, especially if the aim is to mimic the synaptic events occurring between SP-containing primary afferents and their postsynaptic target cells. Finally, it is a formidable task to record from a postsynaptic target cell which is in fact innervated by SP fibers.

Thus, most of what has been done to establish the functional role(s) of SP in the spinal cord has been quite indirect. The slow time course of the excitatory responses as well as the relatively high concentrations needed to produce effects may reflect the barriers posed by the inherent geometry of the spinal cord and/or the fact that electrophysiological assays of SP effects have been carried

Present address: Unité de Neurobiologie des Comportements, Institut National de la Santé et de la Récherche Médicale, U. 176, 33077, Bordeaux, France.
** *Present address:* Helen Scott Playfair Neurobiology Unit, University of Toronto, Toronto, Canada.

out for the most part using the most accessible elements present in the cord (e.g., motoneurons), which may or may not be appropriate target cells for SP-containing afferents. It is clearly too early to eliminate SP as a neurotransmitter substance mediating fast excitatory synaptic events. It is also clear that although biochemical and immunohistochemical evidence show SP-containing fibers to be present and functional in the spinal cord (20,22,23), the electrophysiological observations reported on SP actions do not convincingly demonstrate precise physiological roles for the peptide.

We have used dissociated mouse spinal neurons grown in tissue culture to examine the membrane effects of SP. The preparation grows as a virtual mono-layer and thus has the advantage that individual nerve cells are readily accessible to electrophysiological and micropharmacological techniques. Long-term stable intracellular recordings allow assay of peptide actions at a level of resolution not presently possible *in vivo*. In addition, SP-containing sensory cells and fibers are present in these cultures (7). In this chapter we demonstrate that SP has a variety of effects on cultured mammalian neurons including a rapid excitatory transmitter-like action.

METHODS

Neurons were dissociated from embryonic mouse spinal cords and grown in tissue culture according to methods previously described (3,24). After several months the cells were large enough (ea. $25 = \mu$ diameter cell bodies) to allow application of conventional and voltage clamp techniques (Fig. 1). SP was applied either by iontophoresis from pipettes containing 4mM peptide or by microperfusion using pressure to pipettes containing 10 μM peptide. Similar results were obtained using the two methods of pharmacologic application.

RESULTS

Transmitter-like Events

The accessibility of individual nerve cells allowed discrete delivery of SP to different parts of the cell's surface. SP applied in this manner elicited a nonuniform distribution of responses (Fig. 2). For example, in the cell illustrated, which was recorded using KCl microelectrodes, SP causes both a rapid and slow depolarization of the cell. The slower event occurs over much of the cell's surface, although the response varies in magnitude. The faster event is present only over a circumscribed area of the cell's surface at the level of the cell body. At one site both events could be elicited together (trace at 3 o'clock site on cell body with arrowhead delineating fast from slow events). In contrast, a single time course of response to iontophoresis of glutamate occurs on this cell. The response simply varies in magnitude depending on where it is applied to the cell's surface. Glutamate responses were observed on 100% of the spinal

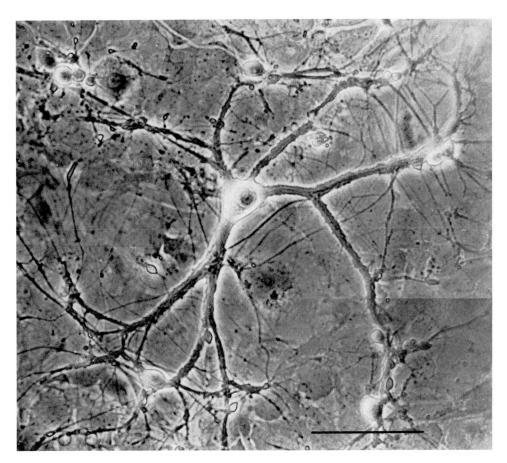

FIG. 1. Phase contrast micrograph of a dissociated spinal neuron growing in tissue culture, typical of those used in the present study. Bar: 50 μm.

cord cells tested (3), while SP-sensitive cells were quite rare, accounting for less than 20% of the spinal cord cell population (26).

The slow event evoked by SP appears to be due primarily to an increase in Cl^- conductance, as reflected in the fact that the "null potential" for the response is similar to that for the putative inhibitory amino acid gamma-aminobutyric acid (GABA), which activates a Cl^- conductance mechanism on these neurons (3). Since GABA responses are found in 100% of the cells tested, it is unlikely that SP activates this inhibitory conductance by engaging GABA receptors. The fast depolarizing event has been compared with the glutamate response in further detail (26). Both peptide and amino acid responses depolarized responsive cells sufficiently to initiate action potential generation (Fig. 3A). The extrapolated null potential for the fast response was about + 20 mV, which is close to the peak of the spike in these cells (Barker et al., *unpublished observa-*

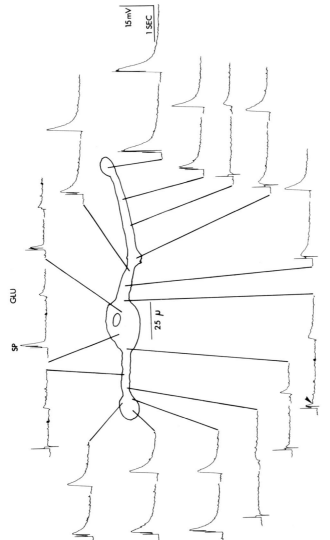

FIG. 2. Nonuniform distribution of membrane responses to SP and glutamate (GLU) on a cultured spinal neuron recorded with a KCl microelectrode. Each membrane potential trace consists of a pair of responses to a 50-msec 40-nA pulse of SP and a 50-msec 50-nA pulse of glutamate iontophoresed from pipettes positioned within 3 μ of the cell's surface at the sites indicated. SP responses always precede glutamate events. The time course and amplitude of the SP responses vary while only the amplitude of glutamate responses varies over the cell's surface. *Arrowhead* delineates fast and slow responses to SP recorded at about 3 o'clock on the cell body. Resting membrane potential: −59 mV.

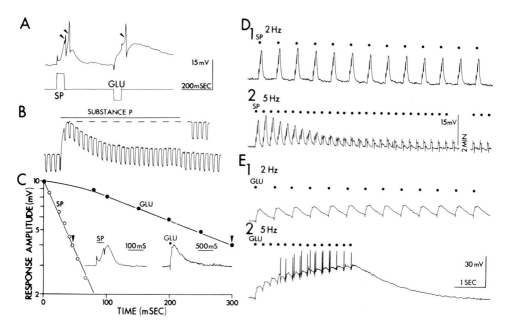

FIG. 3. Excitatory responses to SP and glutamate (GLU) compared on the same cultured spinal neuron. **A:** 50-msec iontophoretic pulses of SP (25 nA) and glutamate (20 nA) rapidly depolarize the cell above threshold for generation of spikes (marked by *arrowheads*), which are attenuated by the frequency response of the pen recorder. Iontophoretic current trace below membrane potential trace. Resting potential: −52 mV. **B:** Sustained application of 40 nA SP (marked by *bar* above trace) leads to depolarization and associated increase in membrane conductance which desensitizes completely. Downward deflections are voltage responses to −0.2 nA current stimuli. *Inset* shows voltage responses at same potential as peak to depolarizing response. The abrupt change in potential at end of the SP iontophoresis is due to the several millivolts coupling artifact between the iontophoretic current and the voltage recording. Membrane potential: −60 mV. **C:** Voltage decays of equal-sized SP and glutamate responses are plotted semilogarithmically. *Downward arrowheads* show time constant of decay, which is about sixfold greater for glutamate response than for SP response. **D1:** Depolarizing responses to 25-nA 50-msec pulses of SP diminish slightly when applied at a frequency of 2 Hz. **D2:** At 5 Hz the responses desensitize completely and remain desensitized for 2 min. **E1:** Depolarizing responses to 20-nA 50-msec pulses of glutamate summate at 2 Hz delivery rate and produce spikes at 5 Hz **(E2)**. Membrane potential **(C–E):** −80 mV. (From Vincent and Barker, ref. 26, with permission.)

tions). Sustained application of SP revealed that the depolarizing response was associated with an increase in membrane conductance (Fig. 3B). Both the voltage response and conductance increase rapidly desensitized in the continued presence of the peptide (Fig. 3B). The time course of the depolarizing response to SP was invariably faster than the kinetics of a comparable depolarization in response to glutamate (Fig. 3C). When the peptide was applied with brief pulses at a relatively slow rate (e.g., 2 Hz) little desensitization of the response occurred. Increasing the application rate to 5 Hz induced a complete and persistent desensitization of the response (Fig. 3D). In contrast, brief pulses of glutamate caused

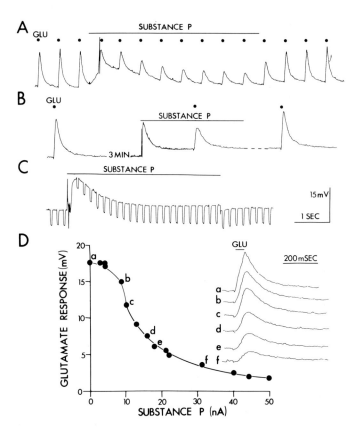

FIG. 4. Modulation of glutamate (GLU) responses by SP. Recordings from two cultured spinal neurons (**A** and **C,D**). **A:** C1 application of 30 nA SP (marked by *bar* above trace) leads to a depolarizing response associated with an increase in membrane conductance both of which desensitize completely. Downward deflections in **C** are voltage responses to −0.15 nA stimuli. The abrupt change in potential at the end of the iontophoresis in **C** is a coupling artifact between the iontophoretic current and the voltage recording. Depolarizing responses to 20-nA 50-msec pulses of glutamate are rapidly and reversibly attenuated by SP **(A).** **B:** SP antagonism of responses to 20-nA 50-msec glutamate pulses does not necessitate activation of glutamate channels immediately preceding SP application, since the peptide depresses glutamate responses as well when a 3-min waiting period is interposed between a control glutamate response and SP iontophoresis (40 nA). Glutamate response on right (with interrupted line serving as artificial base line) shown for visual comparison of control and depressed responses. Apparent residual depolarization during SP iontophoresis is a coupling artifact. Initial part of trace during SP iontophoresis is at one-fifth of recording speed for rest of trace. Membrane potential (mV): −55**(A)**, −65**(B,C)**. **D:** Depression of response to 20-nA 50-msec glutamate pulse by increasing SP iontophoretic current with specimen records on right. A slowing of the glutamate response time course is evident at the higher SP currents. Membrane potential: −80 mV. (From Vincent and Barker, ref. 26, with permission.)

depolarizing responses which summated more as the application rate was increased (Fig. 3D).

Modulation of Postsynaptic Transmitter Responses

A second action of SP observed by pharmacologic application of the peptide to cultured spinal neurons consisted of a rapidly reversible modulation of membrane responses to putative amino acid transmitters in the absence of, or independent of direct actions of the peptide on membrane properties. The most commonly studied interaction has been the depression of glutamate responses by SP (Fig. 4). The time course of the interaction can be seen in Fig. 4A where abrupt application of SP causes a rapidly desensitizing depolarizing response and coincident depression of the depolarizing responses to glutamate. The antagonism of the glutamate voltage response is not due to shunting of the membrane resistance or to a depolarization of the membrane potential, since these returned to control levels as the direct SP response desensitized. The depression of the glutamate response by SP was observed in the absence of any discernible change in membrane properties in the presence of the peptide, as when SP was applied slowly enough to cause desensitization of the fast response or when fast excitatory responses to the peptide were simply not present on the recorded cell. The peptide antagonism of the glutamate response was dose-dependent (Fig. 4D). A similar dose-dependent reversible depression of inhibitory GABA responses has also been found using iontophoretically applied SP (Barker et al., *unpublished observations*). Thus, SP can effectively modulate postsynaptic responses to two common amino acid transmitter substances.

Modulation of Transmitter Release

A third type of pharmacological effect of SP involves stimulation of transmitter release in the presence of elevated Mg^{2+}, which blocks all spontaneously evoked synaptic activity in these cultures (Fig. 5). SP, applied by pressure from pipettes positioned close to the recorded cell, evoked a flurry of discrete excitatory synaptic potentials superimposed on the base line which long outlasted the period of application. This occurred on less than 20% of the cells tested. The stimulation

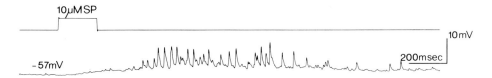

FIG. 5. SP stimulates transmitter release in elevated Mg^{2+}. Intracellular recording of a spinal neuron using a KAc microelectrode. Pressure application of SP (marked by upward deflection on *upper trace*) from a pipette containing 10 μm SP positioned close to the cell surface causes a flurry of synaptic potentials which greatly outlast the application period.

of synaptic activity was similar to that evoked by iontophoresis of glutamate, large currents of which occasionally caused the appearance of synaptic activity. It is unclear whether the stimulated release reflects direct actions of SP on release mechanisms of innervating terminals, or indirect excitatory actions on cell bodies with propagation to, and subsequent release from, innervating terminals. On several occasions SP stimulation of release has been blocked by coincident application of 10 μm leucine-enkephalin (19; Barker et al., *unpublished observation*).

DISCUSSION

Experimental methods used with *in vivo* or *in situ* vertebrate spinal cord preparations have largely precluded any more than an initial level of phenomenology on the pharmacology and physiology of SP. This is due to the relative inaccessibility of the cellular elements in such preparations and, in a number of reports, to the more indirect measures of excitability changes (as in extracellular recordings of changes in spike frequency). The evidence presented in this chapter shows that SP has three functionally distinct actions on the membrane properties of mouse spinal cord cells grown in tissue culture: (a) transmitter-like events including a rapidly desensitizing depolarizing excitatory response and a nondesensitizing inhibitory response involving activation of Cl⁻ conductance; (b) modulation of postsynaptic amino acid responses independent of any other effects of the peptide; and (c) relatively prolonged stimulation of transmitter release.

The rapidly desensitizing depolarizing response and its discrete topography on individual spinal cord cells indicates that SP can mediate rapid post-synaptic excitatory events. This pharmacological response has not been reported from experiments utilizing *in vivo* or *in situ* spinal cord preparations, probably because the peptide has been applied either too slowly, as with bath application, or from iontophoretic pipettes which have diffused sufficient peptide to induce desensitization of the response. Similar rapidly desensitizing depolarizing responses have been observed on cultured spinal neurons with the enkephalins (1,2), the purine nucleoside inosine, and the benzodiazepine flurazepam (17), indicating that this response is not unique to SP. Cross-desensitization among these responses would provide a unique way one substance might alter excitatory events mediated by another, as for example when low maintained level of opioid peptide would markedly attenuate the efficacy of SP-evoked synaptic excitation. The rapidly desensitizing nature of the peptide response would naturally limit the duration and extent of the excitation as well as induce a relative refractory period. This is in marked contrast to the nondesensitizing character of glutamate-mediated responses, which provide a sustained summating type of excitatory synaptic signal. Although physiologically elaborated synaptic events mediated by SP have yet to be observed, rapidly desensitizing excitatory synaptic potentials mediated by acetylcholine (5,9,10,27) and dopamine (18) have been reported in several invertebrate ganglia. It remains to be established if SP mediates primary afferent input into the CNS by generating fast excitatory synaptic events with properties similar to those seen with pharmacologic application of the peptide to cultured spinal neurons.

The modulatory effects of SP on postsynaptic responses to glutamate and GABA independent of other effects on membrane properties is distinctly different from conventional transmitter action which involves alteration in membrane conductance relatively independent of membrane potential. The modulation of the amino acid responses is similar to that observed with leucine- and methionine-enkephalin (1,2). Modulation of transmitter responses by peptides has also been reported *in vivo* (4,6,28). The site of the modulation appears to be at the level of the ionic conductance mechanism in the case of the enkephalin–glutamate interaction (2). The site has not been determined for other peptide–transmitter interactions. Convincing evidence that peptide-mediated modulation has physiological relevance awaits simultaneous recording from a peptidergic neuron and a pair of neurons whose postsynaptic events are a target of peptide action.

We have also observed an apparent presynaptic site of action of SP on cultured neurons. The relatively prolonged nature of stimulated transmitter release is similar to the slowly developing long-lasting excitations observed with iontophoretic applications of the peptide *in vivo*. Presynaptic effects of the peptide have been reported using *in situ* spinal cord (21) and *in vitro* neuromuscular junction preparations (25). Thus, presynaptic regulation of transmitter release may be a widespread and important site of SP action. Detailed investigation of the pharmacology and physiology of this site on central neurons will be difficult.

CONCLUSIONS

Intracellular recordings from dissociated mouse spinal neurons grown in tissue culture have been used to study the effects of SP on neuronal membrane properties. A minority of the cells studied were sensitive to the peptide. Several postsynaptic actions were seen, including a fast excitatory transmitter-like response which rapidly desensitized and a nonsensitizing presumptive increase in Cl^- conductance, as well as modulation of amino acid transmitter responses. An apparent presynaptic stimulation of transmitter release was also seen. The results indicate that the peptide may have multiple functionally distinct sites of action in the CNS. Convincing evidence that these pharmacological actions are physiologically important will require intracellular recordings from identified SP-containing neurons. Dorsal root ganglion cells, which stain positively for SP using immunohistochemical techniques, are present in these spinal cord cultures (7). Thus, this preparation may be useful for examining the physiology of these peptidergic neurons, especially if the neurons can be positively identified while they are still physiologically viable.

ACKNOWLEDGMENT

Jean-Didier Vincent was supported by a grant from the Phillipe Foundation.

REFERENCES

1. Barker, J. L., Gruol, D. L., Huang, L. M., Neale, J. H., and Smith, T. G. (1978): Enkephalin: Pharmacologic evidence for diverse functional roles in the nervous system using primary cultures of dissociated spinal neurons. In: *Characteristics and Functions of Opioids,* edited by L. Terenius and J. Van Ree, pp. 87–88. Elsevier/North-Holland, Amsterdam.
2. Barker, J. L., Neale, J. H., Smith, T. G., and Macdonald, R. L. (1978): Opiate peptide modulation of amino acid responses on cultured mammalian neurons suggests novel form of communication. *Science,* 199:1451–1453.
3. Barker, J. L., and Ransom, B. R. (1978): Amino acid pharmacology of mammalian central neurones grown in tissue culture. *J. Physiol. (Lond.),* 280:331–354.
4. Belcher, G., and Ryall, R. W. (1977): Substance P and Renshaw cells: A new concept of inhibitory synaptic interactions. *J. Physiol. (Lond.),* 272:105–119.
5. Blankenship, J. E., Wachtel, H., and Kandel, E. R. (1971): Ionic mechanisms of excitatory, inhibitory, and dual synaptic actions mediated by an identified interneuron in the abdominal ganglion of *Aplysia. J. Neurophysiol.,* 34:76–92.
6.. Davies, J., and Dray, A. (1976): Changes in amino acid sensitivity during polypeptide 'desensitization.' *Nature,* 262:606–607.
7. Elde, R., Erlandsen, S. L., Barker, J. L., and Neale, J. H. (1979): Characterization of peptidergic neurons in monolayer cultures of spinal cord by immunocytochemistry and scanning electron microscopy. *Soc. Neurosci. Abstr.* 5:526.
8. von Euler, U. S., and Pernow, P., Eds. (1977): *Substance P.* Raven Press, New York.
9. Gardner, D., and Kandel, E. R. (1972): Diphasic post-synaptic potential: A chemical synapse capable of mediating conjoint excitation and inhibition. *Science,* 176:678.
10. Gardner, D., and Kandel, E. R. (1977): Physiological and kinetic properties of cholinergic receptors activated by multiaction interneurons in buccal ganglia of *Aplysia. J. Neurophysiol.,* 40:333–348.
11. Henry, J. L. (1976): Effects of substance P on functionally identified units in cat spinal cord. *Brain Res.,* 14:439–451.
12. Henry, J. L., Krnjevic, K., and Morris, M. E. (1975): Substance P and spinal neurons. *Can. J. Physiol. Pharmacol.,* 53:423–432.
13. Konishi, S., and Otsuka, M. (1974): Effects of substance P and other peptides on spinal neurons of frog. *Brain Res.,* 65:397–410.
14. Konishi, S., and Otsuka, M. (1974): Excitatory action of hypothalamic substance P on spinal motoneurons of newborn rats. *Nature,* 252:734–735.
15. Krivoy, W., Kroeger, D., and Zimmermann, E. (1977): Additional evidence for a role of substance P in modulation of synaptic transmission. In: *Substance P,* edited by U. S. von Euler and B. Pernow, pp. 187–193. Raven Press, New York.
16. Krnjevic, K. (1977): Effects of substance P on central neurons in cats. In: *Substance P,* edited by U. S. von Euler and B. Pernow, pp. 217–230. Raven Press, New York.
17. MacDonald, J. F., Barker, J. L., Skolnick, P., Marangos, P., and Paul, S. (1979): Inosine may be an endogenous ligand for benzodiazepine receptors on cultured spinal neurons. *Science,* 205:715–717.
18. MacDonald, J. F., and Berry, M. S. (1978): Further identification of multiple responses mediated by dopamine in the CNS of *Planorbis comeus. Can. J. Physiol. Pharmacol.,* 56:7–18.
19. Mudge, A. W., Leeman, J. E., and Fischbach, G. D. (1979): Enkephalin inhibits release of substance P from sensory neurons in culture and decreases action potential duration. *Proc. Natl. Acad. Sci. USA,* 76:526–530.
20. Naftchi, J., Abrahams, J. J., St. Paul, H. M., Lowman, E. W., and Schlosser, W. (1978): Localization and changes of substance P in spinal cord of paraplegic cats. *Brain Res.,* 153:507–513.
21. Nicoll, R. A. (1978): The action of thyrotropin-releasing hormone, substance P, and related peptides on frog spinal neurons. *J. Pharm. Exp. Ther.,* 207:817–824.

22. Otsuka, M., and Konishi, S. (1976): Release of substance P-like immunoreactivity from isolated spinal cord of newborn rat. *Nature,* 264:83–84.

23. Pickel, V. M., Reis, D. J., and Leeman, S. E. (1977): Ultrastructural localization of substance P in neurons of rat spinal cord. *Brain Res.,* 122:534–540.

24. Ransom, B. R., Neale, E. H., Henkart, M., Bullock, P., and Nelson, P. G. (1977): The mouse spinal cord in tissue culture. I. Morphology and intrinsic neuronal electrophysiological properties. *J. Neurophysiol.,* 40:1132–1150.

25. Steinacker, A. (1977): Calcium-dependent presynaptic action of substance P at the frog neuromuscular junction. *Nature,* 267:268–270.

26. Vincent, J.-D., and Barker, J. L. (1979): Substance P: Evidence for diverse roles in neuronal function using cultured mouse spinal neurons. *Science,* 205:1409–1412.

27. Wachtel, H., and Kandel, E. R. (1971): Conversion of synaptic excitation to inhibition at a dual chemical synapse. *J. Neurophysiol.,* 34:56–68.

28. Zieglgänsberger, W., and Bayerl, H. (1976): The mechanism of inhibition of neuronal activity by opiates in the spinal cord of the cat. *Brain Res.,* 115:111–128.

Neuropeptides and Neural Transmission,
edited by C. Ajmone Marsan and W. Z. Traczyk.
Raven Press, New York © 1980.

Substance P in Human Plasma

D. Powell, P. Skrabanek, D. Cannon, and A. Balfe

Endocrine Unit, Mater Misericordiae Hospital, Dublin, Ireland

Substance P (SP)-like activity has been detected in plasma in several mammalian species, including man, using bioassays and radioimmunoassays. However, the role of SP in the circulation, the factors that control its secretion or blood levels, and its metabolic fate still remain to be elucidated.

SP-like bioactivity was reported in equine blood by Euler and Gaddum (5), and in acid-alcohol extracts of blood from sheep, rat, guinea-pig, and man by Weissbecker (23).

More recently, immunoreactive SP (ISP) was detected in plasma by radioimmunoassay by several groups. Nilsson et al. (15) found 70 to 299 pmoles/l in man, and 38 to 154 pmoles/l in dogs. Yanaihara et al. (24) found 52 to 622 pmoles/l in human blood. We have previously reported ISP levels averaging 30 pmoles/l in unextracted plasma from blood donors (19). Leeman and Carraway (13) found relatively high apparent ISP levels in rat plasma (424 pmoles/l) and in calf plasma (165 pmoles/l), but only 9 and 18 pmoles/l, respectively, after extraction of the plasma samples with acid acetone. They concluded that non-specific factors were interfering with the assay of ISP in unextracted plasma. Gamse et al. (6) showed that the main source of ISP in feline plasma was the intestine.

In this chapter we shall review our studies on the nature of ISP in human plasma and ISP levels in normal subjects and in patients with various pathological conditions.

NATURE OF ISP IN HUMAN PLASMA

Molecular Size

There is evidence indicating that endogenous circulating ISP is in a molecular form different from the synthetic undecapeptide. Charcoal adsorption studies showed that charcoal can be used to adsorb more than 90% of added synthetic SP from plasma. However, very little, if any, endogenous ISP is adsorbed by charcoal, suggesting that it is attached to a large molecular weight compound (3).

Gel chromatography studies show that while added synthetic SP in plasma elutes in the position corresponding to its molecular weight, endogenous ISP elutes at the void volume on a P-100 column (0.9 × 50 cm), indicating that it is part of a much larger molecule. However, ISP in both acid-acetone and saline extracts of human substantia nigra elutes with labelled Tyr[8]-SP.

In a patient with a SP-secreting ileal carcinoid tumour, we had the opportunity to obtain plasma not only from the peripheral vein (ISP concentration 74 pmoles/l) but also from the mesenteric vein draining the tumour (ISP concentration 274 pmoles/l). During gel chromatography on a P-100 column, ISP from the peripheral sample eluted at the void volume, whereas effluent ISP containing nearly a fourfold concentration of ISP gave two elution peaks: about half of ISP eluted at the void volume and the other half at the position of the co-chromatographed labelled Tyr[8]-SP undecapeptide. These data suggest that SP emerged from the tumour as a small molecular weight substance and subsequently became bound to a large carrier.

DEGRADATION

Endogenous ISP is stable in plasma. However, synthetic SP added to human plasma is rapidly destroyed. The degradation of exogenous SP is temperature-dependent. Moreover, fresh plasma destroys exogenous SP faster than heat-inactivated plasma (19). Circulating SP bioactivity is rapidly degraded in the liver, and Lembeck et al. (14) also found that about 90% of exogenous SP bioactivity is destroyed after 60 min incubation in rat plasma. On the other hand, Bury and Mashford (2) reported that SP-degrading activity is contained not in plasma but in erythrocytes.

Heat inactivation of plasma (60°C, 60 min) reduced the capacity of human plasma to inactivate added exogenous SP by about one-third. However, when a mixture of synthetic SP and human plasma was heated at 60°C for 60 min, only 12% of ISP was recovered, while the same treatment of synthetic SP in assay buffer (containing only 2.5% human plasma) did not affect the recovery of ISP (3).

Lembeck et al. (14) found that bacitracin partially inhibited the degradation of SP bioactivity in rat plasma *in vivo,* though not *in vitro,* and they suggested that SP was degraded by bacitracin-sensitive and bacitracin-insensitive enzymes. The enzymic nature of ISP degradation was further suggested by findings that other enzyme inhibitors, such as teprotide (SQ 20881) in plasma (3) and endothelial cell culture (11), and ethylenediaminetetraacetic acid (EDTA) in whole blood (2), plasma (3), and endothelial cell culture (11), also partially prevented SP degradation. In pregnant sera, both in women (22) and in rats (12), SP bioactivity was inactivated faster than in normal sera. We have shown that in pregnant women there is a significantly lower mean level of plasma ISP (4).

These observations suggest that SP in human blood is degraded by enzymes. Since heat treatment only partially inhibits the degradation of SP, possibly both heat-stable and heat-labile enzymes are involved (3). (For a review of the literature on enzymatic degradation of SP in tissues see ref. 21.)

CLINICAL STUDIES

ISP is detectable in normal human plasma. In 77 normal plasma samples the range of ISP was from < 15 to 93 pmoles/l with a mean of 30 ± 5 pmoles/l ($\pm$ SEM). No correlation was found between ISP levels and blood electrolytes, creatinine, urea, total protein and albumin, calcium, phosphate, cholesterol, uric acid, bilirubin, alkaline phosphatase, lactic dehydrogenase, glutamate-oxalacetate transaminase, and glutamate-pyruvate transaminase (19). In hospital patients with various clinical disorders, no correlation was found between thyroid function and ISP plasma levels. ISP plasma levels in various gastrointestinal disorders were similar to those found in normal subjects (4,19).

Sleep

During nocturnal sleep in 6 human volunteers, plasma ISP was secreted in episodic bursts with about five peaks, when samples were taken every half hour (19). We have studied an additional 8 adult male volunteers in a sleep laboratory. Plasma ISP, growth hormone, prolactin, adrenocorticotrophin, and cortisol were measured at half-hour intervals and EEG was continuously monitored. Plasma ISP ranged from undetectable to 430 pmoles/l with a mean of 77 pmoles/l in 195 plasma samples. The first peak of ISP appeared about 60 to 90 min after sleep onset and subsequent peaks followed at about 90-min intervals, reaching a maximum at about 5 a.m. Plasma ISP was not related to REM or non-REM sleep phases. No correlation was found between plasma ISP and plasma growth hormone, adrenocorticotrophin, and cortisol. However, 30 of 41 peaks of plasma ISP coincided with plasma prolactin peaks (17).

Whether SP plays a role in the physiological regulation of prolactin release in man remain to be seen. We studied ISP plasma levels in awake female patients with hyperprolactinaemia before and after treatment with the dopamine agonist bromocriptine. We have found no correlation between plasma ISP and immuno-reactive prolactin levels in these patients. However, in rats, SP administered intravenously raised plasma prolactin levels (16). Hökfelt et al. (9) found SP-positive nerve fibres in the anterior pituitary in man, suggesting that SP has a role in the control of hormonal secretion from the anterior pituitary.

SP and Carcinoid Tumours

Alumets et al. (1) localised ISP in the cytoplasmic granules of carcinoid tumour cells from a patient with an ileal carcinoid and a high peripheral plasma level of ISP. In 1976 we demonstrated a plasma concentration gradient of ISP across the liver in a patient with metastatic ileal carcinoid (19). Håkanson et al. (7) found ISP immunofluorescence in two carcinoid tumours from patients with high peripheral levels of ISP. Production of ISP by carcinoid tumour *in vitro* was also demonstrated (20). So far, we have studied 9 patients with carcinoid tumours (Table 1). It is interesting that in some patients with carcinoid tumours

TABLE 1. *SP and carcinoid tumours*

Age/sex	Primary site	Urinary 5-HIAA	Plasma SP
56 M	Ileum	↑	↑
65 F	Ileum	↑	↑
60 M	Bronchus	↑	↑
57 F	Ileum	↑	↑
52 M	Ileum	N	N
34 F	Bronchus	N	↑
41 F	Ovary	N	↑
75 F	?	N	↑
56 F	?	N	↑

↑, high; N, normal.

plasma ISP was elevated, while urinary 5-hydroxyindoleacetic acid (5-HIAA) was normal. Ingemansson et al. (10) reported elevated peripheral ISP levels in 3 patients with intestinal carcinoids and in 2 of them they found an intestinal arterio-venous gradient of ISP. In 1 patient, the finding of a postoperative elevation of ISP led to further exploration of the abdomen and to the discovery of two small metastases in the liver.

Since SP can cause flushing, hypotension, tachycardia, increased intestinal peristalsis, and bronchoconstriction, it may contribute to the pathophysiology of the carcinoid syndrome, and ISP may also serve as a carcinoid tumour marker.

SP and Medullary Carcinoma of the Thyroid

Medullary carcinoma of the thyroid (MCT) is morphologically and histochemically related to carcinoid tumours. Several reports have described the carcinoid syndrome in patients with MCT and even in the absence of the carcinoid syndrome, urinary 5-HIAA may be slightly elevated in an occasional patient with MCT.

In 1 patient with MCT we have demonstrated a high content of ISP in the tumour and elevated ISP level in plasma (18). We have since studied an additional 10 patients, including 5 related patients with the familial form of MCT (Table 2). In some of these patients both plasma ISP and calcitonin were elevated, while in other patients plasma ISP and calcitonin levels were dissociated.

SP in Other Malignancies

In a study of 45 patients with various malignancies, plasma ISP levels in the majority of the patients were within normal limits. However, 4 of 8 patients with chronic leukaemia had abnormally high ISP levels. One patient with basaloid carcinoma of the anus had also high plasma ISP level (4).

Harkins et al. (8) reported production of ISP by two murine neuroblastomas in cell culture. We failed to detect any ISP in cell culture from one murine neuroblastoma.

TABLE 2. SP and medullary carcinoma of the thyroid

Sex	Plasma SP (pmoles/l)	Plasma calcitonin (µg/l)
F	155	> 50
F[a]	47	> 50
M	133	50
F	62	32
F[a]	104	14
F	52	1
M[a]	74	0.4
F[a]	56	0.3
M[a]	133	0.3
M[a]	47	< 0.2
M[a]	43	< 0.2

[a] Kindred.

In view of the close relationship between carcinoid tumours and oat-cell carcinomas, we studied 4 human oat-cell carcinoma tumours, but failed to detect any ISP.

CONCLUSION

SP appears to be produced and secreted from tissues as a small molecular weight substance. In the circulation, ISP becomes a large molecular form, possibly by association with a large protein. This association may protect endogenous SP from the fate that befalls exogenously added SP which is rapidly degraded in plasma, probably by both heat-stable and heat-labile enzymes.

In clinical studies in man, ISP is detectable in normal human plasma, and appears to rise and fall during sleep, possibly associated with changes in plasma immunoreactive prolactin levels. ISP is produced by certain malignancies, particularly carcinoid tumours as well as medullary carcinoma of the thyroid. In certain patients the SP produced may contribute to the patient's clinical symptoms.

ACKNOWLEDGMENTS

We thank the Irish Cancer Society, the St. Luke's Fund, and the Medical Research Council of Ireland for generous financial support.

REFERENCES

1. Alumets, J., Håkanson, R., Ingemansson, S., and Sundler, F. (1977): Substance P and 5-HT in granules isolated from an intestinal argentaffin carcinoid. *Histochemistry*, 52:217–222.
2. Bury, R. W., and Mashford, M. L. (1977): The stability of synthetic substance P in blood. *Eur. J. Pharmacol.*, 45:257–260.
3. Cannon, D., Skrabanek, P., and Powell, D. (1979): Difference in behaviour between synthetic

and endogenous substance P in human plasma. *Naunyn Schmiedebergs Arch. Pharmacol.,* 307:251–255.

4. Cusack, D., Cannon, D., Skrabanek, P., and Powell, D. (1979): Substance P plasma levels in pregnancy and in various clinical disorders. *Horm. Metab. Res.,* 11:415–454.

5. Euler, U. S. von, and Gaddum, J. H. (1931): An unidentified depressor substance in certain tissue extracts. *J. Physiol. (Lond.),* 72:74–87.

6. Gamse, R., Mroz, E., Leeman, S., and Lembeck, F. (1978): The intestine as source of immunoreactive substance P in plasma of the cat. *Naunyn Schmiedebergs Arch. Pharmacol.,* 305:17–21.

7. Håkanson, R., Bengmark, S., Brodin, E., Ingemansson, S., Larsson, L. I., Nilsson, G., and Sundler, F. (1977): Substance P-like immunoreactivity in intestinal carcinoid tumours. In: *Substance P,* edited by U. S. von Euler and B. Pernow, pp. 55–58. Raven Press, New York.

8. Harkins, J., Roper, M., Ham, R. G., and Stewart, J. M. (1978): Biosynthesis of substance P in cultured mouse neuroblastoma and rat glioma cells. *Brain Res.,* 147:405–409.

9. Hökfelt, T., Pernow, B., Nilsson, G., Wetterberg, L., Goldstein, M., and Jeffcoate, S. L. (1978): Dense plexus of substance P immunoreactive nerve terminals in eminentia medialis of the primate hypothalamus. *Proc. Natl. Acad. Sci. USA,* 75:1013–1015.

10. Ingemansson, S., Bengmark, S., Nilsson, G., Brodin, E., Larsson, L.-I., and Lunderquist, A. (1977): Aortal, caval, and intestinal vein catheterization for substance-P determination in patients with carcinoid tumours. *Eur. Surg. Res.,* 9:47.

11. Johnson, A. R., and Erdös, E. G. (1976): Peptidases in cultured endothelial cells. In: *Substance P, Nobel Symposium 37.* Stockholm, June 14–16, p. 35 (abstr.).

12. Kocić-Mitrović, D. (1961): Substance P in pregnancy. *Proc. Sci. Soc. Bosnia Herzegovina,* 1:113–115.

13. Leeman, S. E., and Carraway, R. E. (1977): Discovery of a sialogogic peptide in bovine hypothalamic extracts: Its isolation, characterization as substance P, structure, and synthesis. In: *Substance P,* edited by U. S. von Euler and B. Pernow, pp. 5–13. Raven Press, New York.

14. Lembeck, F., Holzer, P., Schweditsch, M., and Gamse, R. (1978): Elimination of substance P from circulation of the rat and its inhibition by bacitracin. *Naunyn Schmiedebergs Arch. Pharmacol.,* 305:9–16.

15. Nilsson, G., Pernow, B., Fischer, G. H., and Folkers, K. (1975): Presence of substance P-like immunoreactivity in plasma from man and dog. *Acta Physiol. Scand.,* 94:542–544.

16. Rivier, C., Brown, M., and Vale, W. (1977): Effect of neurotensin, substance P and morphine on the secretion of prolactin and growth hormone in the rat. *Endocrinology,* 100, 751–754.

17. Skrabanek, P., Cannon, D., Darragh, A., and Powell, D. (1978): Substance P and prolactin secretion during sleep. *Ninth Congress of the International Society for Psychoneuroendocrinology.* Dublin, August 20–24, p. 17 (abstr.).

18. Skrabanek, P., Cannon, D., Dempsey, J., Kirrane, J., Neligan, M., and Powell, D. (1979): Substance P in medullary carcinoma of the thyroid. *Experientia,* 35:1259–1260.

19. Skrabanek, P., Cannon, D., Kirrane, J., Legge, D., and Powell, D. (1976): Circulating immunoreactive substance P in man. *Ir. J. Med. Sci.,* 145:399–408.

20. Skrabanek, P., Cannon, D., Kirrane, J., and Powell, D. (1978): Substance P secretion by carcinoid tumours. *Ir. J. Med. Sci.,* 147:47–49.

21. Skrabanek, P., and Powell, D. (1978): *Substance P, Vol. 1.* Eden Press, Montreal; Churchill Livingstone, Edinburgh; (1980): *Vol. 2, ibid.*

22. Stern, P., Gašparović, I., and Kovač, J. (1961): A factor inactivating substance P present in the serum of pregnant women. *Proc. Sci. Soc. Bosnia Herzegovina,* 1:139–143.

23. Weissbecker, L. (1947): Substanz P im Blut. Ein Beitrag zur Spätgiftproblem. *Naunyn Schmiedebergs Arch. Pharmacol.,* 204:674–688.

24. Yanaihara, C., Sato, H., Hirohashi, M., Sakagami, M., Yamamoto, K., Hashimoto, T., Yanaihara, N., Abe, K., and Kaneko, T. (1976): Substance P radioimmunoassay using *N*-α-tyrosyl-substance P and demonstration of the presence of substance P-like immunoreactivity in human blood and porcine tissue extracts. *Endocrinol. Jap.,* 23:457–463.

Neuropeptides and Neural Transmission,
edited by C. Ajmone Marsan and W. Z. Traczyk.
Raven Press, New York © 1980.

Analgesic and Other Activities of Substance P and Fragments

Robert C. A. Frederickson and Paul D. Gesellchen

Lilly Research Laboratories, Eli Lilly and Company, Indianapolis, Indiana 46285

The evidence has become very convincing that substance P (SP) has a neurotransmitter or neuromodulator role in the central nervous system. In spinal cord it probably serves as the transmitter utilized by primary sensory afferents (12), but its role in higher brain centers is more uncertain. While its probable role in primary sensory afferents might predict that its pharmacology includes algesic activity, surprisingly, it has been reported to produce very potent analgesia, although some controversy exists on this point.

Stewart et al. (18) reported analgesic activity of SP at nanogram doses either intracerebrally or intraperitoneally. This analgesic activity was surprisingly slow in onset (30 min) and long in duration (90–120 min) and could be antagonized by naloxone. Malick and Goldstein (7) found that SP produced dose-related naloxone-reversible analgesia in the rat tail flick test after infusion directly into the periaqueductal gray. These investigators, however, found that much higher doses (several orders of magnitude) of SP were necessary than those used by Stewart et al., and furthermore observed the effect to be of more rapid onset and shorter duration. Starr et al. (15) observed analgesia after intraperitoneal administration; but again the required doses were several orders of magnitude higher than those found effective by Stewart et al. (18). Contrary to the above findings, several groups, have reported that SP produces hyperalgesia (6,11) and antagonizes morphine-induced analgesia (17).

The antagonism of SP analgesia by naloxone suggests a role for opioid receptors, but SP itself does not bind to these receptors (19). It remains possible, nevertheless, that some fragment of SP is the active moiety. Otsuka and colleagues (12) reported that a C-terminal hexapeptide fragment of SP (Glp^6-SP_{6-11}) was more active on neurons in spinal cord than was SP itself. We undertook studies with SP, Glp^6-SP_{6-11}, and other fragments on mouse vas deferens and in the mouse hot plate test in order to examine structure-activity relations and to attempt a clarification of the puzzling controversy over analgesic versus hyperalgesic activity and the possible role of opioid systems. A preliminary account has already been published on this work which indicates dual actions of SP (4).

METHODS

Peptide Synthesis

The tetrapeptide fragment SP_{8-11} was synthesized by the excess mixed anhydride method (20), while the remaining peptide amides were synthesized by solid phase peptide synthesis (8) on a 1% cross-linked benzhydrylamine-polystyrene resin (Beckman, 0.47 mmol N/g N/g resin) using a Beckman 990 automated peptide synthesizer. All amino acid derivatives were coupled in methylene chloride followed by a recouple in 50% methylene chloride-dimethylformamide (21), using 2.5 equivalents of amino acid and 1.25 equivalents of dicyclohexylcarbodiimide (13). The N^α-protecting groups (Boc and Aoc) were removed with 25% trifluoroacetic acid (TFA)-methylene chloride containing 5% triethylsilane as scavenger (Smithwick, *personal communication*). Following attachment of the last residue, the N^α-protecting group was removed with TFA in order to avoid alkylation of the methionine residue during removal of the peptide from the resin in liquid hydrogen fluoride (10).

Peptide Purification

Crude SP, SP_{4-11}, SP_{7-11}, and SP_{8-11} were purified by low pressure reversed-phase liquid chromatography (LP—RPLC) using Michel-Miller[1] glass columns packed with C_{18} silica gel and eluting with an acetonitrile-ammonium acetate buffer system. Following LP-RPLC these peptides were desalted and further purified by chromatography over Sephadex G-10 in dilute aqueous acetic acid. Due to the low solubility of Glp^5-SP_{5-11}, Glp^6-SP_{6-11}, and $AcPhe^7$-SP_{7-11}, these analogs were purified by repeated recrystallization from 50% acetic acid or dimethylformamide-ethyl acetate. All purified peptides were shown to be homogeneous by thin layer chromatography in four solvent systems, elemental analysis (C,H,N), and amino acid analysis.

Mouse Vas Deferens Preparation

Single vas deferens from mature mice (Cox standard, Harlan Industries, 30–40 g) were suspended in 3 ml modified Krebs solution (5), aerated with 95% O_2–5% CO_2, and maintained at 37°C as previously described (4). The field-stimulated twitch (0.15 Hz, 1 msec, 40 V) or drug-induced contractures were recorded on a polygraph via an isometric transducer. Drugs were added in 30-μl aliquots by Hamilton syringe in order to obtain the desired final bath concentration.

---

[1] Michel, K., and Miller, R. (1978): Refillable column for chromatography at elevated pressure U.S. patent No. 4131547, Dec. 26.

Mouse Hot Plate Test for Analgesia

Cox standard mice (20–23 g) were used in these studies. The test utilized an apparatus with an electrically heated, thermostatically controlled (52°C) metal plate (Technilab Instruments, model 475 analgesiometer) and has been described previously (4). A plexiglass cylinder, 12 inches high, 4.75 inches in inner diameter, and open at the top, confined the mice to the hot plate. Hamilton microsyringes bearing 27-gauge needles with stops at 2.5 mm from the needle tip were utilized for intraventricular administration (4,9). The time in seconds from contact with the plate until a hind paw lick occurred was recorded as the response latency. The latency until an escape jump occurred was also recorded. Each mouse was used only once.

RESULTS

Analgesic Activity of SP

SP showed slight but significant analgesic activity at very low doses (1–5 ng/mouse) when placed directly into the lateral ventricles (Fig. 1). The analgesic activity of SP is compared with that of morphine and enkephalins in Fig. 1. SP is clearly very potent but limited in its activity. The threshold dose is about 1 ng, similar to that of the metabolically protected enkephalin analog LY 127623

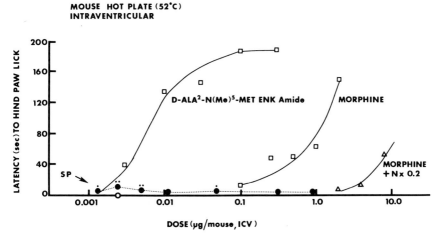

FIG. 1. Dose-response curves of analgesic activity in the mouse hot plate test (hind paw lick) of SP, D-Ala²-N(Me)Met⁵-enkephalin amide, and morphine after i.c.v. administration. The *ordinate* gives the increase in latency (sec) of drug-treated mice compared with mean control latency (saline-treated mice). Latencies were determined at 30 min after SP and morphine and 15 min after D-Ala²-N(Me)Met⁵-enkephalin amide. The *open circle* shows antagonism of the analgesic effect of SP at 2.5 ng/mouse by naloxone (0.2 mg/kg s.c.) injected 15 min before testing. The *open triangles* show antagonism of morphine analgesia by naloxone (0.2 mg/kg s.c.) injected 15 min before testing. (* $p < 0.05$; ** $p < 0.01$).

(D-Ala^2-N(Me)Met^5-enkephalin amide), making these peptides at least 100 times more potent than morphine and four or five orders of magnitude more potent than natural Met-enkephalin. SP, however, differed markedly from the opioids in that the effect was small and did not increase monotonically with increasing doses. In fact, the effect was not seen at doses greater than 10 to 50 ng/mouse. This small analgesic effect of SP, nevertheless, was antagonized by naloxone as was the analgesia produced by the opioids.

Effects of SP and Fragments on Mouse Vas Deferens

The naloxone-reversible analgesia produced by SP suggested activation of opioid receptors, and SP and various analogues were therefore tested on mouse vas deferens to assess any interaction with such receptors. SP had an effect on vas deferens opposite to that of the opioids. The opioids inhibited the electrically induced twitch while SP contracted the tissue and potentiated the twitch (Fig. 2). These effects of SP were not antagonized by naloxone. We next examined if a fragment of SP such as Glp^6-SP$_{6-11}$ might interact with the opioid receptors. Glp^6-SP$_{6-11}$, however, behaved like SP on the vas deferens preparation and showed no opioid-like activity (Fig. 2). The relative potencies of SP and various fragments on the vas deferens are shown in Table 1, which also shows the ranking on guinea pig ileum obtained from the literature (14).

We also examined SP and Glp^6-SP$_{6-11}$ for antagonist properties at the opioid receptors. Indeed, these peptides would reverse an enkephalin-induced depression (4), but this was apparently due to the direct stimulating action rather than to the antagonism of enkephalin receptors since pretreatment of tissues with SP or Glp^6-SP$_{6-11}$ did not diminish the degree of a subsequent depression by enkephalin (Fig. 3). The mouse vas deferens thus appears to contain receptors for SP independent of opioid receptors.

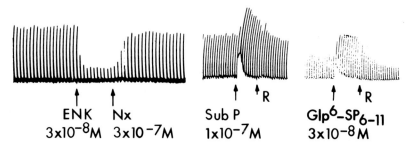

ENK   Nx   Sub P   Glp^6-SP$_{6-11}$
3×10^{-8}M 3×10^{-7}M 1×10^{-7}M 3×10^{-8}M

FIG. 2. Effects of D-Ala^2-Met^5-enkephalin amide (ENK), SP (Sub P), and a hexapeptide fragment of SP (Glp^6-SP$_{6-11}$) on the electrically induced twitch of the mouse vas deferens. Nx, naloxone; R, rinse.

TABLE 1. *Relative potencies of SP and C-terminal fragments*

Peptide[a]	Relative potencies		
	Guinea pig ileum[b]	Mouse vas deferens	Analgesia[c]
SP	1.0	1.0	AAA
SP_{2-11}	0.6–1.0	—	—
SP_{3-11}	0.5–1.7	—	—
SP_{4-11}	0.4–2.6	0.02	A
$Glp^5\text{-}SP_{5-11}$	1.0–4.0	0.02	A
$Glp^6\text{-}SP_{6-11}$	0.8–2.0	0.13	AA
$AcPhe^7\text{-}SP_{7-11}$	—	0.02	HA
SP_{7-11}	0.002–0.05	0.006	NA
SP_{8-11}	0.0002–0.02	<0.001	NA
SP_{9-11}	0.00001	—	—

[a] Glp, pyrrolidone carboxylic acid; SP, H-Arg-Pro-Lys-Pro-Gln-Gln-Phe-Phe-Gly-Leu-Met-NH$_2$.

[b] Ranges of relative potencies determined from four separate studies reported in ref. 15.

[c] Analgesia observed in mouse hot plate assay after i.c.v. injection of peptide. AAA, most active; A, least active; NA, not active; HA, hyperalgesic.

Comparative Analgesic–Hyperalgesic Activity of SP and Fragments

The *in vitro* studies indicated that the hexapeptide fragment $Glp^6\text{-}SP_{6-11}$ was the minimal active structure. The various fragments were tested also in the hot plate test after intraventricular administration to attempt delineation of the structural requirements for analgesic activity. Unfortunately, because of the biphasic nature of the response (4) and the lack of a straightforward dose-response curve, determination of relative ED_{50} and a potency ranking of the

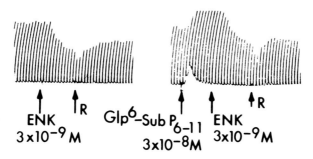

FIG. 3. Example of the lack of antagonism by $Glp^6\text{-}SP_{6-11}$ of the depression of the twitch of the mouse vas deferens by Met-enkephalin (ENK). R, rinse.

various fragments was not possible. The analgesic results are presented in Table 1 by simply indicating whether each fragment was active (A) or not (NA): a substance was considered active for this purpose if it produced a significant analgesic or hyperalgesic effect at any dose level (in the range 1–1,000 ng/mouse i.c.v.) compared with its control group. It appears the hexapeptide is the minimum structure for analgesic activity also.

The comparative activity in the mouse hot plate test of SP, Glp^6-SP_{6-11}, and

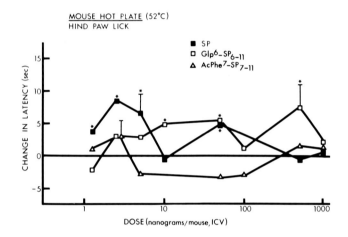

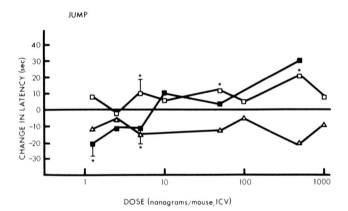

FIG. 4. Comparative dose-response curves of the activity in the mouse hot plate test of SP, Glp^6-SP_{6-11}, and $AcPhe^7$-SP_{7-11}. The *upper graph* gives the change in latency (sec) to hind paw lick compared with the mean control latency (saline-treated animals), and the *lower graph* gives the change in latency to the jump response for each treatment. Latencies were measured at 30 min after the i.c.v. administration of each dose of each compound. Each point represents the mean of two or three separate values determined in separate experiments each utilizing 10 treated and 10 control mice per dose. The lower graph gives the same data for the jump response. * $p < 0.05$.

AcPhe^7-SP$_{7-11}$ in the dose range 1 to 1000 ng/mouse intraventricularly is shown in Fig. 4. SP had a slight analgesic effect (increased latency) on the hind paw lick response (Fig. 4A) at 1.25, 2.5, and 50 ng/mouse. Glp^6-SP$_{6-11}$ had a slight analgesic effect at 10, 50, and 500 ng/mouse while Ac^7-SP$_{7-11}$ had no significant effect at any dose, although there seemed to be a general tendency to reduce the latency (hyperalgesic effect). On the jump response (Fig. 4B) SP had a hyperalgesic effect at 1.25 ng/mouse but none of the other doses produced a significant effect. Glp^6-SP$_{6-11}$ was analgesic at 5, 50, and 500 ng/mouse on the jump response while AcPhe^7-SP$_{7-11}$ lowered the latency to jump at all doses, although only the effect at 5 ng/mouse reached statistical significance. Thus, SP and Glp^6-SP$_{6-11}$ appeared to have analgesic activity with SP being more potent, while AcPhe^7-SP$_{7-11}$ appeared to be hyperalgesic. In general the effects were small, variable, and showed little dose-relationship in the dose range used.

Separation of the Dual Effects of SP with the Use of Antagonists

SP had slight analgesic activity at very low doses, but this activity was lost at higher doses. It seemed that this peculiar dose-response relationship might be due to dual opposing actions of this peptide in brain. We postulated, for example, that at low doses SP might release opioid peptides which mediate the naloxone-reversible analgesia, while at higher doses the direct postsynaptic neuronal stimulatory activity of the substance might counteract the opioid activ-

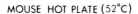

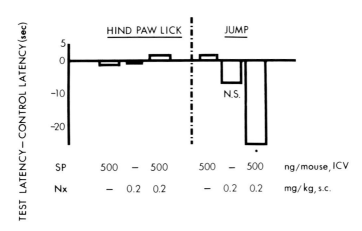

FIG. 5. Hyperalgesic effect of SP (500 ng i.c.v.) plus naloxone (Nx). SP at this dose did not affect latency to hind paw lick when given either alone or with naloxone (0.2 mg/kg s.c.), but did markedly and significantly decrease the latency to jump response when combined with naloxone. Neither SP or naloxone alone at these doses had a significant effect on jump latency. * $p < 0.05$.

ity. We therefore undertook a series of experiments designed to reveal each of these actions separately by selectively antagonizing the other. We treated mice with a combination of either a high dose of SP (500 ng/mouse) plus naloxone to block the effects of any released opioids, or the same high dose of SP plus baclofen (β-[4-chlorophenyl]-gamma-aminobutyric acid, a putative SP antagonist) to oppose the postsynaptic excitatory action. We observed the expected separation of activities and the results are summarized in Figs. 5 and 6. A dose of 500 ng of SP alone had no significant effect on either the hind paw lick or the jump response. In the presence of naloxone (0.2 mg/kg s.c.) this same dose of SP produced a marked and significant hyperalgesic effect (Fig. 5) in the jump response, and in the presence of baclofen (5 mg/kg s.c.) it produced a marked and significant analgesic effect (Fig. 6) on both the hind paw lick and the jump responses.

DISCUSSION

SP and various C-terminal fragments were tested on the mouse vas deferens preparation *in vitro* and in the mouse hot plate test *in vivo*. SP produced a small analgesic effect at very low doses (1–10 ng/mouse i.c.v.), but this effect was lost at higher doses (> 50 ng/mouse i.c.v.). This analgesic activity could be antagonized by naloxone suggesting utilization of opioid receptors, but SP does not bind these receptors (19). We considered the possibility that a metabolite

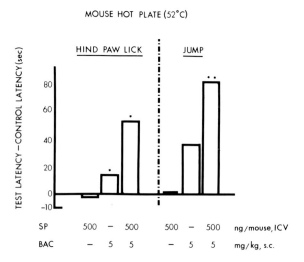

FIG. 6 Analgesic effect of SP (500 ng i.c.v.) plus baclofen (BAC). SP alone at this dose did not affect latency to either hind paw lick or jump. Baclofen alone at 5 mg/kg s.c. slightly increased the response latencies, but only the effect on hind paw lick was statistically significant. The combination of SP plus baclofen produced a significant potentiation of the increase in latencies to both responses. * $p < 0.05$; ** $p < 0.01$.

of SP might mediate this activity and therefore examined SP and a series of C-terminal fragments on the mouse vas deferens and also in the mouse hot plate test. Indeed, Otsuka (12) has reported that a C-terminal hexapeptide, $Glp^6\text{-}SP_{6\text{-}11}$, is even more active than SP itself on neurons in mammalian spinal cord. Neither SP nor any of the fragments demonstrated any agonist or antagonist activity on opioid receptors in the mouse vas deferens, but they did induce contraction of the quiescent tissue presumably by activation of SP receptors in this tissue. The smallest active fragment was the hexapeptide $Glp^6\text{-}SP_{6\text{-}11}$, as has been reported also for guinea pig ileum (14).

Since neither SP nor fragments activated opiate receptors, we presumed the analgesia was probably due to the release of endogenous opioid peptides. The hexapeptide appeared to be the minimal structure with analgesic activity, and indeed, the hexapeptide was more active than the hepta- or octapeptides ($Glp^5\text{-}SP_{5\text{-}11}$, $SP_{4\text{-}11}$). The tetra- and pentapeptides were inactive, although the acylated pentapeptide ($AcPhe^7\text{-}SP_{7\text{-}11}$) showed some hyperalgesic activity. The data are not yet sufficient to attribute the analgesic activity to any one fragment.

The small degree of effect, the high variability, and the lack of a monotonic dose-response relationship raise several questions. These phenomena could be due to several factors such as (a) variations in the actual dose delivered consequent upon the poor solubility of some of the materials; (b) variations in bioavailability; and/or (c) different basal states of experimental animals due, for example, to the diurnal rhythm in availability of opioid peptides for release (3). In particular, we considered that dual opposing effects of SP or fragments may have contributed to the unusual dose-response relationships. Thus we hypothesized that the analgesia at low doses was produced by a release of endogenous opioid peptides, while at higher doses this effect might be opposed by direct postsynaptic stimulatory actions. SP, in fact, has been reported to have both pre- and post-synaptic effects (16) and, furthermore, SP is reported to excite while opioid peptides inhibit neurons involved in transmission of nociceptive information (see, for example, refs. 1,2,4). We were able to reveal each of these activities by selectively antagonizing the other. Thus, SP at a dose that had no effect alone produced a hyperalgesic effect when administered in the presence of naloxone (to block the action of release opioid peptides). To the contrary, in the presence of baclofen to block the postsynaptic excitatory action of SP (12), the same dose that caused hyperalgesia in the presence of naloxone produced marked analgesia. It is not known at this time whether the two actions of SP are mediated by one or more fragments or whether they are due to action on one or more receptor types.

ACKNOWLEDGMENTS

We wish to thank Susan Tafur, Carolyn E. Harrell, Vigo Burgis, and John D. Edwards for technical assistance; John D. Edwards for preparation of the figures; and Arline Scott for typing the manuscript.

REFERENCES

1. Frederickson, R. C. A. (1977): Enkephalin pentapeptides: A review of current evidence for a physiological role in vertebrate neurotransmission. *Life Sci.,* 21:23–42.
2. Frederickson, R. C. A.: Peptide receptors. In: *The Neuroendocrine Functions of the Brain,* edited by M. Motta. Raven Press, New York *(in press).*
3. Frederickson, R. C. A., Burgis, V., and Edwards, J. D. (1977): Hyperalgesia induced by naloxone follows diurnal rhythm in responsivity to painful stimuli. *Science,* 198:756–758.
4. Frederickson, R. C. A., Burgis, V., Harrell, C. E., and Edwards, J. D. (1978): Dual actions of substance P on nociception: Possible role of endogenous opioids. *Science,* 199:1359–1362.
5. Henderson, G., Hughes, J., and Kosterlitz, H. W. (1972): A new example of a morphine-sensitive neuro-effector junction: Adrenergic transmission in the mouse vas deferens. *Br. J. Pharmacol.,* 46:764.
6. Juan, H., and Lembeck, F. (1974). Action of peptides and other algesic agents on paravascular pain receptors of the isolated perfused rabbit ear. *Naunyn Schmiedebergs Arch. Pharmacol.,* 283:151–164.
7. Malick, J. B., and Goldstein, J. M. (1978): Analgesic activity of substance P following intracerebral administration in rats. *Life Sci.,* 23:835–844.
8. Merrifield, R. B. (1963): Solid phase peptide synthesis. I. The synthesis of a tetrapeptide. *J. Am. Chem. Soc.,* 85:2149–2154.
9. Noble, E. P., Wurtman, R. J., and Axelrod, J. (1967): A simple and rapid method for injecting ^{3}H-norepinephrine into the lateral ventricle of the rat brain. *Life Sci.,* 6:281–291.
10. Noble, R. L., Yamashiro, D., and Li, C. H. (1976): Synthesis of a nonadecapeptide corresponding to residues 37–55 of ovine prolactin. Detection and isolation of the sulfonium form of methionine-containing peptides. *J. Am. Chem. Soc.,* 98:2324–2328.
11. Oehme, P., Bergmann, J., Bienert, M., Hilse, H., Piesche, L., Minh Thu, P., and Scheer, E. (1977): Biological action of substance P—its differentiation by affinity and intrinsic efficacy. In: *Substance P, Nobel Symposium, Vol. 37,* edited by U. S. von Euler and B. Pernow. Raven Press, New York.
12. Otsuka, M., and Konishi, S. (1976): Substance P and excitatory transmitter of primary sensory neurons. *Cold Spring Harbor Symp. Quant. Biol.,* 40:135–143.
13. Rebek, J., and Fietler, D. (1974): Mechanism of the carbodiimide reaction. II. Peptide synthesis on the solid phase. *J. Am. Chem. Soc.* 96:1606–1607.
14. Skrobanek, P., and Powell, D. (1978): Substance P. *Annual Research Reviews, Vol. 1,* p. 23. Eden Press, Great Britain.
15. Starr, M. S., James, T. A., and Gaytten, D. (1978): Behavioral depressant and antinociceptive properties of substance P in the mouse: Possible implication of brain monoamines. *Eur. J. Pharmacol.,* 48:203–212.
16. Steinacker, A., and Highstein, S. M. (1976): Pre- and postsynaptic action of substance P at the Mauthner fiber—giant fiber synapse in the hatchet fish. *Brain Res.,* 114:128–133.
17. Stern, P., Huković, S., and Radivojević, M. (1976): The inhibition of the effects of morphine by synthetic substance P. *Experientia,* 32:1326–1327.
18. Stewart, J. M., Getto, C. J., Neldner, K., Reeve, E. B., Krivoy, W. A., and Zimmermann, E. (1976): Substance P and analgesia. *Nature,* 262:784–785.
19. Terenius, L. (1975): Effect of peptides and amino acids on dihydromorphine binding to the opiate receptor. *J. Pharm. Pharmacol.,* 27:450–453.
20. Tilak, M. A. (1970): New solid phase method for quick, quantitative synthesis of analytically pure peptides without intermediate or final purification: I. Synthesis of a nonapeptide. *Tetrahedron Lett.* 11:849–854.
21. Westall, F. C., and Robinson, A. B. (1970): Solvent modification in Merrifield solid-phase peptide synthesis. *J. Org. Chem.,* 35:2842.

Neuropeptides and Neural Transmission,
edited by C. Ajmone Marsan and W. Z. Traczyk.
Raven Press, New York © 1980.

Substance P: Pain Transmission and Analgesia

Z. Szreniawski, A. Członkowski, P. Janicki, J. Libich, and S. W. Gumułka

Departments of Pharmacology and Pharmacodynamics, Institute of Physiological Science, Warsaw Medical School, 00–927 Warsaw, Poland

Although substance P (SP) was discovered 48 years ago (5), its physiological role has not yet been fully elucidated. Radioimmunoassay and bioassay techniques have revealed large amounts of SP in the spinal cord (10–12,14,22,23,27), where the peptide is preferentially localized in the dorsal roots. The largest amount occurs in the dorsal part of the dorsal horns, in the nerve fibers of laminae I–III. Several observations seem to indicate a role for SP as a neurotransmitter or modulator in primary sensory neurons (for a review, see ref. 23). After transection of the spinal cord and by using an immunohistochemical technique, Naftchi et al. (21) observed a sharp increase in the number of SP staining bodies below the section, while the number of stained bodies was decreased above the section. Application of SP as well as of its C-terminal fragments in low concentrations induced depolarization of spinal neurons. Henry et al. (9,10) have demonstrated that electrophoretic application of SP causes excitation of cat spinal neurons that have been activated by noxious stimuli applied to the skin. They also suggested that SP is specifically related to nociception and that it may have an excitatory role in afferent transmission in spinal pain pathways, probably acting at the first afferent synapse. Release of SP from primary afferent fibers may be undergoing an inhibitory control of enkephalinergic interneurons (17,18). In fact, laminae I and II of the dorsal horn contain large quantities of Met-enkephalin. Met-enkephalin in this region is probably localized in the terminals of interneurons, since neither transection of the spinal cord at the thoracic level nor unilateral dorsal rhizotomy at the lumbar and sacral levels produce any change in density of enkephalin-positive nerve terminals in the lumbar spinal cord (14). Enkephalinergic interneurons in the spinal cord were activated by descending pathways that probably orginate in raphe nuclei (14). Activation of these interneurons produced an analgesic effect by preventing release of SP from primary afferent nociceptive fibers (Fig. 1).

In light of the above observations suggesting an excitatory function for SP in spinal cord pain transmission, the discovery of analgesic properties of this peptide following its systemic or intracerebral administration came somewhat as a surprise.

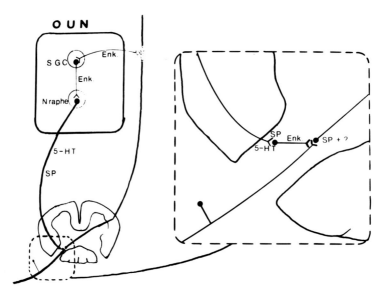

FIG. 1. Diagram illustrating two possible SPergic pathways: descending system (SP-5-HT containing neurones) and ascending system (SP as transmitter at the first synapse in the dorsal horn of spinal cord). SGC, substantia grisea centralis; Enk, enkaphalin.

SP AND ANALGESIA

Stewart et al. (25) reported an analgesic effect for SP in mice evaluated by the hot plate method following both intracerebral and intraperitoneal administration. The analgesic action of SP was of relatively long duration comparable to that of morphine and was completely abolished by naloxone. These observations have been confirmed by Frederickson et al. (6) and Starr et al. (24). Malick and Goldstein (19) have also found a longlasting analgesic effect to SP by the tail flick method in rats. In this study SP was administered into the midbrain periaqueductal gray substance. The analgesic effect produced by SP was significantly antagonized by pretreatment with naloxone.

In contrast to the above results, Growcott and Shaw (7) and Hayes and Tyres (8) failed to demonstrate an analgesic activity for SP in mice and rats. The latter authors even reported a hyperalgesia by the hot plate test after intrathecal administration of SP. In our study (Table 1, Fig. 2) both SP and its shorter C-terminal fragments pyroGlu^6-(SP$_{6-11}$) and SP$_{6-11}$ exerted a marked analgesic action in mouse hot plate and flinch-squeak-jump tests. This analgesic effect was completely abolished by pretreatment with naloxone. Our results agree with observations recently reported by Frederickson *(unpublished data);* nevertheless, it is difficult to account for the disparity with the findings of Growcott and Shaw (7) and Hayes and Tyres (8). The latter authors have suggested that the increase in reaction time in the hot plate test after administration of

TABLE 1. *Effect of SP (180 nmoles/kg) and pyroGlu⁶-(SP₆₋₁₁) (500 nmoles/kg)
on pain thresholds*[a]

Experimental group[b]	N[c]	Flinch	Squeak	Jump
Acetic acid	12	47 (41–54)	199 (156–254)	277 (236–326)
SP	9	95 (78–117)[e]	291 (249–340)	462 (388–549)[e]
Dextran-saline	19	56 (47–66)	302 (250–364)	445 (366–543)
Z-1	15	95 (76–119)[e]	454 (344–599)	766 (595–984)[e]

[a] Stimulus thresholds are expressed in μA; in parentheses are confidence limits (not symmetric since calculated from log values).
[b] Substance P and acetic acid were administered 90 min before testing and Z-1 and dextran-saline 30 min before testing.
[c] N, Number of animals.
[d] $p < 0.05$ as compared with control.
[e] $p < 0.01$ as compared with control.

SP may be due to the known sedative properties of this peptide. In fact, SP and its shorter analogs do decrease locomotor activity, but this effect reaches its peak 30 to 60 min after administration of SP, whereas the analgesic action occurs later, after the sedative effect has disappeared (Figs. 3 and 4). Furthermore, in the hot plate test SP markedly prolongs the reaction time for paw-licking, but shows only a slight effect on jump-off reaction time; it seems highly unlikely that the sedative action of this peptide would increase only the paw-licking reaction time and not the jumping-off reaction time.

In this respect the action of SP and analogs resembles the effect of opiate agonist and antagonistic drugs (e.g., pentazocine) (16). The analgesic properties of SP have also been confirmed by the mouse flinch-squeak-jump method (Table 1) in which potent sedative drugs, i.e., barbiturates and benzodiazepines, showed no analgesic activity. These observations indicate that analgesic and sedative properties of SP and related hexapeptides are two independent phenomena. Pretreatment with naloxone abolished the analgesic action of SP, but failed to antagonize its sedative activity. It must be recognized, however, that the analgesic action of SP in the hot plate test differs from the action of classic analgesic drugs with pure opiate agonistic activity. The latter drugs markedly prolonged the reaction time for both paw-licking and jumping-off, whereas SP significantly prolonged the paw-licking reaction time but had only a weak effect on jumping-off latency.

THE OPIATE RECEPTOR BINDING ACTIVITY OF SP AND RELATED HEXAPEPTIDES

The analgesic properties of SP and its C-terminal analogs with shorter amino acid chains raise the possibility of opiate receptor activity of these drugs. Therefore, we decided to check the binding affinity of SP and both hexapeptides to the ³H-naloxone binding sites in the rat striatum using radiolabeled ³H-naloxone

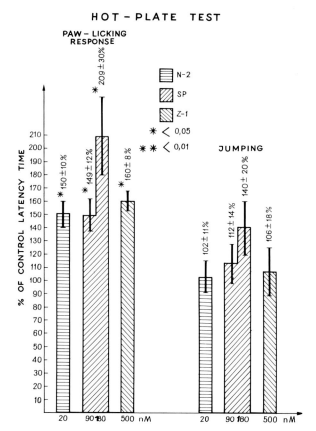

FIG. 2. Analgesic effect of SP_{1-11} (90 and 180 nM/kg i.p.) 45 min prior to the experiment, hexapeptide SP_{6-11} (N-2, 20 nM/kg i.p.) 30 min prior to the experiment, and hexapeptide pyroGlu⁶-(SP_{6-11}) (Z-1, 500 nM/kg, i.p.) 30 min prior to the experiment, as measured on hot plate (55 ± 0.5°C) test in mice. Two different responses were recorded: paw-licking and jumping-off. Ordinate: percentage of control (vehicle pretreated animals) latency time. Vertical bars represent ± SEM. Two-tailed Student's *t*-test was used for statistical analysis. **Significant vs control at $p < 0.01$; *significant vs control at $p < 0.05$. Naloxone (1 mg/kg s.c., 5 min prior to measurement) completely abolished the analgesic action of all three investigated peptides (not shown).

(3). As shown in Fig. 5, SP displayed no receptor binding activity. In contrast to SP, both hexapeptides produced a moderate displacement of specifically bound ³H-naloxone; however, even in concentrations of 10^{-5} M the displacement did not exceed 40%.

The lack of a direct action by SP on opiate receptors is also supported by the observations of Chipkin et al. (2), who found that this peptide does not inhibit contractions by coaxially stimulated guinea pig ileum. On the other hand, Członkowski et al. (3) have reported a moderate opiate receptor binding activity by SP ($IC_{50} = \mu M$) when ³H-labeled ethorphine was used as a specific ligand. In these experiments, the affinity of SP for opiate receptor was of the

LOCOMOTOR ACTIVITY AFTER S.P.

30′ AFTER INJECTION

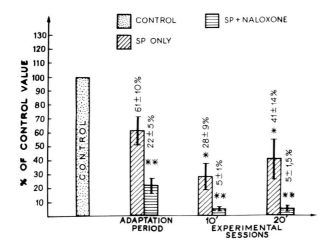

FIG. 3. Effect of SP on locomotor activity in mice (180 nM/kg i.p., 30 min prior to the experiment) was recorded automatically using Knoll actometer, during 5-min adaptation period and two subsequent 10-min experimental sessions. Naloxone (1 mg/kg i.p., 5 min prior to the experiment) was administered. Numbers are means ± SEM. $*p < 0.05$ and $**p < 0.01$ as compared with control group.

LOCOMOTOR ACTIVITY

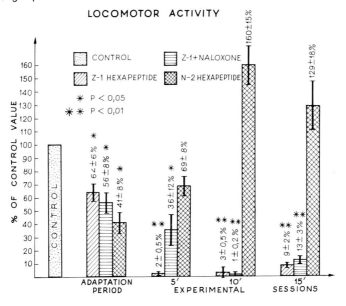

FIG. 4. The locomotor activity of mice directly after i.p. administration of 500 nM/kg of the hexapeptide pyroGlu^6-(SP$_{6-11}$) (Z-1) and 20 nM/kg SP$_{6-11}$ (N-2) measured as described in Fig. 3. Control animals received vehicle only. Naloxone (1 mg/kg s.c.) was administered 5 min prior to the measurement. Numbers are means ± SEM. $*p < 0.05$, and $**p < 0.01$ as compared with control (vehicle-treated animals).

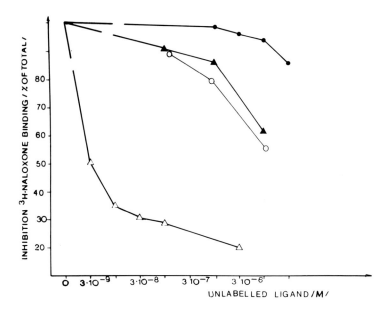

FIG. 5. Displacement of ³H-naloxone by increasing concentrations of the unlabeled ligands in rat's striatal homogenates. Abscissa: the concentration of unlabeled ligand (M). Ordinate: Percentage of total inhibition of ³H-naloxone binding to rat striata. *Closed circles,* Sp$_{1-11}$; *open circles,* pyroGlu^6-(SP$_{6-11}$); *closed triangles,* SP$_{6-11}$; *open triangles,* pentazocine.

same order as the affinity of ACTH$_{1-17}$ and ACTH$_{11-39}$. Some observations also seemed to indicate that SP and enkephalins act on common receptors, at least in vascular smooth muscle and Renshaw cells. In Renshaw cells, SP caused excitation that was blocked by naloxone (4). The excitatory effects of SP were similar to those of the enkephalins and may indicate an action on the same receptors. Moore (20) has found that SP and Met-enkephalin act on a common morphine-sensitive receptor in vascular smooth muscle.

In view of the above findings and the possibility suggested by several authors that there exists various opiate receptor types, the possibility of a direct action by SP on at least one population of opiate receptors cannot be completely ruled out.

SP AND THE SEROTONINERGIC SYSTEM

Autoradiographic, fluorescence-histochemic, microspectrofluorimetric, and immunofluorimetric studies have disclosed the presence of SP in certain serotonin (5-HT)-containing neurons in the CNS (1). Numerous cell bodies localized in the raphe nuclei (the n. raphe magnus, n. raphe obscurus, and n. raphe pallidus), parts of the n. reticularis gigantocellularis, and the n. interfascicularis hypoglossi contain both SP and 5-HT immunoreactive materials (13). According to the hypothesis advanced by Hökfelt et al. (14), a descending projection to the spinal cord, which originates in the raphe nuclei and contains SP and 5-HT as transmitter, plays an essential role in stimulation-produced analgesia, activating enkephalin interneurons in the dorsal horn and in the spinal trigeminal nucleus. Some biochemical observations indicate that SP can influence the activity of the serotoninergic system within the CNS (15,24). The serotoninergic system seems to be involved in pain transmission and in the analgesic effect of morphine and related opiate-like drugs (26).

It was therefore of interest to investigate the effect of the 5-HT depletor parachlorophenylalanine (PCPA) on the antinociceptive action of SP and its shorter analog pyroGlu^6-(SP$_{6-11}$) in mice. As shown in Fig. 6, pretreatment with PCPA methylester (300 mg/kg/day for 3 subsequent days) completely abolished the analgesic activity of both SP and pyroGlu^6-(SP$_{6-11}$). This finding indicates that 5-HT is involved in the antinociceptive action of SP. As mentioned above the serotoninergic system seems to play an important role in the analgesic activity of drugs that belong to various pharmacological groups, such as morphine, some other narcotic analgesics, and the cholinomimetics. On the basis of these findings one may speculate that the serotoninergic system perhaps constitutes a common site for the antinociceptive action of various centrally acting drugs.

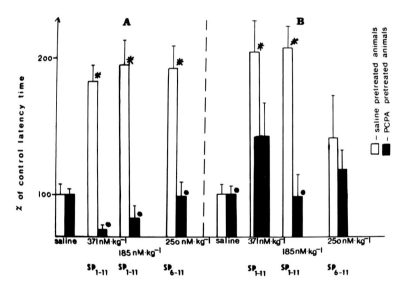

FIG. 6. Effect of PCPA pretreatment on analgesic action of SP$_{1-11}$ and pyroGlu^6-(SP$_{6-11}$) hexapeptide as measured in mouse hot plate test (55 ± 0.5°C). *Open column,* saline pretreated mice; *shaded column,* PCPA pretreated (300 mg/kg/day i.p. for 3 days) mice. Values represent the mean latency time of paw-licking response (panel **A**) and jumping-off response (panel **B**). Vertical bars represent ± SEM. Because of maximal effects, analgesic action of SP and pyroGlu^6-(SP$_{6-11}$) are measured 60 and 30 min, respectively, after drug administration. For the statistical analysis two-tailed Student's *t*-test was used. *$p < 0.05$ with respect to appropriate controls (vehicle-treated animals); *circles,* $p < 0.05$ with respect to saline (without PCPA) pretreated animals.

CONCLUSIONS

SP seems to play a complex role in pain transmission. Administered systemically, it produces a long-lasting antinociceptive effect that is completely antagonized by the pure opiate anatagonist naloxone. The analgesic properties of SP are not connected with its sedative action.

The mode of SP's analgesic action seems to differ from those of the narcotic analgesics, the enkephalins, and the endorphins, since SP possesses no opiate receptor binding activity. On the other hand, central serotoninergic neurons may be involved in SP-induced antinociception, since pretreatment with PCPA completely abolishes the analgesic effect of SP and its C-terminal fragment pyroGlu^6-(SP$_{6-11}$). This shorter C-terminal peptide derivative of SP exerts effects similar to those of SP central action; however, this peptide is about six times less potent by molar weight, and its central action appears somewhat sooner.

REFERENCES

1. Chan-Polay, V., Jonsson, G., and Polay, S. L. (1978): On the coexistence of serotonin and substance P in neurons of the rat's central nervous system. *Proc. Natl. Acad. Sci. USA,* 75:1582–1586.
2. Chipkin, R. E., Stewart, J. M., and Morris, D. H. (1978): Substance P and opioid interaction on stimulated and non-stimulated guinea-pig ileum. *Eur. J. Pharmacol.,* 53:21–27.
3. Członkowski, A., Höllt, V., and Herz, A. (1978): Binding of opiates and endogenous opioid peptides to neuroleptic receptor sites in the corpus striatum. *Life Sci.,* 22:953–962.
4. Davies, J., and Dray, A. (1977): Substance P and opiate receptors. *Nature,* 268: 351–355.
5. Euler, U. S. von, and Gaddum, J. H. (1931): An unidentified depressor substance in certain tissue extracts. *J. Physiol., (Lond.),* 72:74–87.
6. Frederickson, R. C. A., Burgis, V., Harrell, C. E., and Edwards, J. D. (1978): Dual actions of substance P on nociception—possible role of endogenous opioids. *Science,* 199:1359–1361.
7. Growcott, J. W., and Shaw, J. S. (1979): Failure of substance P to produce analgesia in the mouse. *Br. J. Pharmacol.,* 66:129P.
8. Hayes, A. G., and Tyres, M. B. (1979): Effect of intrathecal and intracerebroventricular injection of substance P on nociception in the rat and mouse. *Br. J. Pharmacol.,* 66:2P.
9. Henry, J. L. (1976): Effect of substance P on functionally identified units in cat spinal cord. *Brain Res.,* 114:439–451.
10. Henry, J. L. Krnjevic, K., and Morris, M. E. (1975): Substance P and spinal neurones. *Can. J. Physiol. Pharmacol.,* 53:423–432.
11. Hökfelt, T., Kellerth, J. O., Nilsson, G., and Pernow, B. (1975): Substance P localization in the central nervous system and in some primary sensory neurons. *Science,* 190:889–890.
12. Hökfelt, T., Kellerth, J. O., Nilsson, G., and Pernow B. (1975): Experimental immunohistochemical studies on localization and the distribution of substance P in cat primary sensory neurones. *Brain Res.,* 100:234–252.
13. Hökfelt, T., Ljungdahl, Å., Steinbusch, H., Verhofstad, A., Nilsson, G., Brodin, E., Pernow, B., and Goldstein, M. (1978): Immunohistochemical evidence of substance P-like immunoactivity in some 5-hydroxytryptamine-containing neurons in the rat central nervous system. *Neuroscience,* 3:517–538.
14. Hökfelt, T., Ljungdahl, Å., Terenius, L., Elde, R., and Nilsson, G. (1977): Immunochemical analysis of peptide pathways possibly related to pain and analgesia: Encefalin and substance P. *Proc. Natl. Acad. Sci. USA,* 74:3081–3085.
15. James, T. A., and Starr, M. S. (1979): Effects of substance P injected into the substantia nigra. *Br. J. Pharmacol.,* 65:423–429.
16. Janicki, P., and Libich, J. (1979): Detection of antagonist activity for narcotic analgesics in mouse hot-plate test. *Pharmacol. Biochem. Behav.,* 10:623–626.

17. Jessell, T. M. (1977): Opiate inhibition of substance P release from the rat trigeminal nucleus, in vitro. *J. Physiol. (Lond.),* 4:270:50–70.
18. Jessell, T. M., and Iversen, L. L. (1977): Opiate analgesics inhibit substance P release from rat trigeminal nucleus. *Nature,* 268:549–551.
19. Malick, J. S., and Goldstein, J. M. (1978): Analgesic activity of substance P following intracerebral administration in rats. *Life Sci.,* 23:835–844.
20. Moore, A. F. (1979): The interaction of enkephalins with substance P on vascular smooth muscle. *Res. Commun. Chem. Pathol. Pharmacol.,* 23:233–242.
21. Naftchi, N. E., Abrahams, S. J., Paul, H. M. St., Lowman, E. W., and Schlosser, W. (1978): Localization and changes of substance P in spinal cord of paraplegic cats. *Brain Res.,* 153:507–513.
22. Otsuka, M., Konishi, S., and Takahashi, T. (1972): The presence of a motoneurone-depolarising peptide in bovine dorsal roots of spinal nerves. *Proc. Jap. Acad.,* 48:342–346.
23. Otsuka, M., and Takahashi, T. (1977): Putative peptide neurotransmitters. *Annu. Rev. Pharmacol. Toxicol.,* 17:425–439.
24. Starr, M. S., James, T. A., Gayten, D. (1978): Behavioural depressant and antinociceptive properties of substance P in the mouse: Possible implication of brain monoamines. *Eur. J. Pharmacol.,* 48:203–212.
25. Stewart, J. M., Getto, C. J., Neldner, K., Reeve, E. B., Krivoy, W. A., and Zimmermann, E. (1976): Substance P and analgesia. *Nature,* 262:784–785.
26. Surgue, M. F. (1979): On the role of 5-hydroxytryptamine in drug-induced antinociception. *Br. J. Pharmacol.,* 65:677–681.
27. Takahashi, T., and Otsuka, M. (1975): Regional distribution of substance P in the spinal cord and nerve roots of the cat and the effect of dorsal root section. *Brain Res.,* 87:1–11.

Neuropeptides and Neural Transmission,
edited by C. Ajmone Marsan and W. Z. Traczyk.
Raven Press, New York © 1980.

An Examination of Desensitization as a Basis for Defining Substance P-like Agonist Activity

C. C. Jordan

*Department of Pharmacology, University College London,
London, WC1E 6BT, United Kingdom*

The availability of a specific antagonist for substance P (SP) would greatly assist in testing the assumption that analogues of this peptide act through the same receptors. In the absence of such an antagonist, the phenomenon of desensitization has been adopted by some authors as a means of distinguishing, at least to some extent, between SP-containing extracts and other smooth muscle stimulants. Gaddum (8) found a degree of specificity in the desensitizing effects of SP-containing extracts on intestinal smooth muscle, although some cross-desensitization was apparent between the peptide and tryptamine. In contrast to this, Lembeck and Fischer (9) concluded that desensitization between the "tachykinins" SP, physalaemin and eledoisin was group-specific in that there was little cross-desensitization between these peptides and the kinins bradykinin and kallidin. Bergmann and colleagues have used cross-desensitization between various peptide derivatives of SP as a basis for determining structure-activity relationships in terms of affinity and intrinsic activity (2,3). This approach assumes that the presence of a given concentration of one (desensitizing) agonist peptide will reduce the fraction of non-desensitized receptors available for interaction with a second agonist. Thus, the desensitizing agonist is used to produce an effect analogous to that of an irreversible antagonist.

All these studies have employed different experimental designs, but an assumption implicit in all is that the "specific" desensitization involves a change in conformation of the receptors with which the peptides interact, although there appears to be no direct evidence that this is the case. We report here some preliminary attempts to examine this assumption by analysing desensitization in the guinea-pig ileum on the basis of a model proposed by Rang (11) and Rang and Ritter (12) for cholinergic receptors in chick and frog skeletal muscle.

The model assumes that the receptor can exist in two forms, R being the normal conformation and R' the desensitized conformation. Either form can bind drug molecules but with different dissociation constants, and transition between the two forms $R \rightleftharpoons R'$ is slow. Two predictions of the model are that (a) the degree of desensitization produced by an agonist is dependent on its relative affinities for R and R', and that (b) the time-course of recovery from desensitization should be exponential and should be the same irrespective of the nature of the desensitizing agent.

If this model satisfactorily accounted for desensitization in the guinea-pig ileum, it might be possible to use the rate constant for recovery from desensitization as an index predictive of SP-like activity.

METHODS

Segments of guinea pig ileum, approximately 40 mm in length, were suspended in 2-ml organ baths containing Tyrode solution of the following composition: Na^+ 149.2 mM, K^+ 2.7 mM, Ca^{2+} 1.8 mM, Mg^{2+} 2.1 mM, Cl^- 145.3 mM, $H_2PO_4^-$ 0.4 mM, HCO_3^- 11.9 mM, and glucose 5 mM. The temperature was maintained at 32°C and the bathing medium was bubbled continuously with oxygen–carbon dioxide (95:5%). Contractions were recorded isotonically and displayed on Servoscribe 1s potentiometric recorders.

In pilot experiments, dose cycles of 2, 5, 10, and 15 min were compared using a randomized block design, each block consisting of three (sub-maximal) dose levels. For a given dose level, it was found that the variance of the response was minimized when a 10-min dose cycle was employed, and so this was used for all experiments in this study. Taking the moment of drug administration as time 0, the preparation was washed at 20, 35, 300, and 570 sec.

The volume of the bathing medium was 1.8 ml and all drugs were added in a volume of 0.2 ml by means of plastic syringes. All glassware was silanized before use (Dimethyldichlorosilane, B.D.H.).

The basic protocol common to all experiments was as follows. A serial dose-response curve was first obtained for the test agent. Where cross-desensitization between two compounds was to be investigated, an additional dose-response curve was obtained for the desensitizing agent so that desensitizing doses could be expressed as multiples of the calculated EC_{50}. Three doses were then selected from the linear part of the log dose-response curve such that the middle and higher doses were two and four times the lowest dose (c.f. Schild, ref. 13). These doses were then administered as three randomized blocks (each dose occurring once in a given block), in order to obtain a standard log dose-response curve. Ten minutes after completing this series of doses, the desensitizing agent was administered and left in contact for 10 min. The preparation was then washed and the recovery from desensitization was followed by administering doses of test agent at various post-desensitization intervals and then returning to the 10-min dose cycle thereafter. Post-desensitization dose ratios were obtained by interpolation from the log dose-response regression line. Only those post-desensitization responses encompassed by the standard curve were used for estimating dose ratios. The fraction of receptors in the desensitized conformation (P_d) at time t after removing the desensitizing agent was estimated from the relationship:

$$P_d = \frac{x - 1}{x}$$

where x = dose ratio at time t (12)

In order to distinguish combinations of drugs in various experiments, desensitizing agents are labelled thus: $SP_{(D)}$.

Synthetic SP, eledoisin-related peptide (ERP), physalaemin, and SP-octapeptide (SP-OCT) were obtained from Beckman (Geneva). Other drugs were obtained as follows: acetylcholine iodide (ACh), histamine acid phosphate, and 5-hydroxytryptamine creatinine sulphate (5-HT), B.D.H., Poole; atropine sulphate, Sigma.

RESULTS

Specificity of Desensitization with SP as Test Agonist

ACh, 5-HT, and histamine all proved capable of desensitizing the actions of SP, but the time-course of recovery differed in each case. The effect of ACh was studied in most detail. When plotted as $\ln(P_d)$ versus t [where P_d = fraction of receptors desensitized and t = time after removal of desensitizing agent (see Rang and Ritter, ref. 12)], the recovery appeared to have two components. An initial slow phase gave way to a subsequent fast phase with a delay which appeared to be determined by the magnitude of the desensitizing dose (see Fig. 1, left). A similar pattern was observed when ACh was used as both desensitizing and test agent (Fig. 1, right). The desensitizing action of ACh against SP and ACh was blocked by atropine.

Desensitization Induced by SP

SP produced marked desensitization against itself, recovery having only a single component. In addition, it produced varying degrees of desensitization against ACh, histamine, and 5-HT. The effect against ACh was least marked, dose ratios of less than 2 being observed at t = 3 min following a desensitizing dose of SP (2 μM).

During the course of initial experiments, it was noted that the response to "desensitizing" doses of SP showed a gradual decline over the 10-min exposure period. Superimposed on this falling response was a marked increase in spontaneous rhythmic activity of the preparation (Fig. 2a), suggesting the release of an endogenous smooth muscle stimulant. Addition of atropine (0.1 μM) to the bath before administration of the desensitizing dose produced a change in the nature of the response. The rhythmic activity was substantially reduced or abolished and the overall response declined more rapidly towards base line (Fig. 2b), the rate of decline being greatest with large doses of SP. These responses

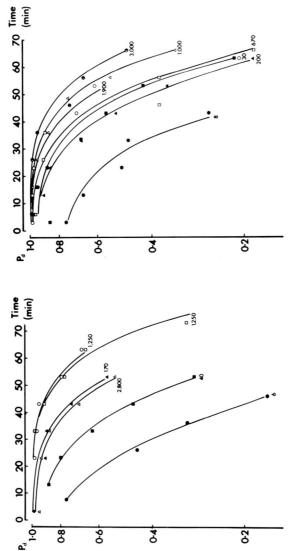

FIG. 1. Left: Recovery of responses to SP following desensitization with various doses of ACh (25 nM–20 μM) left in contact with the ileum for 10 min. Each curve represents results from a single experiment and the desensitizing doses, expressed as multiples of the EC_{50}, are indicated adjacent to each line. The points were fitted by eye and it is not intended to imply a particular quantitative relationship. **Right:** Similar experiments to those just described, but ACh was used both as desensitizing and test agonist.

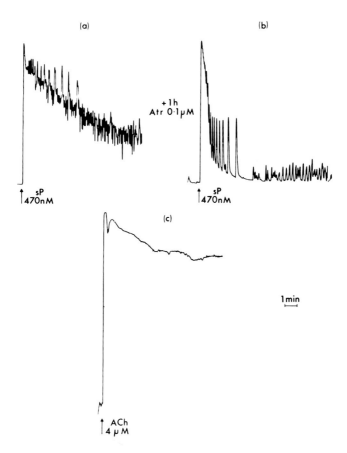

FIG. 2. Contractile responses of guinea-pig ileum during exposure to "desensitizing agents." **(a)** SP (470 nM) was administered at the *arrow* and left in contact for 10 min. **(b)** Same preparation as in **(a)** but response to SP was obtained in the presence of atropine (100 nM). Note the rapid decline in the overall response and the absence of high frequency rhythmic activity compared with **(a).** The low frequency spikes seen in the presence of atropine were due to contraction of the circular muscle and were observed in a number of preparations with SP and other peptides. **(c)** Response to a desensitizing dose of ACh (4 μM) in another preparation showing the prolonged contraction obtained with this agonist. Histamine produced responses of a similar nature.

contrasted with those to ACh or histamine whereby the response was maintained at 70 to 80% of the initial peak (Fig. 2c).

Since release of ACh thus appeared to be an important component in the response to desensitizing doses of SP, it seemed possible that it might also contribute to the desensitization process. The effect of atropine (1 μM) on desensitization was thus studied. In the presence of atropine, cross-desensitization was no longer observed for the combinations $SP_{(D)}$ versus 5-HT, $5-HT_{(D)}$ versus SP, $ACh_{(D)}$ versus SP, and $SP_{(D)}$ versus histamine with concentrations of desensitizing agent up to SP (2 μM), 5-HT (200 μM), and ACh (100 μM). However,

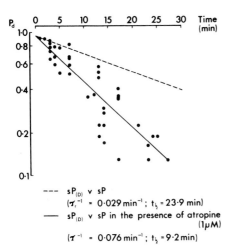

FIG. 3. Recovery of responses to SP following desensitization with SP in guinea-pig ileum. *Broken line* indicates the mean regression line for semi-logarithmic plot of proportion of receptors in desensitized state (P_d) against time (t) in the absence of atropine (individual points not shown). *Solid line* indicates the mean regression line for results from experiments in which atropine (1 μM) was present throughout.

desensitization was still observed for the combination histamine(D) versus SP. In addition, the time-course of recovery for SP(D) versus SP was altered, the recovery half-time for the relationship ln (P_d) versus t indicating a more rapid recovery in the presence than in the absence of atropine (Fig. 3). The time constant in the absence of atropine was calculated from the mean regression line to be 23.9 min (six experiments, $r = -0.813$, $p < 0.001$), although there was a wide variation between experiments. In the presence of atropine the equivalent figure was 9.2 min (14 experiments, $r = -0.892$, $p < 0.001$).

Cross-Desensitization Between SP and Peptide Analogues

Cross-desensitization between SP and the structurally related peptides ERP, SP-OCT, and physalaemin was studied with atropine present throughout the experiments. The results are summarized in Table 1. The interaction of SP and SP-OCT is illustrated in more detail in Fig. 4. Figure 4 (left) shows recovery from the desensitizing action of SP-OCT against SP. The fraction of receptors desensitized declined as a single exponential with a half-time of 8.7 min. Increasing the desensitizing dose from 200 nM to 2 μM produced no further increase in the degree of desensitization. Lowering the dose, however, resulted in smaller post-desensitization dose ratios. When SP was used as desensitizing agent and SP-OCT as test agent, a single exponential recovery phase was again obtained, but the rate constant indicated a slower process ($t_{1/2} = 23.7$ min). Increasing the desensitizing dose resulted in larger dose ratios but the recovery rate constant was unchanged.

On the basis of the recovery rate constants obtained for the combinations of desensitizing and test agents studied so far, the results may be divided roughly into two groups. Where SP was used as test agent, a similar recovery rate was seen irrespective of the desensitizing agent (SP, ERP, SP-OCT), a mean half-time of 9.2 min being obtained. A similar time-course was seen for the

TABLE 1. *Cross-desensitization between SP and related peptides in guinea-pig ileum*

Desensitizing agent	Test agent	τ_r^{-1} (min^{-1})	$t_{1/2}$ (min)	N	p
SP	SP	0.076	9.2	14	<0.001
ERP	SP	0.072	9.6	3	<0.001
SP-OCT	SP	0.080	8.7	6	<0.001
SP-OCT	SP-OCT	0.069	10.0	6	<0.001
SP	SP-OCT	0.029	23.7	6	<0.001
SP	ERP	0.034	20.4	5	<0.001
SP	PHYS	0.036	19.3	5	<0.001

Quantitative measures of recovery from desensitization induced by SP and related peptides in the guinea-pig ileum. Recovery rate constants (τ_r^{-1}) and the recovery half-times ($t_{1/2}$) were obtained from the mean regression line for N experiments in each case; p values relate to regression coefficients. For the purposes of this comparison "supra-maximal" desensitizing doses (usually 100 nM) were used in all experiments.

Abbreviations: ERP, eledoisin-related peptide; PHYS, physalaemin; SP, Substance P; SP-OCT, SP-octapeptide.

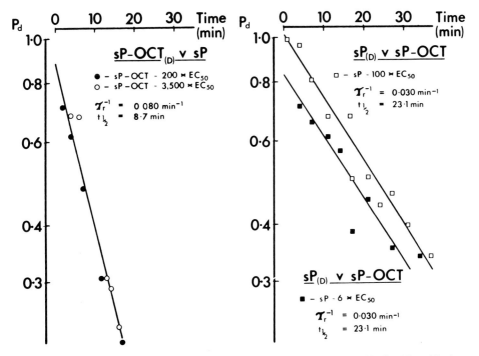

FIG. 4. Cross-desensitization between SP and SP-OCT. **Left:** SP-OCT$_{(D)}$ vs SP. Semi-logarithmic plot as in Fig. 3. Results from six preparations in which SP-OCT (200 or 3,500 $\times$ EC$_{50}$) was used as desensitizing agent. No difference was observed in the degree of desensitization produced by the two dose levels. The rate constant is the value obtained for the mean regression line from the six preparations. **Right:** SP$_{(D)}$ vs SP-OCT. Similar experiments to those in **(a)** but using two dose levels of SP (6 or 100 $\times$ EC$_{50}$). Data from three preparations at each dose level. The higher dose caused an increased degree of desensitization (i.e., larger post-desensitization dose ratios), but the recovery rate was unchanged ($t_{1/2}$ = 23.1 min in each case).

combination SP-OCT$_{(D)}$ versus SP-OCT (10.0 min). However, when SP was used as desensitizing agent against ERP, SP-OCT, or physalaemin, the recovery rate was considerably reduced, the average time constant being 21.1 min. Attempts to determine the rate of recovery from physalaemin as desensitizing agent using SP as test agent have been largely unsuccessful since, in most preparations, spasm of the circular muscle lasting several minutes after washing out the desensitizing dose has prevented estimation of dose ratios for the immediate post-desensitization period.

DISCUSSION

Cross-desensitization between SP and other (non-peptide) smooth muscle stimulants has been reported previously by Gaddum (8) and its occurence may, at least to some extent, be a consequence of the experimental design. For example, a substantially shorter period of exposure to the desensitizing agent may have reduced the atropine-sensitive indirect component. We have made no attempt to elucidate the mechanism of action of SP in releasing ACh, but the peptide is known to interact with other cholinergic systems such as the motoneurone collateral–Renshaw cell synapse in the mammalian spinal cord (1). Here, SP was found to depress the excitatory effects of ACh on Renshaw cells although, on some occasions, a cholinomimetic effect was observed. The authors suggested that this excitatory action may result from ACh release, whilst the inhibitory effect may involve some allosteric interaction with nicotinic receptors.

In the guinea-pig ileum SP might, therefore, cause a release of ACh by a direct effect on cholinergic terminals. However, an alternative possibility is that it may mimic the effects of a capsaicin-sensitive sensory system impinging on cholinergic ganglion cells (14).

Since cross-desensitization between ACh and SP was essentially uni-directional (i.e., ACh$_{(D)}$ versus SP) and was blocked by atropine, it appears that the effect is mediated entirely through a cholinergic mechanism. The process underlying cross-desensitization is likely to involve post-receptor events since atropine has no effect on normal SP dose-response relationships. One possibility is that prolonged exposure to ACh results in a depletion of intracellular calcium, the response to muscarinic agonists being highly sensitive to calcium levels (4–7).

A similar mechanism might apply in the desensitizing effect of histamine against SP, since Schild (13) has demonstrated that at least part of the desensitization produced by histamine against itself is calcium-dependent. In a different system, the rat parotid gland, cross-desensitization occurs between the potassium releasing actions of SP, carbachol, and phenylephrine and this again is a calcium-dependent phenomenon (10).

The interaction between the small number of peptide analogues of SP so far investigated is not readily described by the model proposed by Rang and Ritter (12), although only the time-course of recovery from desensitization has been considered in the present series of experiments. Nevertheless, it is clear from the group of peptides summarised in Table 1 that the prediction of identical recovery rates independent of the nature of the desensitizing agent does not apply. Furthermore, there are difficulties in proposing alternative mechanisms in view of the apparent inconsistency in the behaviour of SP itself. Thus, with SP as test agonist, there was reasonable agreement in the recovery rates when SP, ERP, or SP-OCT were used as desensitizing agents, but when SP was used as desensitizing agent against SP-OCT, ERP, or physalaemin, the recovery rate was approximately halved. The interaction SP-OCT$_{(D)}$ versus SP-OCT produced a recovery rate similar to that obtained with SP as test agonist.

Thus, the recovery rate constant does not appear to be simply related either to the nature of the desensitizing or the test agent. Before rejecting the cyclic model (12) for this system, however, the possibility that additional factors may be influencing recovery should be considered. It was noted that, in the absence of atropine, the release of endogenous ACh appeared to reduce the rate of post-desensitization recovery for the combination SP$_{(D)}$ versus SP. The release of an additional mediator might influence the rate of recovery, for example when using SP (but not ERP and SP-OCT) as desensitizing agents, but there remains the exceptional case of SP$_{(D)}$ versus SP which has a relatively rapid recovery rate.

Clearly it is necessary to examine the interaction between other permutations of the peptides studied so far and to extend the study to other peptide analogues in order to establish an overall pattern. However, the present study does indicate that a simple qualitative test of cross-desensitization is not an adequate criterion for classifying a substance as being "SP-like," although it remains possible that a quantitative index of desensitization could be obtained on which to base such a judgement.

ACKNOWLEDGMENTS

I am greatly indebted to Mr. Paul Gater for his contribution to the experiments. I am pleased to acknowledge also the assistance of Mr. Mike Bovingdon with initial experiments, and Dr. D. G. Haylett and Dr. D. H. Jenkinson for helpful discussions.

REFERENCES

1. Belcher, G., and Ryall, R. W. (1977): Substance P and Renshaw cells: A new concept of inhibitory synaptic interactions. *J. Physiol. (Lond.)*, 272:105–119.
2. Bergmann, J., Oehme, P., Bienert, M., and Niedrich, H. (1974): Differenzierung der biologischen Aktivität von Eledoisin- und Substanz P-Analogen in Affinität und Wirkaktivität am isolierten Meerschweinchen-Ileum und Vergleich mit der Aktivität am Ratten-Colon. *Experientia*, 30:1315–1317.
3. Bergmann, J., Oehme, P., Bienert, M., and Niedrich, H. (1975): Studien zum Wirkungsmechanismus glattmuskulär angreifender Peptide. II. Differenzierung der biologischen Aktivität von Tachykininen in Affinität und intrinsic activity. *Acta. Biol. Med. Ger.*, 34:475–481.
4. Chang, K.-J., and Triggle, D. J. (1973): Quantitative aspects of drug-receptor interactions. I.

Ca^{2+} and cholinergic receptor activation in smooth muscle: A basic model for drug-receptor interactions. *J. Theor. Biol.*, 40:125–154.

5. Chang, K.-J., and Triggle, D. J. (1973): Quantitative aspects of drug-receptor interactions. II. The role of Ca$^{2+}_{mem}$ in desensitization and spasmolytic activity. *J. Theor. Biol.*, 40:155–172.

6. Durbin, R. P., and Jenkinson, D. H. (1961): The calcium dependence of tension development in depolarized smooth muscle. *J. Physiol. (Lond.)*, 157:90–96.

7. Fastier, F. N., Purves, R. D., and Taylor, K. M. (1973): Observations on 'fade': A complication of the contractile response of smooth muscle to a large dose of an agonist. *Br. J. Pharmacol.*, 49:490–497.

8. Gaddum, J. H. (1953): Tryptamine receptors. *J. Physiol. (Lond.)*, 119:363–368.

9. Lembeck, F., and Fischer, G. (1967): Gekreuzte Tachyphylaxie von Peptiden. *Naunyn Schmiedebergs Arch. Pharmacol. Exp. Pathol.*, 258:452–456.

10. Putney, J. W. (1977): Muscarininc, alpha-adrenergic and peptide receptors regulate the same calcium influx sites in the parotid gland. *J. Physiol. (Lond.)*, 268:139–149.

11. Rang, H. P. (1973): *Receptor mechanisms.* (Fourth Gaddum Memorial Lecture, School of Pharmacy, University of London, 1973.) *Br. J. Pharmacol.*, 48:475–495.

12. Rang, H. P., and Ritter, J. M. (1970): On the mechanism of desensitization at cholinergic receptors. *Mol. Pharmacol.*, 6:357–382.

13. Schild, H. O. (1973): An effect of calcium on histamine desensitization of guinea-pig ileum. *Br. J. Pharmacol.*, 49:717–719.

14. Szolcsányi, J., and Barthó, L. (1978): New type of nerve-mediated cholinergic contractions of the guinea-pig small intestine and its selective blockade by capsaicin. *Naunyn Schmiedebergs Arch. Pharmacol.*, 305:83–90.

Neuropeptides and Neural Transmission,
edited by C. Ajmone Marsan and W. Z. Traczyk.
Raven Press, New York © 1980.

Effect on the Estrous Cycle of Female Rats of Implantation of Substance P Fragment SP$_{6-11}$ into the Diencephalon

Elżbieta Kacprzak and Władysław Z. Traczyk

Department of Physiology, Institute of Physiology and Biochemistry, School of Medicine in Lodz, 90–131 Lodz, Poland

It has been well established that steroid hormones regulate gonadotropin secretion. Systemic estrogen administration has been found to cause estrogen-induced sterility that is particularly prominent at the vaginal cornification stage (14). Contrary to this is the finding that ventral hypothalamus and preoptic area stimulation induces ovulation in female rats (1). Stimulation applied to the preoptic-suprachiasmatic or the arcuate-ventromedial nucleus regions in male rats results in an increase of both plasma luteinizing hormone (LH) and prolactin levels (7). Implantation of estrogen in the same area inhibits ovulation and altered gonadotropin secretion and reproductive behaviour (22,25–28,30,33), and monoamines are known to be involved in this estrogen effect (23).

The anterior deafferentation of the medial basal hypothalamus induces persistent estrus and elevates serum LH and serum prolactin (2,3). Complete deafferentation of the medial basal hypothalamus causes constant diestrus and very low serum LH and serum prolactin at low diestrous levels (2,3).

Systemic and topical estrogen application, electrical stimulation, and hypothalamus deafferentation influence the release of LH-releasing hormone (LH-RH). The nerve fibers containing LH-RH were found in the median eminence (15) and in the cell bodies in the arcuate region (17). The highest concentrations of LH-RH were found in the median eminence, and were lower by one-half in the arcuate nucleus (31). LH-RH immunoreactive fibers were demonstrated only in the tuberoinfundibular tract (36), but LH-RH containing cell bodies were also found in the suprachiasmatic area after anterior deafferentation of the hypothalamus (37). LH-RH fluctuations in the hypothalamus were also found during the rat estrous cycle (34).

A high concentration of Substance P (SP) was found in the hypothalamus (32) and was isolated from this structure in pure form (6). The role of SP in the physiology of the hypothalamohypophyseal system has not been established. The role of SP in LH-RH release from the hypothalamus is also still unknown. The high content of SP in the hypothalamus (9), its presence in the nerve fibers of this structure (8), and its potassium-evoked calcium-dependent release from the tissue (19,35) suggest that this peptide may also be involved in LH-

RH release as a neurotransmitter or neuromodulator in the hypothalamus. Investigations carried out on rat pituitaries *in vitro* indicate that SP, only when added to the incubation medium in very high concentration, releases LH and follicle-stimulating hormone (FSH) (10). Injections into cerebral ventricles of SP and the hexapeptide C-terminal derivatives of SP indicate that one of these peptides, SP$_{6-11}$, prolonged the estrous cycle during which the injection was made (18). The biological activity of undecapeptide SP and shorter chain peptides of the C-terminal partial sequence of SP exerted different activities depending on which tissue served as indicator (4,43,44). Some shorter chain peptides possess an even higher biological activity than SP.

The influence of SP$_{6-11}$ injected into cerebral ventricles on the length of the estrous cycle requires further confirmation. In the following experiments chemitrodes containing the investigated compounds on their tips were implanted over the medial basal hypothalamus in such a way as to avoid partial damage of LH-RH containing cell bodies and nerve fibers.

MATERIALS AND METHODS

Animals

The experiments were performed on female rats, weighing 200 to 280 g and were selected from a larger group of animals according to the regularity of the length of their estrous cycle. The rats were F$_1$ generation cross strains bred in our department of male Buffalo with female Wistar rats from the stock of the Institute of Oncology in Gliwice. The animals were kept in standard conditions of a 14-hr light:10-hr darkness cycle and received standard rat pellets and water *ad libitum.*

Determination of Estrous Cycles

Daily vaginal smears were taken at 9 a.m., which was 3 hr after the light was switched on. The appearance in the smears of cornified cells with only a few or no leukocytes was recognized as estrus and the first day of the estrous cycle. Two weeks before chemitrode implantation vaginal smears were taken over at least three complete consecutive estrous cycles. The 4-day-cycle animals with well-pronounced vaginal cornification were selected for chemitrode implantation. After implantation no less than three cycles were observed, and the animals were sacrificed only if the regularity was not disturbed. In the case of prolongation of the estrus or diestrus, vaginal smears were taken every day until two regular cycles reappeared.

Chemitrodes

The chemitrodes were made from glass capillaries about 0.5 mm in external diameter and 0.2 mm in internal diameter, diagonally cut at the tip. The lumen of the capillaries was filled with dental cement, except for a space about 0.5 mm from the tip which was filled with stilboestrol, hexapeptide SP_{6-11}, or tripeptide SP_{9-11}—the C-terminal partial sequences of undecapeptide SP. The peptides were synthesized by the conventional method at the Faculty of Chemistry, University of Warsaw (24). Stilboestrol was heated and when it had melted, the tips of the capillaries were filled. The peptides were moistened with a minute volume of dimethylformamide and were put on the tips of the capillaries in dense liquid state. They were later kept for 24 hr in a high vacuum to remove the dimethylformamide. About 250 µg of the peptide or stilboestrol was placed on the tip of each glass capillary. Since SP_{6-11} dissolves poorly in water (39), it should be kept on the tip of the chemitrode for some time when implanted into the brain.

Chemitrode Implantation

For implantation of the chemitrodes during estrus, the rats were anesthetized with hexobarbital (80 mg/kg body weight intraperitoneally); in the stereotaxic instruments two symmetrical chemitrodes were implanted into the diencephalon over the medial basal hypothalamus. The stereotaxic coordinates for the tip of the chemitrode were chosen according to De Groot's stereotaxic atlas (16) 6 mm anterior from the frontal zero plane, 1 mm lateral from the sagittal zero plane, and 6 mm down from the skull surface.

The chemitrodes were implanted in a position such that the diagonally cut surface with the active compound faced the sagittal zero plane (Fig. 1). The chemitrodes were fixed to the external surface of the skull by means of dental acrylic cement.

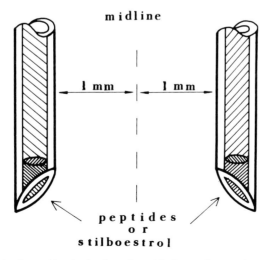

FIG. 1. Chemitrodes in position for implantation with diagonally cut glass capillary at the tip.

Histological Verification

After completion of the estrous cycle determination the animals were sacrificed by a lethal dose of hexobarbital, and the heads put into 10% formalin solution for 2 weeks. After fixation in formalin, the brains were removed from the skull, dehydrated in alcohol, embedded in celloidin, and cut on a microtome into coronal slices 60 μm thick. The slices were stained for myelin by the method of Weil.

Localization of the tips of the chemitrodes in the diencephalon of each animal was marked on schematic coronal sections of rat brain according to De Groot's stereotaxic atlas (16).

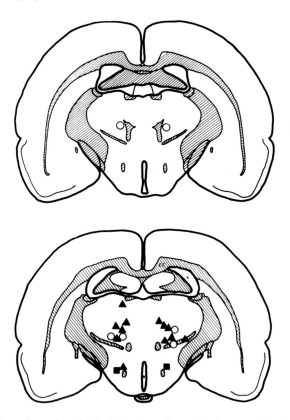

FIG. 2. Coronal sections of rat brain indicating stilboestrol placement in diencephalon (10 rats) and effect on estrous cycles. *Open circles* indicate no influence; *black triangles,* prolongation of the diestrous phase; *black squares,* prolongation of the estrous phase. Schematic coronal sections in Figs. 2–4 according to De Groot's stereotaxic atlas (16).

——————————————————▶

FIG. 3. Coronal sections of rat brain indicating SP$_{9-11}$ placement in diencephalon (10 rats) and effect on estrous cycles. *Open circles* indicate no influence; *black triangles,* prolongation of the diestrous phase; *black squares,* prolongation of the estrous phase.

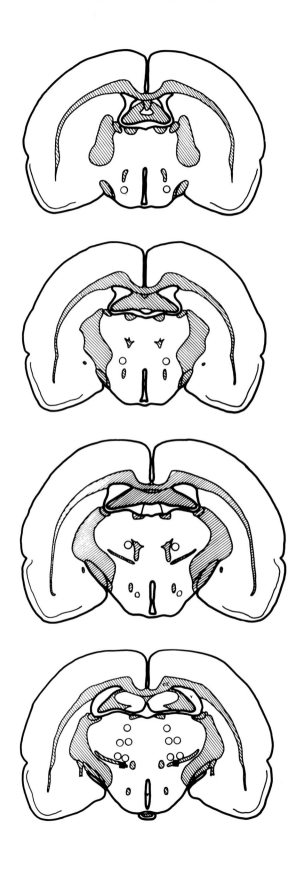

RESULTS

Effect of Stilboestrol Implantation

Chemitrodes with stilboestrol were implanted in 10 animals. The estrous cycle, during which the implantation was performed in 6 out of 10 animals, was prolonged to more than 2 days in the diestrous phase. In this group of animals the estrus appeared after 7 to 15 days; on the average, prolongation of estrous cycles amounted to 10 days. After that, two normal-length estrous cycles were observed.

In 3 animals the implantation of a chemitrode failed to change the length of the estrous cycles, and in 1 animal the next estrous phase took longer than 2 days. The distribution in the diencephalon of tips of chemitrodes is shown in Fig. 2.

Effect of SP_{9-11} Implantation

In 9 out of 10 animals with implanted tripeptide, the estrous cycle during which the implantation was performed and the two successive cycles were normal as before the operation. In only 1 animal was the first estrous phase after SP_{9-11} implantation longer than 2 days. The distribution in the diencephalon of tips of chemitrodes in this group of animals is shown in Fig. 3.

Effect of SP_{6-11} Implantation

Chemitrodes with the hexapeptide SP_{6-11} were implanted in 20 animals. In 13 animals the next estrous phase after implantation was longer than 2 days; that is, it lasted from 3 to 8 days with the average being 5 days. After that, two normal-length cycles with a 1-day estrous phase were observed. In 7 animals the estrous cycle during which the implantation was performed as well as the two successive cycles were normal with a 1-day estrous phase. The distribution of the tips of chemitrodes in the diencephalon is shown in Fig. 4.

DISCUSSION

Stilboestrol implanted into the diencephalon over the medial basal hypothalamus affected the length of the estrous cycle by prolonging the diestrous phase of the cycle. This result is in agreement with the data reported by Lisk (25,26) who found, after implantation of a small amount of oestrogen into the hypothala-

---------------------------►

FIG. 4. Coronal sections of rat brain indicating SP_{6-11} placement in diencephalon (20 rats) and effect on estrous cycles. *Open circles* indicate no influence; *black triangles*, prolongation of the diestrous phase; *black squares*, prolongation of the estrous phase.

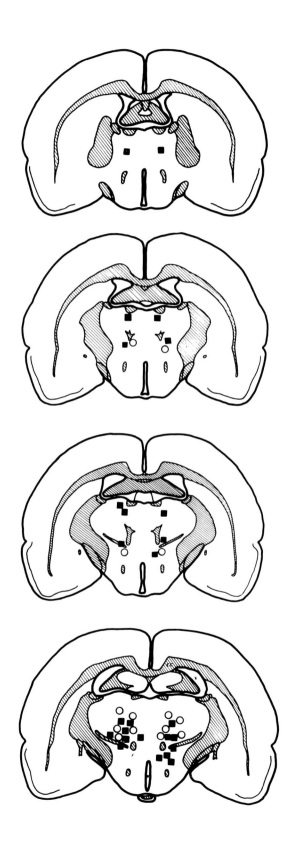

mus, a prolongation of diestrous or proestrous-diestrous phase according to vaginal smear records in female rats.

The tripeptide SP$_{9-11}$, which is biologically inactive (4,43,44), does not affect the estrous cycle. On the contrary, the hexapeptide SP$_{6-11}$, which possibly is more resistant to brain enzymes than SP (29), affected the length of the estrous phase of the cycle by prolonging it.

Several peripheral and central factors are involved in controlling the estrous cycle. One essential factor is the feedback exerted by estrogen, progesterone, and gonadotropins on hypothalamic and extrahypothalamic neurons. Brain mediators such as dopamine, noradrenaline, and 5-hydroxytryptamine may affect the LH-RH release into primary capillaries of hypophyseal portal vessels. There is still no agreement on the interaction between the known factors involved in the estrous cycle control, and new factors have been suggested (41).

The electrochemical stimulation of the medial preoptic area or median eminence-arcuate region on the first day of diestrus produced only a slight elevation of plasma LH, and on the proestrus day produced the highest elevation (20,21). However, other results suggest a decrease of hypothalamic sensitivity to stimulation during proestrous (40).

Repeated daily injections of estradiol to ovariectomized rats induced a fivefold increase in dopamine turnover in the medial and lateral palisade zone of the median eminence and a reduction of noradrenaline turnover in the subependymal layer of the median eminence (11). The inhibitory feedback of estradiol on LH secretion seems partly to involve an increase in dopamine turnover in the median eminence and a reduction in hypothalamic noradrenaline turnover (13). A facilitatory hypothalamic noradrenergic mechanism and an inhibitory dopaminergic mechanism in the median eminence controlling LH-RH secretion are postulated (12,38). The lesion of the median raphe or dorsal raphe nuclei induced prolongation of the estrous phase, which can be explained by a decrease in forebrain 5-hydroxytryptamine concentration (42). Persistent estrus was also obtained by anterior hypothalamic deafferentation (2,3).

Considering that SP injected into cerebral ventricles stimulates both the synthesis and utilization of dopamine, noradrenaline, and 5-hydroxytryptamine in rat brain (5), this could possibly be the mechanism through which SP$_{6-11}$ induces estrous phase prolongation. This mechanism should be rather diffuse as, in spite of some dispersion of SP$_{6-11}$ placement in the diencephalon, the results are similar.

ACKNOWLEDGMENTS

We wish to acknowledge the valuable assistance of Mrs. K. Sadzińska in experiments and histology. We are very grateful to Professor S. Drabarek from the Faculty of Chemistry, University of Warsaw, for kindly making available synthetic peptides SP$_{6-11}$ and SP$_{9-11}$. The study was conducted under Contract

10.4.2.01.5.12 with the Polish Academy of Sciences and supported by the Ford Foundation, New York, Grant 770-0540.

REFERENCES

1. Barraclough, C. A. (1966): Modifications in the CNS regulation of reproduction after exposure of prepubertal rats to steroid hormones. *Recent Prog. Horm. Res.,* 22:503–539.
2. Blake, C. A., Weiner, R. I., Gorski, R. A., and Sawyer, C. H. (1972): Secretion of pituitary luteinizing hormone and follicle stimulating hormone in female rats made persistently estrous or diestrous by hypothalamic deafferentation. *Endocrinology,* 90:855–861.
3. Blake, C. A., Weiner, R. I., and Sawyer, C. H. (1972): Pituitary prolactin secretion in female rats made persistently estrous or diestrous by hypothalamic deafferentation. *Endocrinology,* 90:862–866.
4. Bury, R. W., and Mashford, M. L. (1976): Biological activity of C-terminal partial sequences of Substance P. *J. Med. Chem.,* 19:851–856.
5. Carlsson, A., Magnusson, T., Fisher, G. H., Chang, D., and Folkers, K. (1977): Effects of synthetic Substance P on central monoaminergic mechanisms. In: *Substance P,* edited by U. S. von Euler and B. Pernow, pp. 201–205. Raven Press, New York.
6. Chang, M. M., and Leeman, S. E. (1970): Isolation of a sialogogic peptide from bovine hypothalamic tissue and its characterization as Substance P. *J. Biol. Chem.,* 245:4784–4790.
7. Colombo, J. A. (1978): Prolactin and LH release after stimulation of the preoptic-suprachiasmatic and arcuate-ventromedial n. regions in male rats under pentobarbital anesthesia. *Neuroendocrinology,* 26:150–162.
8. Cuello, A. C., and Kanazawa, I. (1978): The distribution of Substance P immunoreactive fibres in the rat central nervous system. *J. Comp. Neurol.,* 178:129–156.
9. Duffy, M. J., Mulhall, D., and Powell D. (1975): Subcellular distribution of Substance P in bovine hypothalamus and substantia nigra. *J. Neurochem.,* 25:305–307.
10. Fisher, G. H., Humphries, J., Folkers, K., Pernow, B., and Bowers, C. Y. (1974): Synthesis and some biological activities of Substance P. *J. Med. Chem.,* 17:843–846.
11. Fuxe, K., Hökfelt, T., Löfström, A., Johansson, O., Agnati, L., Everitt, B., Goldstein, M., Jeffcoate, S., White, N., Eneroth, P., Gustafsson, J.-Å., and Skett, P. (1976): On the role of neurotransmitters and hypothalamic hormones and their interactions in hypothalamic and extrahypothalamic control of pituitary function and sexual behavior. In: *Subcellular Mechanisms in Reproductive Neuroendocrinology,* edited by F. Naftolin, K. J. Ryan, and J. Davies, pp. 193–246. Elsevier, Amsterdam.
12. Fuxe, K., Löfström, A., Agnati, L., Hökfelt, T., Johansson, O., Eneroth, P., Gustavsson, J. Å., Skett, P., Jeffcoate, S., and Fraser, H. (1977): Functional morphology of the median eminence. In: *Progress in Reproductive Biology, Vol. 2: Clinical Reproductive Neuroendocrinology,* edited by P. O. Hubinont, M. L'Hermite, and C. Robyn, pp. 41–53. Karger, Basel.
13. Fuxe, K., Löfström, A., Eneroth, P., Gustafsson, J.-Å., Hökfelt, T., Scett, P., Wuttke, W., Fraser, H., and Jeffcoate, S. (1976): Interactions between hypothalamic catecholamine nerve terminals and LRF containing neurons. Further evidence for an inhibitory dopaminergic and a facilitatory noradrenergic influence. In: *Basic Applications and Clinical Uses of Hypothalamic Hormones,* edited by A. L. Charro Salgado, R. Fernández-Durango, J. G. López Del Campo, F. J. Ebling, and I. W. Henderson, pp. 165–177. Excerpta Medica, Amsterdam, Oxford.
14. Gorski, R. A. (1963): Modification of ovulatory mechanisms by postnatal administration of estrogen to the rat. *Am. J. Physiol.,* 205:842–844.
15. Goldsmith, P. C., and Ganong, W. F., (1975): Ultrastructural localization of luteinizing hormone-releasing hormone in the median eminence of the rat. *Brain Res.,* 97:181–193.
16. De Groot, J. (1963): *The Rat Forebrain in Stereotaxic Coordinates.* N. V. Noord-Hollandsche Uitgevers Maatschappij, Amsterdam.
17. Hoffman, G. E., Melnyk, V., Hayes, T., Bennett-Clarke, C., and Flower, E. (1978): Immunocytology of LHRH neurons. In: *Brain-Endocrine Interaction III. Neural Hormones and Reproduction,* edited by D. E. Scott, G. P. Kozlowski, and A. Weindl, München, pp. 67–82. Karger, Basel.
18. Jakubowska-Naziembło, B., Włodzimierska, B., and Traczyk, W. Z. (1979): The effect of intraventricular administration of Substance P and its hexapeptide fragments on the oestrus cycle

in female rats. Proceedings of the 14th Congress of the Polish Physiological Society, September 11–13, 1978, Lodz. *Acta Physiol. Pol.,* 30:83.

19. Jessell, T., Iversen, L. L., and Kanazawa, I. (1976): Release and metabolism of Substance P in rat hypothalamus. *Nature,* 264:81–83.

20. Kalra, S. P., and McCann, S. M. (1973): Variations in the release of LH in response to electro-chemical stimulation of preoptic area and of medial basal hypothalamus during the estrous cycle of the rat. *Endokrinology,* 93:665–669.

21. Kalra, S. P., Krulich, L., and McCann, S. M. (1973): Changes in gonadotropin-releasing factor content in the rat hypothalamus following electrochemical stimulation of anterior hypothalamic area and during the estrous cycle. *Neuroendocrinology,* 12:321–333.

22. Kawakami, M., and Visessuvan, S. (1977): The modes of the anterior hypothalamic area as the regulatory center for the gonadotropin release. *Endokrinologie,* 70:225–235.

23. Kendall, D. A., and Narayana, K. (1978): Effect of oestradiol-17β on monoamine concentrations in the hypothalamus of anoestrous ewe. *J. Physiol. (Lond.),* 282:44P–45P.

24. Lipkowski, A., Majewski, T., Drabarek, S., and Traczyk, W. Z. (1975): Synthesis of the biologi-cally active hexapeptide fragment of Substance P, *Third Conference on Chemistry of Amino Acids and Peptides,* p. 31. University of Warsaw, Warsaw, 16–18 October, 1975.

25. Lisk, R. D. (1962): Diencephalic placement of estradiol and sexual receptivity in the female rat. *Am. J. Physiol.,* 203:493–496.

26. Lisk, R. D. (1965): Reproductive capacity and behavioural oestrus in the rat bearing hypo-thalamic implants of sex steroids. *Acta Endocrinol.,* 48:209–219.

27. Lisk, R. D., and Ferguson, D. S. (1973): Neural localization of estrogen-sensitive sites for inhibition of ovulation in the golden hamster *Mesocricetus auratus. Neuroendocrinology,* 12:153–160.

28. Lisk, R. D., and Newlon, M. (1963): Estradiol: Evidence for its direct effect on hypothalamic neurons. *Science,* 139:223–224.

29. Marks, N. (1976): Biodegradation of hormonally active peptides in the central nervous system. In: *Subcellular Mechanisms in Reproductive Neuroendocrinology,* edited by F. Naftolin, K. J. Ryan, and J. Davies, pp. 129–147. Elsevier, Amsterdam.

30. Palka, Y. S., Ramirez, V. D., and Sawyer, C. H. (1966): Distribution and biological effects of tritiated estradiol implanted in the hypothalamo-hypophysial region of female rats. *Endocrinology,* 78:487–499.

31. Palkovits, M., Arimura, A., Brownstein, M., Schally, A. V., and Saavedra, J. M. (1974): Luteiniz-ing hormone-releasing hormone (LH-RH) content of the hypothalamic nuclei in rat. *Endocrinology,* 96:554–558.

32. Pernow, B. (1953): Studies on Substance P. Purification, occurrence and biological action. *Acta Physiol. Scand.,* 29(Suppl. 105):1–90.

33. Ramirez, V. D., Abrams, R. M., and McCann, S. M. (1964): Effect of estradiol implants in the hypothalamo-hypophysial region of the rat on the secretion of luteinizing hormone. *Endocrinology,* 75:243–248.

34. Ramirez, V. D., and Sawyer, C. H. (1965): Fluctuations in hypothalamic LH-RF (luteinizing hormone releasing factor) during the rat estrous cycle. *Endocrinology,* 76:282–289.

35. Schenker, C., Mroz, E. A., and Leeman S. E. (1976): Release of Substance P from isolated nerve endings, *Nature,* 264:790–792.

36. Sétáló, G., Vigh, S., Schally, A. V., Arimura, A., and Flerkó, B. (1975): LH-RH-containing neural elements in the rat hypothalamus. *Endocrinology,* 96:135–142.

37. Sétáló, G., Vigh, S., Schally, A. V., Arimura, A., and Flerkó, B. (1976): Immunohistological study of the origin of LH-RH-containing nerve fibers of the rat hypothalamus. *Brain Res.,* 103:597–602.

38. Simpkins, J. W., Advis, J. P., Hodson, C. A., and Meites, J. (1979): Blockade of steroid-induced luteinizing hormone release by selective depletion of anterior hypothalamic norepineph-rine activity. *Endocrinology,* 104:506–509.

39. Traczyk, W. Z. (1977): Circulatory effects of Substance P, SP$_{6-11}$ and [pGlu^6]SP$_{6-11}$ hexapeptides. In: *Substance P,* edited by U. S. von Euler and B. Pernow, pp. 297–309. Raven Press, New York.

40. Turgeon, J. L., and Barraclough, C. A. (1976): The existence of a possible short-loop negative feedback action of LH in proestrous rats. *Endocrinology,* 98:639–644.

41. Vijayan, E., and McCann, S. M. (1978): The effects of intraventricular injection of γ-aminobu-

tyric acid (GABA) on prolactin and gonadotropin release in conscious female rats. *Brain Res.,* 155:35–43.

42. Waloch, M., Kostowski, W., Szreniawski, Z., Bidziński, A., and Hauptmann, M. (1978): The effect of raphe nuclei lesions on the rat ovarian cycle. *Acta Physiol. Pol.,* 29:413–422.
43. Yajima, H., Kitagawa, K., and Segawa, T. (1973): Studies on peptides. XXXVIII. Structure-activity correlations in Substance P. *Chem. Pharm. Bull. (Tokyo),* 21:2500–2506.
44. Yanaihara, N., Yanaihara, C., Hirohashi, M., Sato, H., Iizuka, Y., Hashimoto, T., and Sakagami, M. (1977): Substance P analogs: Synthesis, and biological and immunological properties. In: *Substance P,* edited by U. S. von Euler and B. Pernow, pp. 27–33. Raven Press, New York.

Neuropeptides and Neural Transmission,
edited by C. Ajmone Marsan and W. Z. Traczyk.
Raven Press, New York © 1980.

SP-Like Immunoreactivity in Cerebrospinal and Perfusing Cerebral Ventricle Fluid in Rats

D. Cannon, D. Powell, P. Skrabanek, *E. Strumiłło-Dyba, and *W. Z. Traczyk

*Endocrine Unit, Mater Misericordiae Hospital, Dublin 7, Ireland; and *Department of Physiology, Institute of Physiology and Biochemistry, School of Medicine in Lodz, 90–131 Lodz, Poland*

The isolation of Substance P (SP) from bovine hypothalami in pure form (4) and the determination of its chemical structure (5) allows further studies on its distribution in the central nervous system (1,2,21) and presence in neuronal bodies and nerve fibers (11,12).

SP is released *in vitro* from isolated nerve endings (26), hypothalamic slices (16), isolated substantia nigra (14), isolated trigeminal nucleus (15), and isolated spinal cord of newborn rat (24). SP is also present in human cerebrospinal fluid (22) where it probably appears from the extracellular space to which SP-reactive granules are discharged, according to the immunocytochemical studies done on rat spinal cord (6).

The purpose of the present experiments was to check if SP-like radioimmune material appears in rat cerebrospinal fluid in a detectable concentration and if it could be released *in vivo* into the fluid perfusing cerebral ventricles. The release of SP-like radioimmune material after peripheral stimulation was also studied.

MATERIALS AND METHODS

The experiments with ventriculo-cisternal perfusion were performed on 10 male rats, weighing from 300 to 360 g, F_1 generation cross strains bred in our department of male August with female Wistar rats from the stock of the Institute of Oncology in Warsaw. Animals were kept in standard conditions of a 14-hr light:10-hr darkness cycle and received standard rat pellets and water *ad libitum*. Urethane anaesthesia, 1.0 g/kg body weight, was injected intraperitoneally.

Using a simple stereotaxic instrument for rats the following points were marked on the cranial bones: 5 mm anterior to the frontal zero plane and 3 mm lateral from the sagittal zero plane (10). Holes were made with a dental drill in cranial bones through which cannulae of stainless steel of external diameter 0.6 mm were inserted into both lateral cerebral ventricles to a depth of 4 mm from the surface of the skull. The cannulae were connected to a vessel containing perfusion fluid consisting of McIlwain-Rodnight's solution (20). The outflow cannula was inserted into the cerebellomedullar cistern, according to the method described elsewhere (18) with some further modification (19). The right sciatic nerve was exposed, cut, and the central segment placed on bipolar platinum electrodes. The central segment of the sciatic nerve was stimulated with square pulses of 0.2 msec duration, 300 Hz frequency, and amplitude up to 15 V, generated for 30 min by a Grass Stimulator Model S 4 K in 30-sec trains separated by 30-sec intervals.

The first portion obtained from the cerebellomedullar cistern was 0.2 ml of cerebrospinal fluid. Next, three 30-min portions of the fluid perfusing cerebral ventricles were collected. The cerebrospinal fluid and the perfusion fluid were collected in polyethylene tubes kept in a bath at 0°C. All collected portions were centrifuged, poured into ampoules with dextrane (110,000 MW), lyophilized, and kept in sealed ampoules until the radioimmunoassay. During the 30 min of collection of the fourth portion of the perfusion fluid, the central end of the sectioned sciatic nerve was electrically stimulated.

Immunoreactive SP was measured in the first portions of cerebrospinal fluid and in the third and fourth portions of perfusion fluid. SP was measured by radioimmunoassay as described previously (23), using antiserum 1-3-H of high affinity whose primary recognition site is the carboxy-terminal pentapeptide portion of the SP molecule (3). An SP analogue with tyrosine substituted for phenylalanine at position 8 was labelled with ^{125}I and used as tracer. The sensitivity of the assay is 1.5 fmoles (23).

RESULTS

In the first collected portion of cerebrospinal fluid the concentration of immunoreactive SP was 0.7 to 5.0 ng/ml. The second portions sampled during ventriculo-cisternal perfusion were discarded, as they may have contained McIlwain-Rodnight's solution mixed with some volume of residual cerebrospinal fluid in the cerebral ventricles. The third portion of perfusion fluid collected contained 45.71 ± 13.30 (mean $\pm$ SEM) percentage activity of SP detected in the first portion of cerebrospinal fluid (Fig. 1). The fourth portion of perfusion fluid collected during stimulation of the central end of cut sciatic nerve contained 123.81 ± 50.07 (mean $\pm$ SEM) percentage activity of SP in the first portion. The increase of SP activity in the fourth portion as compared with the SP activity in the third portion was significant ($p < 0.05$).

DISCUSSION

Sciatic nerve stimulation (7) or caudate nucleus stimulation (8) increased acetylcholinesterase concentration in the cerebrospinal fluid sampled from the

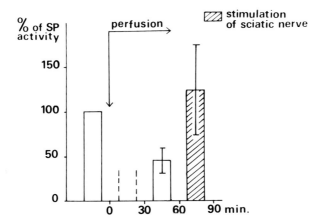

FIG. 1. Concentration of immunoreactive SP in fluids collected from cisterna magna during ventriculo-cisternal perfusion. The first left bar represents SP concentration in the cerebrospinal fluid expressed as 100% SP activity. Second sampled portions (0–30 min) were discarded. The SP concentration in the third (30–60 min.) and fourth (60–90 min) portions of perfusion fluid were expressed as mean ± SEM as percentage of activity of the first portion of cerebrospinal fluid. During sampling of the fourth portions, stimulation was applied to the cut central end of the sciatic nerve.

cisterna magna of rabbits anaesthetized with urethane. External factors also changed the release of prostaglandins into the cerebral ventricles in the dogs (13).

The concentration of SP found in the human cerebrospinal fluid was rather low (22,25), but the degradation of SP may have occurred in the fluid collected from a lumbar puncture. In the reported experiments the concentration of SP in the cerebrospinal fluid was much higher, but the fluid was collected from the cisterna magna and the cerebral ventricles. The high level of SP in the fluid sampled during ventriculo-cisternal perfusion indicates that SP is continuously released into cerebral ventricles. A significant increase in SP concentration in the perfusion fluid following sciatic nerve stimulation is evidence that afferent nerve impulses could change this release.

The source of SP which appeared in the cerebral ventricles are probably the SP-positive cell bodies and nerve terminals present in the periaqueductal central gray matter, in the nucleus raphe magnus (12), and in other structures (2,11,12). The release of SP from structures neighbouring cerebral ventricles could probably be modulated, as opiates (15) and gamma-aminobutyric acid (14) affected SP release from brain tissue *in vitro*.

The role of SP in the cerebrospinal fluid is still obscure. Application of SP on neurons in the nucleus locus coeruleus (9) and in the nucleus cuneatus (17) elicited their excitation. According to these data it is possible that SP acting from the cerebrospinal fluid on superficial structures of the medulla oblongata could modulate neural transmission.

ACKNOWLEDGMENTS

We wish to acknowledge the valuable assistance of Mrs. Z. Sędzińska. This study was conducted under Contract 10.4.2.01.5.12 with the Polish Academy of Sciences and supported by the Ford Foundation, New York, Grant 770–0540.

REFERENCES

1. Barber, R. P., Vaughn, J. E., Slemmon, J. R., Salvaterra, P. M., Roberts, E., and Leeman, S. E. (1979): The origin, distribution and synaptic relationships of Substance P axons in rat spinal cord. *J. Comp. Neurol.,* 184:331–351.
2. Brownstein, M. J., Mroz, E. A., Kizer, J. S., Palkovits, M., and Leeman, S. E. (1976): Regional distribution of Substance P in the brain of the rat. *Brain Res.,* 116:299–311.
3. Cannon, D., Skrabanek, P., Powell, D., and Harrington, M. G. (1977): Immunological characterization of two Substance P antisera with Substance P fragments and analogues. *Biochem. Soc. Trans.,* 5:1736–1738.
4. Chang, M. M., and Leeman, S. E. (1970): Isolation of sialogogic peptide from bovine hypothalamic tissue and its characterization as Substance P. *J. Biol. Chem.,* 245:4784–4790.
5. Chang, M. M., Leeman, S. E., and Niall, H. D. (1971): Amino-acid sequence of Substance P. *Nature (New Biol.),* 232:86–87.
6. Chan-Palay, V., and Palay, S. L. (1977): Ultrastructural identification in rat sensory ganglia and their terminals in the spinal cord by immunocytochemistry. *Proc. Natl. Acad. Sci. USA,* 74:4050–4054.
7. Chubb, I. W., Goodman, S., and Smith, A. D. (1974): Increased concentration of an isoenzyme of acetylcholinesterase in rabbit cerebrospinal fluid after peripheral stimulation, *J. Physiol. (Lond.),* 242:118P–120P.
8. Greenfield, S. A., and Smith, A. D. (1976): Changes in acetylcholinesterase concentration in rabbit cerebrospinal fluid following central electrical stimulation, *J. Physiol. (Lond.),* 258:108P–109P.
9. Guyenet, P. G., and Aghajanian, G. K. (1977): Excitation of neurons in the nucleus locus coeruleus by Substance P and related peptides. *Brain Res.,* 136:178–184.
10. De Groot, J. (1963): *The Rat Forebrain in Stereotaxic Coordinates.* N. V. Noord-Hollandsche Uitgevers Maatschappij, Amsterdam.
11. Hökfelt, T., Kellerth, J. O. Nilsson, G., and Pernow, B. (1975): Substance P: Localization in the central nervous system and in some primary sensory neurons. *Science,* 190:889–890.
12. Hökfelt, T., Ljungdahl, Å., Terenius, L., Elde, R., and Nilsson, G. (1977): Immunohistochemical analysis of peptide pathways possibly related to pain and analgesia: Enkephalin and Substance P. *Proc. Natl. Acad. Sci. USA,* 74:3081–3085.
13. Holmes, S. W. (1970): The spontaneous release of prostaglandins into the cerebral ventricles of the dog and the effect of external factors on this release. *Br. J. Pharmacol.,* 38:653–658.
14. Jessell, T. M. (1977): Inhibition of Substance P release from the isolated rat substantia nigra by GABA. *Br. J. Pharmacol.,* 59:486P.
15. Jessel, T. M., and Iversen, L. L. (1977): Opiate analgesics inhibit Substance P release from rat trigeminal nucleus. *Nature,* 268:549–551.
16. Jessell, T., Iversen, L. L., and Kanazawa, I. (1976): Release and metabolism of Substance P in rat hypothalamus. *Nature,* 264:81–83.
17. Krnjević, K., and Morris, M. E. (1974): An excitatory action of Substance P on cuneate neurones. *Can. J. Physiol. Pharmacol.,* 52:736–744.
18. Leśnik, H., and Traczyk, W. Z. (1978): Effect of increased concentration of Ca^{++} and Mg^{++} in the fluid perfusing the cerebral ventricles, and hypoxia on evoked tongue jerks. *Acta Physiol. Pol.,* 29:27–35.
19. Łuczyńska, M., and Traczyk, W. Z. (1980): Influence of cerebral ventricles perfusion with hexapeptide derivatives of Substance P on evoked tongue jerks in rats. *Brain Res. (in press).*
20. McIlwain, H., and Rodnight, R. (1962): *Practical Neurochemistry,* Churchill, London. Citation

after Daniel, A. R., and Lederis, K. (1967): Release of neurohypophysial hormones in vitro. *J. Physiol. (Lond.),* 190:171–187.

21. Mroz, E. A., Brownstein, M. J., and Leeman, S. E. (1977): Distribution of immunoassayable Substance P in the rat brain: Evidence for the existence of Substance P-containing tracts. In: *Substance P,* edited by U. S. von Euler and B. Pernow, pp. 147–154, Raven Press, New York.

22. Nilsson, G., Pernow, B., Fischer, G. H., and Folkers, K. (1977): Radioimmunological determination of Substance P. In: *Substance P,* edited by U. S. von Euler and B. Pernow, pp. 41–48. Raven Press, New York.

23. O'Connell, R., Skrabanek, P., Cannon, D., and Powell D. (1976): High-sensitivity radioimmunoassay for Substance P. *Irish J. Med. Sci.,* 145:392–398.

24. Otsuka, M., and Konishi, S. (1976): Release of Substance P-like immunoreactivity from isolated spinal cord of newborn rat. *Nature,* 264:83–84.

25. Powell, D., Skrabanek, P., and Cannon, D. (1977): Substance P: radioimmunoassay studies. In: *Substance P,* edited by U. S. von Euler and B. Pernow, pp. 35–40. Raven Press, New York.

26. Schenker, Ch., Mroz, E. A., and Leeman, S. E. (1976): Release of Substance P from isolated nerve endings. *Nature,* 264:790–792.

Neuropeptides and Neural Transmission,
edited by C. Ajmone Marsan and W. Z. Traczyk.
Raven Press, New York © 1980.

Effect of Substance P Analogue on Chronic Deprivation of Sleep of Wistar Rats Under Stress

K. Hecht, *P. Oehme, **I. A. Kolemetseva, **I. P. Lyovshina, M. Poppei, and **M. G. Airapetjanz

*Humboldt-Universit Charité, Psychiatric Hospital, Department of Neuropathophysiology, Berlin, GDR; *Academy of Sciences of the GDR, Institute of Drug Research, Berlin-Friedrichsfelde, GDR; and **Academy of Sciences of the USSR, Institute of Higher Nervous Activity and Neurophysiology, Moscow, USSR*

A nonapeptide that elicits a number of characteristics of orthodox sleep, following application to rabbits, was isolated by Monnier et al. (7) from blood dialysates of rabbit brain after stimulation of hypnogenic areas of the thalamus. The occurrence of sleep spindles and δ-waves was one such characteristic phenomenon and was responsible for the denotation of this peptide as δ-sleep-inducing peptide (DSIP). In addition to DSIP two more sleep-inducing peptides of much lower molecular weights were also isolated (4,8). Those two sleep factors are probably not identical with DSIP, nor are they degradation products of the nonapeptide. A fourth sleep peptide of structural similarity to oxytocin and vasopressin, neurohormones of the pituitary, was described by Pavel et al. in 1977 (13).

The present authors and/or their associates have studied for some time the peripheral and central effects of substance P (SP) and other tachykinins (1,2,9–11). SP, an undecapeptide, was found to be present in various cerebral regions and also outside the central nervous system (for review, see ref. 3). The role of SP as a potential transmitter or modulator is currently under discussion since its mechanism of action and physiological importance have not yet been fully elucidated. The authors feel inclined to define SP as a *regula*tor pept*ide* (regulide) with reference to their own findings, according to which the action of SP on the stress-affected animals proved stronger than on the clinically intact animal (5,6). Thus, the real SP action would seem to depend on the original condition of the animal concerned (12), while intraperitoneal application of the same peptide has been reported to result in a complete normalisation of most various stress-induced disorders, for example, in processes of learning or in blood pressure regulation (13).

Against this background, it appeared justified to expect that SP might be capable of normalizing stress-induced sleep disorders as well. However, a shortened analogue (Lys-*Phe-Ile-Gly-Leu-Met-NH₂*) rather than SP was chosen by the authors for these experiments, since previous studies had shown that analogue (SP-A) produces the same normalising effect on various stress models (5,6).

That analogue is structurally derived from SP (Arg-Pro-Lys-Pro-Gln-Gln-*Phe-Phe-Gly-Leu-Met-NH₂*) or even more from eledoisin, a peptide of cold-blooded animals (PGL-Pro-Ser-Lys-Asp-Ala-*Phe-Ile-Gly-Leu-Met-NH₂*). SP-A is similar to both tachykinins with regard to the essential COOH-terminal penta-peptide sequence.

METHODS

The SP-A analogue was intraperitoneally applied as an aqueous solution at the dose of 250 µg/kg. Control animals received the solvent (saline solution), and female Wistar rats were used for experimentation.

Rats were four months of age when testing started, their body weights being between 200 and 250 g. Twenty animals were exposed to immobilisation stress in a plastic tube over 4 weeks, with alternating periods of 24 hr of fixation and 24 hr of free movement (15). Ten animals were used as controls. The wake–sleep cycle was followed-up through EEG recordings from electrodes implanted in the optic cortex and hippocampus. (Stereotactic coordinates for the latter structures being: 4.0 mm frontal, 2.5 mm lateral, and 3.5 mm horizontal). The electroencephalographic recordings were taken once a day in the freely moving animal between 9 a.m. and 11 a.m., which is during the minimum of circadian rhythm of spontaneous locomotor activity, on 5 consecutive days. A

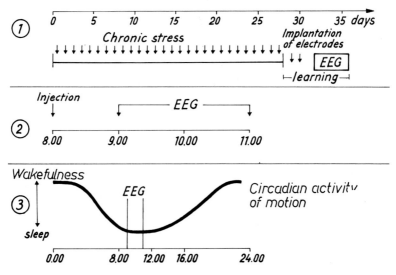

FIG. 1. Diagram of experiment. **1.** Chronic stress; **2.** injection and examination intervals; **3.** injection and examination intervals, depending on the circadian rhythm of spontaneous locomotor activity.

TABLE 1. *Characterisation of wake–sleep stages*

Stage	Behaviour	EEG
I. Active wakefulness	Locomotor activity	Desynchronisation
II. Passive wakefulness	No locomotor	Desynchronisation
III. Superficial sleep	Sleep	Syncronisation α-θ-δ-activity
IV. Deep slow sleep	Sleep	δ-activity
V. Paradoxical sleep	Sleep	Desynchronisation θ-activity

daily dose of 250 μg/kg SP-A was intraperitoneally applied, 1 hr before testing. A diagram of the experimental arrangement is given in Fig. 1.

The EEG was evaluated by means of a Type MB 5204 frequency analyser and the stages of the sleep–wake cycle were defined as in Table 1. The periods of sleep usually were interrupted two to four times by 2- to 5-min phases of paradoxical sleep. Blood pressure as well as respiratory and heart rates were also tested.

RESULTS

The controls were awake for 23.7% of the 2-hr testing period (stages I and II) and were asleep for 76.3% (stages III–V). Animals under chronic stress were characterised by deprivation of sleep, the wake period accounting for 51.3%

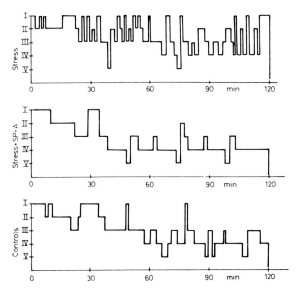

FIG. 2. Proportionate amounts of wake and sleep phases of controls, animals under stress without SP-A, and animals under stress with SP-A treatment on 4 consecutive days. *Ordinate:* sleep phases; *Abscissa:* time in minutes.

TABLE 2. *Wake–sleep phases of rats under stress, with and without SP-A*

Phase	Controls ($N = 40$)	Stress ($N = 40$)	Stress + SP-A ($N = 40$)
I	19.0 ± 0.08	33.8 ± 2.0 Δ	18.5 ± 2.0
II	9.5 ± 0.5	27.8 ± 3.6 Δ	9.8 ± 0.45
III	30.5 ± 1.3	26.4 ± 3.8	22.0 ± 3.0
IV	50.3 ± 1.5	27.7 ± 3.1 Δ	60.5 ± 5.2
V	10.7 ± 0.4	4.3 ± 0.37 Δ	9.2 ± 1.4

Mean values in min ($\bar{x} \pm$ SEM) for different stages. Stress group vs controls, $p < 0.001$ Δ. Stress vs stress + SP-A group, $p < 0.001$ Δ.

and the sleep period for 48.7%. Sleeping time of animals exposed to stress began to be normalised as early as the first application of SP-A and was almost identical with that of the controls (76.5% of sleep period, 23.5% of wake period) after four applications.

The average amounts of wake and sleep periods of each individual animal (Fig. 2) were summarised by groups of 10 animals each for 4-day period. The results may be seen from Table 2. The effect recorded from sleep EEG 24 hr after 4-day SP-A treatment was almost identical with the effect recorded from direct action of the peptide.

Also tested were the latencies up to the first occurrence of a characteristic sign of a given sleep phase. These were delayed or extended with statistical significance in animals under chronic stress, as of phase III, in comparison with the controls. Such prolongation of latency was eliminated by SP-A treat-

TABLE 3. *Latencies of rats under stress, with and without SP-A*

Phase	Controls ($N = 40$)	Stress ($N = 40$)	Stress + SP-A ($N = 40$)
II	5.4 ± 0.6	5.1 ± 2.2	6.3 ± 1.36
III	13.1 ± 1.8	28.3 ± 5.9 Δ	16.5 ± 2.7
IV	27.8 ± 4.9	59.4 ± 7.1 Δ	22.0 ± 4.0
V	55.5 ± 6.2	79.8 ± 11.8 Δ	62.9 ± 8.8

Mean values in min ($\bar{x} \pm$ SEM) for the different latencies. Stress group vs controls, $p < 0.001$ Δ. Stress group vs stress + SP-A group, $p < 0.001$ Δ.

TABLE 4. *Vegetative functions of rats under stress with and without SP-A*

	Controls ($N = 20$)	Stress ($N = 20$)	Stress + SP-A ($N = 20$)
Blood pressure (mm Hg)			
(Torr)	116 ± 6	163 ± 14 Δ	125 ± 11
Respiratory rate (per min)	77 ± 8	150 ± 12 Δ	75 ± 8
Heart rate (per min)	308 ± 46	588 ± 42 Δ	298 ± 38

Stress group vs controls, $p < 0.001$ Δ. Stress group vs stress + SP-A group, $p < 0.001$ Δ.

ment, and the latencies then recorded were similar to those of the controls, as may be seen from Table 3.

SP-A treatment not only normalised sleep but it also reversed the physiological standard changes in vegetative function that had been caused by chronic stress. Findings to this effect are given in Table 4.

DISCUSSION

With regard to hypnogenic action of DSIP, there is basically one common denominator that results from a comparison between the results reported by Monnier et al. (7) and the findings described in this chapter: SP-A, just as DSIP, acts primarily on the delta-sleep portion of the EEG. On the other hand, there are certain differences between the two studies which are due to methodological problems: Monnier's experiments were based on acute conditions in intact cats and the authors experiments were based on chronic conditions in rats exposed to stress. In other words, normal sleep was induced, more or less, from a wake phase by DSIP. The authors, however, produced sleep deprivation with considerable changes to the functional sleep structure and then eliminated that condition by means of SP-A. Consequently, the authors of this chapter, have induced an impairment of sleep and have then restored it to normal. This normalisation applied not only to delta sleep but to paradoxical sleep as well. The latter case was in some way related to results reported by Urban and de Wied (15) who succeeded in controlling paradoxical sleep by means of $ACTH_{4-10}$.

No changes in blood pressure were recorded by Monnier et al. (7). Yet, in the present experiments sleep deprivation was accompanied by arterial hypertension, and that hypertension was changed to normal pressure. DSIP, as used by Monnier et al. caused bradycardia, whereas SP-A succeeded in changing tachycardia to normal rhythm. These differences appeared to depend on the original condition of the animals at the time of peptide application.

Condition-dependent action of SP and SP-A has been realised by the authors also in another context (12). Unspecific modulating function is considered to be characteristic of the SP analogue used by the authors which, like SP, normalised other functions as well, both vegetative and those of the central nervous system (5,6). The authors would like to propose the term of "regulator peptide" to denote that peptide with such action quality (Oehme et al., *this volume*).

Further studies will be required to substantiate the physiological relevance of the type of action described.

SUMMARY

Reduced or otherwise impaired delta activity and paradoxical sleep periods of sleep EEG taken of Wistar rats under stress proved to be restorable by injection of 250 μg/kg of an SP analogue (Lys-Phe-Ile-Gly-Leu-Met-NH$_2$). SP thus has been proved to have modulating function, and the authors propose to denote it by the name of "regulator peptide."

REFERENCES

1. Bergmann, J., Bienert, M., Niedrich, H., Mehlis, B., and Oehme, P. (1974): Uber den Einfluss der Kettenlängen bei C-terminalen Sequenzen der Substanz P—im Vergleich mit analogen Physalaemin- und Eledoisin-Peptiden—auf die Wirksamkeit am Meerschweinchen-Ileum. *Experientia,* 30:401–403.
2. Bienert, M., Mehlis, B., Kühler, M., Bergman, J., and Niedrich, H. (1978): Synthese von Halogenacetyl- und Chlorambucil-Peptiden des Eledoisins, Physalaemin und der Substanz P als potentielle Affinitätsmarker. *Journal f. prakt. Chemie,* 320:261–269.
3. Bury, R. W., and Mashford, M. L. (1977): Substance P: Its pharmacology and physiological roles. *Austr. J. Exp. Biol. Med. Sci.,* 55:671–735.
4. Fencl, V., Koski, G., and Pappenheimer, J. (1971): Factors in cerebro spinal fluid from goats that affect sleep and activity in rats. *J. Physiol. (Lond.),* 216:565–589.
5. Hecht, K., Oehme, P., and Poppei, M. (1979): A substance P analogue—its effects upon learning and memorising processes, behavioral patterns, and blood pressure in neurotic hypertensive rats. *Pharmazie,* 34:45–49.
6. Hecht, K., Oehme, P., Poppei, M., and Hecht, T. (1979): Conditioned-reflex learning of normal juvenile and adult rats exposed to action of substance P and of an SP analogue. *Pharmazie,* 34:419–423.
7. Minone, S., and Uckizono, K. (1974): The presence of a sleep promoting material in the brain of sleep deprived rats. *Proc. Jap. Acad.,* 50:214–246.
8. Monnier, M., Dudler, L., Gächter, R., and Schoenenberger, G. A. (1975): Humoral transmission of sleep. IX. Activity and concentration of the sleep peptide delta in cerebral and systemic blood fractions. *Pfluegers Arch.,* 360:225–242.
9. Niedrich, H., Bienert, M., Mehlis, B., Bergman, J., and Oehme, P. (1975): Studien zum Wirkungsmechanismus glattmuskulär angreifender Peptide. III. Der Einfluss der N-azylierung auf die Wirksamkeit von C-terminalen Teilsequenzen des Eledoisins, des Physalaemins und der Substanz P am Meerschweinchen-Ileum. *Acta Biol. Med. Germ.,* 34:483–489.
10. Oehme, P., Bergmann, J., Bienert, M., Hilse, H., Piesche, L., Minh Thu, P., and Scheer, E. (1977): Biological action of substance P—its differentiation by affinity and intrinsic efficacy. In: *Substance P,* edited by U. S. von Euler and B. Pernow, pp. 327–335. Raven Press. New York.
11. Oehme, P., Bergmann, J., Niedrich, H., Jung, F., and Menzel, G. (1970): Zur Pharmakologie von Hydrazinocarbonsäuren, Hydrazinopeptiden und anderen Hydrozinderivaten. VII. Pharmakologische Untersuchungen herterologer Eledoisin-Sequenzen. *Acta Biol. Med. Germ.,* 25:613–625.
12. Oehme, P., Hecht, K., Piesche, L., and Hilse, H. (1978): Substance P—pharmacology, properties and mode of action. *Abstracts of the 7th International Congress of Pharmacology.* Paris, p. 130. Pergamon, London.
13. Pavel, S., Psatta, D., and Goldstein, R. (1977): Slow-wave sleep induced in cats by extremely small amounts of synthetic and pineal vasotocin injected into the third ventricle of the brain. *Brain Res. Bull.,* 2:251–254.
14. Poppei, M., and Hecht, K. (1971): Der Einfluss einer wiederholten Bewegungseinschränkung der lokomotorischen Reaktion auf den systolischen Blutdruck von Albinoratten. *Acta Biol. Germ.,* 27:297–306.
15. Urban, J., and de Wied, D. (1978): Neuropeptides: Effects on paradoxical sleep and theta rhythm in rats. *Pharmacol., Biochem. Behav.,* 8:51–59.

Neuropeptides and Neural Transmission,
edited by C. Ajmone Marsan and W. Z. Traczyk.
Raven Press, New York © 1980.

Activity of Medullary Centers After Perfusion with [pGlu⁶]SP$_{6-11}$ Hexapeptide, a Derivative of Substance P, Through Cerebral Ventricles

Władysław Z. Traczyk and Maria Łuczyńska

Department of Physiology, Institute of Physiology and Biochemistry, School of Medicine in Lodz, 90–131 Lodz, Poland

The existence of some direct humoral control of neural centers has attracted the attention of many investigators for a long time. The brain intercellular and the cerebrospinal fluids circulating through the cerebral ventricles can be regarded as the humoral pathway through which the brain centers can also communicate. The humoral communication between centers neighbouring on the cerebral ventricular system form, what has been called by Feldberg (30), the "inner brain surface," and requires further consideration.

In the structures that can be classified as belonging to the "inner brain surface," the concentration of some active compounds is higher than in others. In the rat brain Substance P (SP) originating from the caudate nucleus and putamen was accumulated in the highest concentration in the reticular part of the substantia nigra (13,34). Apart from their presence in the spinal dorsal horns (41), SP immunoreactive fibers in the rat brain run in a longitudinal rostro-caudal direction in the periventricular and periaqueductal gray matter and are also found in the locus coeruleus, in the nucleus principalis nervi trigemini and, in a very high density in the substantia gelatinosa of the nucleus tractus spinalis nervi trigemini (24,42).

The level of SP was markedly lowered in the dorsal horn after sectioning the dorsal root in cats, but only slightly diminished around the central canal of the spinal cord (86). SP remains in fibers from local circuit interneurons and in the longitudinal bundle found immediately ventral to the central canal in rats, and it can probably affect the release of other neuroactive compounds into the cerebrospinal fluid (7). In the rat spinal cord it was also found that SP-reactive granules were discharged into the extracellular space, and in this way they may act on neighbouring cells (20).

In the rat brain methionine-enkephalin (Met-Enk) and leucine-enkephalin (Leu-Enk) were found (82). In the periaqueductal central gray matter, in the nucleus raphe magnus, and in the substantia gelatinosa of the nucleus tractus spinalis nervi trigemini, SP-positive and also Met-Enk-positive cell bodies and nerve terminals were observed (43). A dense distribution of Met-Enk and Leu-Enk fibers and terminals was seen in the nucleus tractus spinalis nervi trigemini throughout the reticular formation and in the motor nuclei of IV, VII, X, and XII cranial nerves (75).

SP and enkephalins could be released from rat brain tissue *in vitro*. SP was released from rat hypothalamus slices (51), isolated spinal cord (71), and isolated nerve endings (77), and the enkephalins were released *in vitro* from corpus striatum (39), globus pallidus (46), substantia nigra (48), and trigeminal nucleus (49,50). Gamma-aminobutyric acid (GABA), which is generally accepted to be a potent inhibitory mediator, was released from various brain structures (3,47,53). Opiate analgesics (49,50,66) and GABA (48) exerted their inhibitory effect on SP release from brain tissue.

In the cerebrospinal fluid of patients suffering from various mental disorders SP was very low, 3 pmoles/liter on the average (67), but the degradation of SP may have occurred in the cerebrospinal fluid obtained from a lumbar puncture. Endorphins (44,80,91) and GABA (29,72) were also found in cerebrospinal fluid.

It is likely that SP, enkephalins, and GABA released in minute amounts, but continuously, into cerebrospinal fluid circulating through cerebral ventricles (92) may compete in exerting their effects on the medullary neural centers neighbouring the IVth cerebral ventricle.

Highly purified natural SP was introduced into rabbit and cat cerebral ventricles by von Euler and Pernow (28), and they described some effects on the respiration rate and arterial blood pressure. Effects, even opposite in nature may depend on the SP dose introduced intraventricularly.

Somatic medullary reflexes seem to be a better indicator of the influence on medullary centers of the active compound present in ventricular fluid. The morphological and functional organisation of the sensory trigeminal nuclei was intensively studied in cat (27,65,84,97) as well as in rat (4,68,69,81). The inhibition of the spinal trigeminal nucleus by the locus coeruleus nucleus (76) and the inhibition of the latter nucleus by the dorsal raphe nucleus (78) was studied. Special attention was given to the tooth pulp afferents and to their medullary projection in the cat (12,25,31,35,60,61,73,90,95,96), in the rhesus monkey (87), and in the rat (45).

In the pulpal cross-sections of the cat's canine tooth 81% of non-myelinated fibers were found (8), and in the pulp perfusate a high concentration of SP appeared (70). Tooth pulp stimulation was used to study the jaw opening reflex (5) and the stimulation of the trigeminal nerve for the orthodromical activation of hypoglossal motoneurons (36,37).

The trigemino-hypoglossal reflex (85) facilitation or inhibition could be evaluated according to the amplitude of retractive movements of the tongue (58), as stretching the tongue had no influence on hypoglossal motoneurons (37). The absence of proprioceptors in the tongue muscles of the cat was confirmed by morphological and physiological studies (11).

SP isolated from bovine hypothalamus, having an established amino acid sequence of undecapeptide (19) and obtained by chemical synthesis, has a strong vasodilator activity (14,15,88). The C-terminal hexapeptide of SP, according to the assays on smooth muscle of digestive tracts, possesses a higher activity (14) and the derivative of C-terminal hexapeptide [pGlu⁶]SP₆₋₁₁ the highest (93,94). The latter hexapeptide was found to exert a strong action on the brain centers when injected into the cerebral ventricles (56,89) or perfused through them (63), and was therefore chosen for the studies reported herein.

For the study of SP influence on medullary centers and its interaction with enkephalins and GABA, the polysynaptic medullary reflex was performed. The intensity of the evoked tongue movements was the indicator of the influence of SP, penetrating from the lumen of the IVth cerebral ventricle into the medulla, on secondary sensory neurons, on interneurons, as well as on hypoglossal motoneurons.

The effects of SP on respiration and arterial blood pressure were also studied, but mainly for the determination of the threshold concentration of the active compounds in the fluid perfusing cerebral ventricles, since in respiration and blood pressure control several related peripheral and central mechanisms are involved.

MATERIALS AND METHODS

Animals

The experiments were performed on male rats, weighing 290 to 370 g (330 g on the average), about 5 months old, F_1 generation cross strains bred in our department of male August with female Wistar rats from the stock of the Institute of Oncology in Warsaw. The animals were kept in standard conditions of a 14-hr light:10-hr darkness cycle and received standard rat pellets and water *ad libitum.*

The animals chosen for arterial blood pressure recording were anaesthetized with urethane (1.0 g/kg body weight i.p.), and for evoked tongue jerks or respiration recording were anaesthetized with chloralose (150 mg/kg body weight i.p.). In animals prepared for arterial blood pressure recording, the skin on the neck was cut in the midline and a polyethylene tube was inserted into the trachea.

Perfusion of Cerebral Ventricles

After general anaesthesia had set in, the head of the animal was immobilized in a simple stereotaxic instrument specially adapted for perfusion of cerebral ventricles in rats. Perfusion was carried out according to the method previously described (58) with some further modification (62,63) which consisted in fixation of the animal's head in the stereotaxic instrument in a position that widens the space between the occipital bone of the cranium and the first cervical vertebrae. The palatum durum just behind the upper incisors was 20 mm below the interauricular axis. This position of the animal's head allows the introduction of a cannula into the cerebellomedullar cistern and its fixation in rigid position in the cannula holder attached to the ear bars (Fig. 1).

The skin on the animal's head was incised in the midline and the bones of the skull were exposed. Two holes were drilled in the skull 5 mm anteriorly to the frontal interaural zero plane and 3 mm laterally on either side of the sagittal zero plane, and two stainless steel cannulas with an external diameter 0.6 mm were inserted into the lateral ventricles to a depth of 4 mm from the surface of the skull. The cannulas were connected to a vessel with perfusion fluid, that is with McIlwain-Rodnight's solution composed according to Daniel and Lederis (64) as follows (millimoles per litre): NaCl, 120.0; KCl, 4.8; KH_2PO_4. 1.2; $MgSO_4$, 1.3; $CaCl_2 + 2\ H_2O$, 2.8; $NaHCO_3$, 2.6; and glucose, 10.0.

The cannula for the cerebellomedullar cistern consisted of two tubes; an outer guide tube and an inner tube of external diameter 0.6 mm, both of stainless steel. The outer tube was inserted through the skin and muscles to the atlantooccipital membrane which was punctured by the inner tube, the tip of which was introduced into the cistern. The vessels with the inflow and outflow perfusion fluid were kept in such a position above and below the rat's head, respectively, to obtain a perfusion volume from 0.3 to 0.8 ml per 10 min during the whole experiment.

The record noted during cerebral ventricles perfusion with McIlwain-Rod-

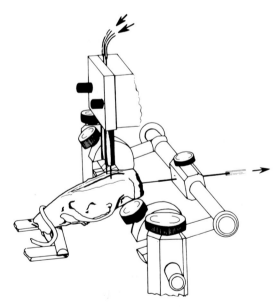

FIG. 1. Position of rat's skull in a stereotaxic instrument adapted for ventriculo-cisternal perfusion. The inflow cannulas for lateral ventricles are fixed vertically and the outflow cannula for the cerebellomedullar cistern is fixed almost horizontally in the cannula holder.

night's solution was regarded as the control. Perfusion fluids were also composed with active compounds dissolved in McIlwain-Rodnight's solution. These were: a hexapeptide $[pGlu^6]SP_{6-11}$, the C-terminal derivative of SP, in concentrations of 500 pmoles, 5 nmoles, and 50 nmoles/ml; 50 nmoles Leu-Enk/ml; 10 μmoles GABA/ml; and 10 μmoles GABA with 50 nmoles $[pGlu^6]SP_{6-11}$/ml. The $[pGlu^6]SP_{6-11}$ and Leu-Enk were dissolved and then lyophilized with a carrier—dextrane 40,000 MW as described elsewhere (88)—to obtain a form that would be soluble in McIlwain-Rodnight's solution. The concentration of dextrane in the perfusion fluid was 2%.

The peptides $[pGlu^6]SP_{6-11}$ (59) and Leu-Enk were synthesized by the conventional method of peptide synthesis at the Faculty of Chemistry, University of Warsaw.

Respiratory Movements and Blood Pressure Recording

The respiratory movements were recorded in animals anaesthetized with chloralose (150 mg/kg body weight i.p.). The skin on the side of the rat's thorax was connected by a silk thread to a lever of an isotonic transducer and the respiratory movements of the thorax were recorded by means of a Kovo Line Recorder TZ 21 S.

The arterial blood pressure was recorded in animals anaesthetized with urethane (1.0 g/kg body weight i.p.). A polyethylene tube filled with saline and heparine was introduced into the left femoral artery and the mean arterial blood pressure was recorded on a kymograph with the aid of a mercury manometer constructed according to the USA Pharmacopeia sixteenth revision.

Recording of Evoked Tongue Jerks

Evoked tongue jerks (ETJ) were recorded in animals anaesthetized with chloralose (150 mg/kg body weight i.p.) in which the mouth was kept open by fixing the mandible to the stereotaxic instrument. The tip of the tongue was connected by a silk thread to a lever of an isotonic transducer, and distinct sharp backward movements of the stretched tongue were recorded by means of a Kovo Line Recorder TZ 21 S. The amplitude of electric pulses stimulating the infraorbital nerve or the tooth pulp was adjusted so that each stimulation evoked a distinct tongue jerk. Throughout the whole experiment the tongue was stretched with the same force by the lever of a transducer and the amplitude of the electric pulses was not changed. The amplitudes of ETJ recorded on the tape during each 10-min period were measured in millimeters and the mean amplitude of ETJ was obtained.

Stimulation of Infraorbital Nerve and Tooth Pulp

The skin below the left eye of the animal was incised, and the infraorbital nerve was exposed and placed on a thin bipolar silver electrode connected to a Grass stimulator model S 4 K. The nerve was stimulated bipolarly with electric pulses at a frequency of 6/min, duration 3 msec, and amplitude up to 10 V to obtain the recorded amplitude of ETJ about 20 mm.

Both lower incisors were cut little by little with a dental separating disk until the pulp cavity was reached. A fine single stainless steel electrode was introduced into the pulp cavity of both incisors. The electrodes were fixed by means of dental cement. The stimulation was performed bipolarly through the pulp of both incisors and consisted of a volley of four square electric pulses of 3 msec duration, separated by 2-msec intervals, amplitude up to 10 V, and repeated six times per minute. The amplitude of electric pulses was adjusted to record a distinct amplitude of ETJ after each volley of pulses. The electrodes in the pulp cavities were connected to a Grass stimulator S 4 K with a pulse generator as external control.

At the end of each experiment 1% trypan blue solution was perfused through the cerebral ventricles, and after decapitation the rat's head was kept in 10% formalin for 1 week. The brain was then taken out of the skull cavity and the distribution of the dye in the cerebral ventricles and the staining of the ependyma were checked under a dissecting stereomicroscope. Only those results obtained on animals with a clear staining of the ependyma of the lateral, third, and fourth ventricles were taken into account.

Mean values of respiratory movements, of arterial blood pressure, and of ETJ during control perfusion and perfusion with active compounds were compared by the paired *t*-test.

RESULTS

Changes of Respiratory Movement Rate and Arterial Blood Pressure During Perfusion of Cerebral Ventricles

During control perfusion of cerebral ventricles with McIlwain-Rodnight's solution the respiration rate per minute was 51.3 ± 4.5 (mean $\pm$ SEM). Successive perfusion of cerebral ventricles in the same animals with [pGlu⁶]SP₆₋₁₁ in increasing concentrations of 500 pmoles/ml, 5 nmoles/ml, and 50 nmoles/ml decreased the respiration rate per minute to 48.3 ± 4.6, 41.5 ± 3.6, and 35.7 ± 2.9, respectively (Fig. 2). Only perfusion with 50 nmoles/ml significantly decreased ($p < 0.01$) the respiration rate as compared with control perfusion at the beginning of the experiment. The decrease of respiration rate was simultaneously accompanied by an increase in the amplitude of the respiratory movements of the thorax.

Successive perfusions of cerebral ventricles in the same animals with control solution and solution containing [pGlu⁶]SP₆₋₁₁ in increasing concentrations had little effect on arterial blood pressure. During the 5th and 10th min of perfusion with McIlwain-Rodnight's solution and 500 pmoles/ml [pGlu⁶]SP₆₋₁₁, the mean arterial blood pressure insignificantly decreased as compared with the 1st min

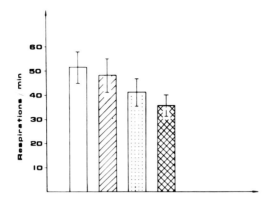

FIG. 2. Respiration rate per minute (mean ± SEM) in rats in chloralose anaesthesia (N = 9) during successive ventriculo-cisternal perfusion with McIlwain-Rodnight's solution and with [pGlu⁶]SP₆₋₁₁ in concentrations of 500 pmoles, 5 nmoles, and 50 nmoles/ml. □ Control sol, ▨ 500 pmol/ml [pGlu⁶]SP₆₋₁₁, ▦ 5 nmol/ml [pGlu⁶]SP₆₋₁₁, ▩ 50 nmol/ml [pGlu⁶]SP₆₋₁₁.

of perfusion (Fig. 3). Higher concentrations of [pGlu⁶]SP₆₋₁₁ in the perfusion fluid transiently but insignificantly ($p > 0.05$) elevated the blood pressure.

A significant increase in mean arterial blood pressure ($p < 0.01$) was recorded at the 5th and 10th min of cerebral ventricle perfusion with highest concentration of 50 nmoles/ml of [pGlu⁶]SP₆₋₁₁ (Fig. 4). Perfusion of ventricles immediately afterwards with 50 nmoles/ml Leu-Enk decreased the blood pressure to the control level. This decrease could be regarded as being related to the diminution of [pGlu⁶]SP₆₋₁₁ concentration in the ventricular fluid rather than to the presence of Leu-Enk. In the next group of animals (Fig. 5) the preceding perfusion with 50 nmoles/ml Leu-Enk had no effect on the arterial blood pressure increase induced by the following perfusion with 50 nmoles/ml [pGlu⁶]SP₆₋₁₁.

The arterial blood pressure decreased insignificantly ($p < 0.05$) during ven-

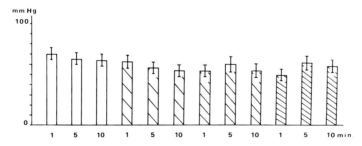

FIG. 3. Blood pressure (mean ± SEM) in rats in urethane anaesthesia (N =10) during 1st, 5th, and 10th min of successive ventriculo-cisternal perfusion with McIlwain-Rodnight's solution and with [pGlu⁶]SP₆₋₁₁ in concentrations of 500 pmoles, 5 nmoles, and 50 nmoles/ml. □ Control sol, ◪ 500 pmol/ml [pGlu⁶]SP₆₋₁₁, ◪ 5 nmol/ml [pGlu⁶]SP₆₋₁₁, ◪ 50 nmol/ml [pGlu⁶]SP₆₋₁₁.

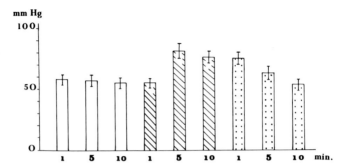

FIG. 4. Blood pressure (mean ± SEM) in rats in urethane anaesthesia (*N* = 12) during 1st, 5th, and 10th min of successive ventriculo-cisternal perfusion with McIlwain-Rodnight's solution, 50 nmoles/ml [pGlu⁶]SP₆₋₁₁, and 50 nmoles/ml Leu-Enk. □ McIlwain sol, ◩ 50 nmol/ml [pGlu⁶]SP₆₋₁₁, ⊡ 50 nmol/ml Leu-Enk.

tricular perfusion with 10 μmoles/ml GABA. The presence of 10 μmoles/ml GABA together with 50 nmoles/ml [pGlu⁶]SP₆₋₁₁ did not prevent a significant ($p < 0.01$) blood pressure elevation caused by the hexapeptide (Fig. 6).

Changes in Amplitude of ETJ by Infraorbital Nerve Stimulation During Cerebral Ventricle Perfusion

Ventricular perfusion with successively increased concentrations of [pGlu⁶]SP₆₋₁₁ (5 and 50 nmoles/ml) significantly increased the amplitude of ETJ ($p < 0.05$ and $p < 0.02$, respectively) as compared with the amplitude of ETJ during control perfusion with McIlwain-Rodnight's solution (Fig. 7).

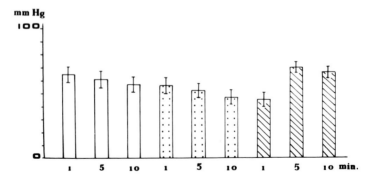

FIG. 5. Blood pressure (mean ± SEM) in rats in urethane anaesthesia (*N* = 11) during 1st, 5th, and 10th min of successive ventriculo-cisternal perfusion with McIlwain-Rodnight's solution, 50 nmoles/ml Leu-Enk, and 50 nmoles/ml [pGlu⁶]SP₆₋₁₁. □ McIlwain sol, ◩ 50 nmol/ml [pGlu⁶]SP₆₋₁₁, ⊡ 50 nmol/ml Leu-Enk.

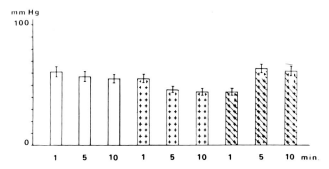

FIG. 6. Blood pressure (mean ± SEM) in rats in urethane anaesthesia (*N* = 11) during 1st, 5th, and 10th min of successive ventriculo-cisternal perfusion with McIlwain-Rodnight's solution, 10 μmoles/ml GABA, and 10 μmoles/ml of GABA together with 50 nmoles/ml [pGlu⁶]SP₆₋₁₁. □ McIlwain sol, ⊞ 10 μmol/ml GABA, ▨ 10 μmol/ml GABA, + 50 nmol/ml [pGlu⁶]SP₆₋₁₁.

Changes in Amplitude of ETJ by Tooth Pulp Stimulation During Cerebral Ventricle Perfusion

Successive perfusion of cerebral ventricles in the same animals with control solution and solutions containing [pGlu⁶]SP₆₋₁₁ in increasing concentrations had little effect on the amplitude of ETJ due to tooth pulp stimulation (Fig. 8).

Application of highest concentration of [pGlu⁶]SP₆₋₁₁ 50 nmoles/ml just after the control perfusion also had little effect on the amplitude of ETJ due to tooth pulp stimulation, as was the case with subsequent perfusion with 50 nmoles/ml Leu-Enk (Fig. 9).

Successive ventricular perfusion with 50 nmoles/ml Leu-Enk and 50 nmoles/ml [pGlu⁶]SP₆₋₁₁ did not change significantly the amplitude of ETJ due to tooth pulp stimulation (Fig. 10).

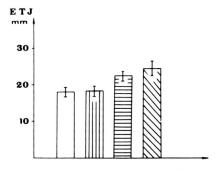

FIG. 7. Amplitude of ETJ due to infraorbital nerve stimulation (mean ± SEM) in rats in chloralose anaesthesia (*N* = 16), recorded during successive 10-min of ventriculo-cisternal perfusion with McIlwain-Rodnight's solution and with [pGlu⁶]SP₆₋₁₁ in concentrations of 500 pmoles, 5 nmoles, and 50 nmoles/ml with intervals for the exchange of the fluid in cerebral ventricles. □ Control sol, ▥ 500 pmol/ml [pGlu⁶]SP₆₋₁₁, ▤ 5 nmol/ml [pGlu⁶]SP₆₋₁₁, ▧ 50 nmol/ml [pGlu⁶]SP₆₋₁₁.

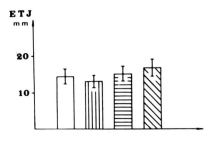

FIG. 8. Amplitude of ETJ due to tooth pulp stimulation (mean ± SEM) in rats in chloralose anaesthesia ($N = 6$), recorded during successive 10-min of ventriculo-cisternal perfusion with McIlwain-Rodnight's solution and with [pGlu⁶]SP₆₋₁₁ in concentrations of 500 pmoles, 5 nmoles, and 50 nmoles/ml. ☐ Control sol, ▥ 500 pmol/ml [pGlu⁶]SP₆₋₁₁, ▤ 5 nmol/ml [pGlu⁶]SP₆₋₁₁, ▨ 50 nmol/ml [pGlu⁶]SP₆₋₁₁.

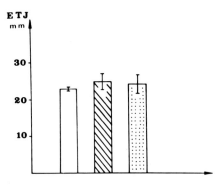

FIG. 9. Amplitude of ETJ due to tooth pulp stimulation (mean ± SEM) in rats in chloralose anaesthesia ($N = 10$), recorded during successive 10-min of ventriculo-cisternal perfusion with McIlwain-Rodnight's solution, 50 nmoles/ml [pGlu⁶]SP₆₋₁₁, and 50 nmoles/ml Leu-Enk. ☐ Control sol, ▦ 50 nmol/ml Leu-Enk, ▨ 50 nmol/ml [pGlu⁶]SP₆₋₁₁.

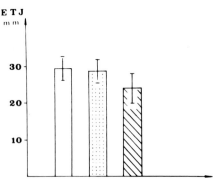

FIG. 10. The amplitude of ETJ due to tooth pulp stimulation (mean ± SEM) in rats in chloralose anaesthesia ($N = 7$), recorded during successive 10-min of ventriculo-cisternal perfusion with McIlwain-Rodnight's solution, 50 nmoles/ml Leu-Enk, and 50 nmoles/ml [pGlu⁶]SP₆₋₁₁, ☐ Control sol, ▦ 50 nmol/ml Leu-Enk, ▨ 50 nmol/ml [pGlu⁶]SP₆₋₁₁.

DISCUSSION

Cerebral ventricle perfusion with [pGlu⁶]SP₆₋₁₁ in increasing concentrations decreased the respiration rate. The effect was dose-dependent but significant only for the highest concentration. Injections into the third ventricle of natural highly purified SP in small and medium doses induced hyperpnea (28). High doses of SP lowered the respiratory frequency.

Our result with a decrease of the respiration rate indicates only that a concentration of 50 nmoles/ml [pGlu⁶]SP₆₋₁₁ in perfusion fluid affects the brain centers. The mechanism of decrease of the respiration rate is not connected with H⁺ which changed the neuronal activity in the surface layer of the rat medulla oblongata (32,33). [pGlu^6]SP$_{6-11}$ was present only in a minute amount as compared with other compounds of the McIlwain-Rodnight's solution which stabilize the H$^+$ concentration.

The value of blood pressure at the 5th and 10th min of perfusion was taken into consideration because at that time the maximum of the pressor response usually appeared. A significant blood pressure increase was obtained during perfusion with the highest [pGlu^6]SP$_{6-11}$ concentration. A stepwise increase of [pGlu^6]SP$_{6-11}$ concentration in periods of time longer than 10 min gave a moderate nonsignificant response. The repetition of intraventricular injections of [pGlu^6]SP$_{6-11}$ at 15-min intervals also diminished successive responses (89).

Elevation of blood pressure was usually obtained by SP injections into cerebral ventricles in rabbits (28), cats (28), and rats (89). Intraventricular injection of other peptides such as angiotensin II (79), bradykinin (21), and thyrotropin-releasing hormone (52) also increased arterial blood pressure. The pressor responses were elicited by electrical stimulation of brain structures, some of which neighboured the cerebral ventricle system. Stimulation of the septum in rats produced hypertension (16) and local administration of bradykinin into the lateral septal area also increased arterial blood pressure in rats (22,23). On the other hand, the injection of SP into the same septal area caused no change in blood pressure (22).

The iontophoretic application of SP excited the great majority of neurons in the locus coeruleus (38) composed in the rat almost exclusively of noradrenaline-containing cells which have wide afferent projections (18). Intraventricular injections of SP stimulate both synthesis and utilization of dopamine, noradrenaline, and 5-hydroxytryptamine (17), and in this way may influence the medullary cardiovascular reflexes (74) which may be affected by the area postrema in rat (98).

The blood pressure response to SP could not be connected only with medullary centers as bilateral vagotomy (89), and cross-section of the spinal cord in the lower cervical segment (56) did not affect significantly the blood pressure response to intraventricular administration of [pGlu^6]SP$_{6-11}$. The activation by SP of the hypothalamo-neurohypophyseal system in the rat (6) should be considered, but in our experiments GABA did not inhibit the pressor response, as could have been expected according to the results of other authors (2,26,83). Leu-Enk perfusion of the cerebral ventricles did not prevent the pressor response in spite of the high density of opiate receptors in some brain structures neighbouring cerebral ventricles (10). The molar concentration of Leu-Enk equal to that of [pGlu^6]SP$_{6-11}$ is too low to abolish the activity of the latter peptide.

The excitatory action of SP on spinal motoneurons (54), cuneate neurons (55), nucleus locus coeruleus neurons (38), and neurons of other structures except Renshaw cells (9) is now firmly established. The exacerbation of ETJ by infraorbital nerve stimulation during cerebral ventricle perfusion with [pGlu^6]SP$_{6-11}$ is in agreement with the general view on the role of SP. The [pGlu^6]SP$_{6-11}$ used for perfusion in the same concentration has little effect on the amplitude of ETJ due to tooth pulp stimulation. The amplitude of ETJ was so pronounced in both groups of animals in which infraorbital nerve and tooth pulp were stimulated that some differences in the stimulus used should have no significant influence on the results.

The hexapeptide may exert a direct excitatory action on neurons constituting the trigemino-hypoglossal reflex arc or on the indirect inhibitory activity from the periaqueductal gray matter or dorsal raphe nucleus. Electrical stimulation of both structures in decerebrate cats reduced or abolished the jaw-opening reflex response evoked by stimulation of either the tooth pulp or infraorbital nerve (1). The hexapeptide can also activate some inhibitory interneurons, as it was found in the spinal cord or in other brain mechanisms which inhibit ETJ (57).

The amplitude of ETJ due to tooth pulp stimulation was not affected significantly by the Leu-Enk perfusion which preceded or followed in equal molar concentration the [pGlu⁶]SP₆₋₁₁. It is possible that significant changes in ETJ could be elicited by higher Leu-Enk concentrations, as more potent Met-Enk applied iontophoretically inhibited single neuron activity in the caudal medulla of rat (40).

According to the reported results, it can be postulated that SP and its derivatives acting from the lumen of cerebral ventricles exacerbates the medullary reflexes in which most of the primary afferent fibers are not the SP-containing ones. On the contrary, the noxious stimuli which induce nerve pulses in many of SP-containing primary afferent fibers are not exacerbated by SP and its derivative acting from the ventricular fluid. Whether in physiological conditions the brain centers can communicate through the cerebrospinal fluid by way of SP, its derivatives, or other active compounds remains to be elucidated by further studies.

ACKNOWLEDGMENTS

The authors are grateful for the technical assistance of Mrs. Anna Kliszko, Mrs. Krystyna Sadzińska, and Mr. Aleksy Sobczyk. This study was conducted under Contract 10.4.2.01.5.12 with the Polish Academy of Sciences and supported by Grant M76.01C from the Population Council, Biomedical Division, New York.

REFERENCES

1. Andersen, R. K., Lund, J. P., and Puil, E. (1978): Excitation and inhibition of neurons in the trigeminal nucleus caudalis following periaqueductal gray stimulation. *Can. J. Physiol. Pharmacol.,* 56:157–161.
2. Antonaccio, M. J., Kerwin, L., and Taylor, D. G. (1978): Effects of central GABA receptor agonism and antagonism on evoked diencephalic cardiovascular responses. *Neuropharmacology,* 17:597–603.
3. Assumpção, J. A., Bernardi, N., Dacke, C. G., and Davidson, N. (1979): Evidence for a neuronal release of isotopically labelled γ-amino-*n*-butyric acid (GABA) from the rat dorsal medulla in vivo. *Experientia,* 35:225–227.

4. Ayliffe, S. J., and Hill, R. G. (1979): Responses of cells in the trigeminal subnucleus caudalis of the rat to noxious stimuli. *J. Physiol. (Lond.),* 287:18P–19P.
5. Azerad, J., and Woda, A. (1976): Tooth pulp projection to the trigeminal complex and jaw opening reflex in the cat. *J. Biol. Buccale,* 4:109–115.
6. Baertschi, A. J., and Dreifuss, J. J. (1979): Effects of enkephalins and of Substance P on the hypothalamo-neurohypophysial system of the rat. *J. Physiol. (Lond.),* 289:56P–57P.
7. Barber, R. P., Vaughn, J. E., Slemmon, J. R., Salvaterra, P. M., Roberts, E., and Leeman, S. E. (1979): The origin, distribution and synaptic relationships of Substance P axons in rat spinal cord. *J. Comp. Neurol.,* 184:331–351.
8. Beasly, W. L., and Holland, G. R. (1978): A quantitative analysis of the innervation of the pulp of the cat's canine tooth. *J. Comp. Neurol.,* 178:487–494.
9. Belcher, G., and Ryall, R. W. (1977): Substance P and Renshaw cells: A new concept of inhibitory synaptic interactions. *J. Physiol. (Lond.),* 272:105–119.
10. Bird, S. J., Atweh, S. F., and Kuhar, M. J. (1976): Microiontophoretic study of the effects of opiates on autoradiographically localized opiate receptors. In: *Opiates and Endogenous Opioid Peptides,* edited by H. W. Kosterlitz, pp. 199–204. North-Holland, Amsterdam, New York, Oxford.
11. Blom, S. (1960): Afferent influences on tongue muscle activity. A morphological and physiological study in the cat. *Acta Physiol. Scand.,* 49(Suppl. 170):1–97.
12. Brookhart, J. M., Livingston, W. K., and Haugen, F. P. (1953): Functional characteristics of afferent fibers from tooth pulp of cat. *J. Neurophysiol.,* 16:634–642.
13. Brownstein, M. J., Mroz, E. A., Kizer, J. S., Palkovits, M., and Leeman, S. E. (1976): Regional distribution of Substance P in the brain of the rat. *Brain Res.,* 116:299–311.
14. Bury, R. W., and Mashford, M. L. (1976): Biological activity of C-terminal partial sequences of Substance P. *J. Med. Chem.,* 19:854–856.
15. Bury, R. W., and Mashford, M. L. (1977): Cardiovascular effects of synthetic Substance P in several species. *Eur. J. Pharmacol.,* 45:335–340.
16. Calaresu, F. R., and Mogenson, G. J. (1972): Cardiovascular responses to electrical stimulation of the septum in the rat. *Am. J. Physiol.,* 223:777–782.
17. Carlsson, A., Magnusson, T., Fisher, G. H., Chang, D., and Folkers, K. (1977): Effect of synthetic Substance P on central monoaminergic mechanisms. In: *Substance P,* edited by U.S. von Euler and B. Pernow, pp. 201–205. Raven Press, New York.
18. Cedarbaum, J. M., and Aghajanian, G. K. (1978): Afferent projections to the rat locus coeruleus as determined by a retrograde tracing technique. *J. Comp. Neurol.,* 178:1–16.
19. Chang, M. M., Leeman, S. E., and Niall, H. D. (1971): Amino-acid sequence of Substance P. *Nature (New Biol.),* 232:86–87.
20. Chan-Palay, V., and Palay, S. L. (1977): Ultrastructural identification of Substance P cells and their processes in rat sensory ganglia and their terminals in the spinal cord by immunocytochemistry. *Proc. Natl. Acad. Sci. USA,* 74:4050–4054.
21. Corrêa, F. M. A., and Graeff, F. G. (1974): Central mechanisms of the hypertensive action of intraventricular bradykinin in the unanaesthetized rat. *Neuropharmacology,* 13:65–75.
22. Corrêa, F. M. A., and Graeff, F. G. (1975): Central site of the hypertensive action of bradykinin. *J. Pharmacol. Exp. Ther.,* 192:670–676.
23. Corrêa, F. M. A., and Graeff, F. G. (1976): On the mechanism of the hypertensive action of intraseptal bradykinin in the rat. *Neuropharmacology,* 15:713–717.
24. Cuello, A. C., and Kanazawa, I. (1978): The distribution of Substance P immunoreactive fibers in the rat central nervous system. *J. Comp. Neurol.,* 178:129–156.
25. Davies, W. I. R., Scott, Jr. D., Vesterstrøm, K., and Vyklický, L. (1971): Depolarization of the tooth pulp afferent terminals in the brain stem of the cat. *J. Physiol. (Lond.),* 218:515–532.
26. Dyball, R. E. J., and Shaw, F. D. (1979): Inhibition by GABA of hormone release from the neurohypophysis in the rat. *J. Physiol. (Lond.),* 289:78P–79P.
27. Eisenman, J., Landgren, S., and Novin, D. (1963): Functional organization in the main sensory trigeminal nucleus and in the rostral subdivision of the nucleus of the spinal trigeminal tract in the cat. *Acta Physiol. Scand.,* 59 (Suppl. 214):1–44.
28. von Euler, U. S., and Pernow, B. (1956): Neurotropic effects of Substance P. *Acta Physiol. Scand.,* 36:265–275.
29. Faull, K. F., DoAmaral, J. R., Berger, P. A., and Barchas, J. D. (1978): Mass spectrometric

identification and selected ion monitoring quantitation of γ-amino-butyric acid (GABA) in human lumbar cerebrospinal fluid. *J. Neurochem.,* 31:1119–1122.

30. Feldberg, W. (1963): *A Pharmacological Approach to the Brain from its Inner and Outer Surface.* Edward Arnold, London.

31. Fields, R. W., Tache, R. B., and Savara, B. S. (1975): The origin of trigeminal response components elicited by electrical stimulation of the tooth pulp of the cat. *Arch. Oral Biol.,* 20:437–443.

32. Fukuda, Y., Honda, J., Schläfke, M. E., and Loeschcke, H. H. (1978): Effect of H⁺ on the membrane potential of silent cells in the ventral and dorsal surface layers of the rat medulla in vitro. *Pflüegers Arch.,* 376:229–235.

33. Fukuda, Y., and Loeschcke, H. H. (1977): Effect of H⁺ on spontaneous neuronal activity in the surface layer of the rat medulla oblongata in vitro. *Pflüegers Arch.* 371:125–134.

34. Gale, K., Hong, J. S., and Guidotti, A. (1977): Presence of Substance P and GABA in separate striatonigral neurons. *Brain Res.,* 136:371–375.

35. Goldberg, L. J., and Browne, P. A. (1974): Differences in the excitability of two populations of trigeminal primary afferent central terminals. *Brain Res.,* 77:195–209.

36. Green, J. D., De Groot, J., and Sutin, J. (1957): Trigemino-bulbar reflex pathways. *Am. J. Physiol.,* 189:384–388.

37. Green, J. D., and Negishi, K. (1963): Membrane potentials in hypoglossal motoneurons. *J. Neurophysiol.,* 26:835–856.

38. Guyenet, P. G., and Aghajanian, G. K. (1977): Excitation of neurons in the nucleus locus coeruleus by Substance P and related peptides. *Brain Res.,* 136:178–184.

39. Henderson, G., Hughes, J., and Kosterlitz, H. W. (1978): In vitro release of Leu- and Met-enkephalin from the corpus striatum. *Nature,* 271:677–678.

40. Hill, R. G., Pepper, C. M., and Mitchell, J. F. (1976): The depressant action of iontophoretically applied met-enkephalin on single neurones in rat brain. In: *Opiates and Endogenous Opioid Peptides,* edited by H. W. Kosterlitz, pp. 225–230. North-Holland, Amsterdam, New York, Oxford.

41. Hökfelt, T., Elde, R., Johansson, O., Luft, R., Nilsson, G., and Arimura, A. (1976): Immunohistochemical evidence for separate populations of somatostatin-containing and Substance P-containing primary afferent neurons in the rat. *Neuroscience,* 1:131–136.

42. Hökfelt, T., Kellerth, J. O., Nilsson, G., and Pernow, B. (1975): Substance P: Localization in the central nervous system and in some primary sensory neurons. *Science,* 190:889–890.

43. Hökfelt, T., Ljungdahl, Å., Terenius, L., Elde, R., and Nilsson, G. (1977): Immunohistochemical analysis of peptide pathways possibly related to pain and analgesia: Enkephalin and Substance P. *Proc. Natl. Acad. Sci. USA,* 74:3081–3085.

44. Hosobuchi, Y., Rossier, J., Bloom, F. E., and Guillemin, R. (1979): Stimulation of human periaqueductal gray for pain relief. Increases immunoreactive β-endorphin in ventricular fluid. *Science,* 203:279–281.

45. Igarashi, S., Sasa, M., and Takaori, S. (1979): Input from tooth pulp to locus coeruleus neurons. *Electroencephalogr. Clin. Neurophysiol.,* 47:6P.

46. Iversen, L. L., Iversen, S. D., Bloom, F. E., Vargo, T., and Guillemin, R. (1978): Release of enkephalin from rat globus pallidus in vitro. *Nature,* 271:679–681.

47. Iversen, L. L., Mitchell, J. F., and Srinivasan, V. (1971): The release of γ-aminobutyric acid during inhibition in the cat visual cortex. *J. Physiol. (Lond.),* 212:519–534.

48. Jessel, T. M. (1977): Inhibition of Substance P release from the isolated rat substantia nigra by GABA. *Br. J. Pharmacol.,* 59:486P.

49. Jessell, T. M. (1977): Opiate inhibition of Substance P release from the rat trigeminal nucleus, in vitro. *J. Physiol. (Lond.),* 270:56P–57P.

50. Jessel, T. M., and Iversen, L. L. (1977): Opiate analgesics inhibit Substance P release from rat trigeminal nucleus, *Nature,* 268:549–551.

51. Jessell, T. M., Iversen, L. L., and Kanazawa, I. (1976): Release and metabolism of Substance P in rat hypothalamus. *Nature,* 264:81–83.

52. Koivusalo, F., Paakkari, I., Leppäluoto, J., and Karppanen, H. (1979): The effect of centrally administered TRH on blood pressure, heart rate and ventilation in rat. *Acta Physiol. Scand.,* 106:83–86.

53. Kondo, Y., and Iwatsubo, K. (1978): Increased release of preloaded ³H GABA from substantia nigra in vivo following stimulation of caudate nucleus and globus pallidus. *Brain Res.,* 154:395–400.

54. Konishi, S., and Otsuka, M. (1974): Excitatory action of hypothalamic Substance P on spinal motoneurones of newborn rats. *Nature,* 252:734–735.
55. Krnjević, K., and Morris, M. E. (1974): An excitatory action of Substance P on cuneate neurones. *Can. J. Physiol. Pharmacol.,* 52:736–744.
56. Kubicki, J. (1980): Studies on mechanism of pressor response into cerebral ventricles by administration of Substance P and hexapeptide [pGlu⁶]SP₆₋₁₁ in rats. *Acta Physiol. Pol. (in press).*
57. Leśnik, H. (1978): Effect of vasopressin and oxytocin perfusion of the cerebral ventricles on evoked tongue jerks. *Acta Physiol. Pol.,* 29:307–315.
58. Leśnik, H., and Traczyk, W. Z. (1978): Effect of increased concentration of Ca^{++} and Mg^{++} in the fluid perfusing the cerebral ventricles, and hypoxia on evoked tongue jerks. *Acta Physiol. Pol.,* 29:27–35.
59. Lipkowski, A., Majewski, T., Drabarek, S., and Traczyk, W. Z. (1975): Synthesis of the biologically active hexapeptide fragment of Substance P. *Third Conference on Chemistry of Amino Acids and Peptides,* October 16–18, 1975, p. 31. University of Warsaw, Warsaw.
60. Lisney, S. J. W. (1978): Evidence for primary afferent depolarization of tooth pulp afferents following stimulation of other trigeminal afferents in the cat. *J. Physiol. (Lond.),* 282:12P–13P.
61. Lisney, S. J. W. (1978): Some anatomical and electrophysiological properties of tooth-pulp afferents in the cat. *J. Physiol. (Lond.),* 284:19–36.
62. Łuczyńska, M., (1978): Inhibition of evoked tongue jerks during the rat's cerebral ventricles perfusion with gamma-aminobutyric acid and beta-phenyl-gamma-aminobutyric acid. *Acta Physiol. Pol.,* 29:231–236.
63. Łuczyńska, M., and Traczyk, W. Z. (1980): Influence of cerebral ventricles perfusion with hexapeptide derivatives of Substance P on evoked tongue jerks in rats. *Brain Res. (in press).*
64. McIlwain, H., and Rodnight, R. (1962): *Practical Neurochemistry,* Churchill, London. Citation after: Daniel, A. R., and Lederis, K. (1967): Release of neurohypophysial hormones in vitro, *J. Physiol. (Lond.),* 190:171–187.
65. McKinley, W. A., and Magoun, H. W. (1942): The bulbar projection of the trigeminal nerve. *Am. J. Physiol.,* 137:217–224.
66. Mudge, A. W., Leeman, S. E., and Fischbach, G. D. (1979): Enkephalin inhibits release of Substance P from sensory neurons in culture and decreases action potential duration. *Proc. Natl. Acad. Sci. USA,* 76:526–530.
67. Nilsson, G., Pernow, B., Fisher, G. H., and Folkers, K. (1977): Radioimmunological determination of Substance P. In: *Substance P,* edited by U. S. von Euler and B. Pernow, pp. 41–48. Raven Press, New York.
68. Nord, S. G. (1967): Somatotropic organization in the spinal trigeminal nucleus, the dorsal column nuclei and related structures in rat. *J. Comp. Neurol.,* 130:343–356.
69. Nord, S. G., and Kyler, H. J. (1968): A single unit analysis of trigeminal projections to bulbar reticular nuclei of the rat. *J. Comp. Neurol.,* 134:485–494.
70. Olgart, L., Gazelius, B., Brodin, E., and Nilsson, G. (1977): Release of Substance P-like immunoreactivity from the dental pulp. *Acta Physiol. Scand.,* 101:510–512.
71. Otsuka, M., and Konishi, S. (1976): Release of Substance P-like immunoreactivity from isolated spinal cord of newborn rat. *Nature,* 264:83–84.
72. Perlow, M. J., Enna, S. J., O'Brien, P. J., Hoffman, H. J., and Wyatt, R. J. (1979): Cerebrospinal fluid gamma-aminobutyric acid: Daily pattern and response to haloperidol. *J. Neurochem.,* 32:265–268.
73. Pfaffmann, C. (1939): Afferent impulses from the teeth due to pressure and noxious stimulation. *J. Physiol. (Lond.),* 97:207–219.
74. Reis, D. J., and Cuénod, M. (1965): Central neural regulation of carotid baroreceptor reflexes in the cat. *Am. J. Physiol.,* 209:1267–1277.
75. Sar, M., Stumpf, W. E., Miller, R. J., Chang, K. J., and Cuatrecasas, P. (1978): Immunohistochemical localization of enkephalin in rat brain and spinal cord. *J. Comp. Neurol.,* 181:17–38.
76. Sasa, M., and Takaori, S. (1973): Influence of the locus coeruleus on transmission in the spinal trigeminal nucleus neurons. *Brain Res.,* 55:203–208.
77. Schenker, C., Mroz, E. A., and Leeman, S. E. (1976): Release of Substance P from isolated nerve endings. *Nature,* 264:790–792.
78. Segal, M. (1979): Serotonergic innervation of the locus coeruleus from the dorsal raphe and its action on responses to noxious stimuli. *J. Physiol. (Lond.),* 286:401–415.

79. Severs, W. B., Daniels, A. E., and Buckley, J. P. (1967): On the central hypertensive effect of angiotensin II. *Int. J. Neuropharmacol.,* 6:199–205.
80. Sjölund, B., Terenius, L., and Eriksson, M. (1977): Increased cerebrospinal fluid levels of endorphins after electro-acupuncture. *Acta Physiol. Scand.,* 100:382–384.
81. Smith, R. L. (1973): The ascending fiber projections from the principal sensory trigeminal nucleus in the rat. *J. Comp. Neurol.,* 148:423–446.
82. Smith, T. W., Hughes, J., Kosterlitz, H. W., and Sosa, R. P. (1976): Enkephalins: Isolation, distribution and function. In: *Opiates and Endogenous Opioid Peptides,* edited by H. W. Kosterlitz, pp. 57–62. North-Holland, Amsterdam, New York, Oxford.
83. Srimal, R. C., Gulati, K., and Dhawan, B. N. (1977): On the mechanism of central hypotensive action of clonidine. *Can. J. Physiol. Pharmacol.,* 55:1007–1014.
84. Stewart, W. A., and King, R. B. (1963): Fiber projections from the nucleus caudalis of the spinal trigeminal nucleus. *J. Comp. Neurol.,* 121:271–282.
85. Sumino, R., and Nakamura, Y. (1974): Synaptic potentials of hypoglossal motoneurons and a common inhibitory interneuron in the trigemino-hypoglossal reflex. *Brain Res.,* 73:439–454.
86. Takahashi, T., and Otsuka, M. (1975): Regional distribution of Substance P in the spinal cord and nerve roots of the cat and the effect of dorsal root section. *Brain Res.,* 87:1–11.
87. Tamarova, Z. A., Shapovalov, A. I., and Vyklický, L. (1973): Projection of the tooth pulp afferents in the brain stem of rhesus monkey. *Brain Res.,* 64:442–445.
88. Traczyk, W. Z. (1977): Circulatory effects of Substance P, SP₆₋₁₁ and [pGlu⁶]SP₆₋₁₁ hexapeptides. In: *Substance P,* edited by U. S. von Euler and B. Pernow, pp. 297–301. Raven Press, New York.
89. Traczyk, W. Z., and Kubicki, J. (1980): Pressor response to Substance P and hexapeptide [pGlu⁶]SP₆₋₁₁ injections into cerebral ventricles in rats. *Neuropharmacology (in press).*
90. Vyklický, L., Keller, O., Jastreboff, P., Vyklický, L., Jr., and Butkhuzi, S. M. (1977): Spinal trigeminal tractotomy and nociceptive reactions evoked by tooth pulp stimulation in the cat. *J. Physiol. (Paris),* 73:379–386.
91. Wahlström, A., Jahansson, L., and Terenius, L. (1976): Characterization of endorphins (endogenous morphine-like factors) in human CSF and brain extracts. In: *Opiates and Endogenous Opioid Peptides,* edited by H. W. Kosterlitz, pp. 49–56. North-Holland, Amsterdam, New York, Oxford.
92. Woodward, D. L., Reed, D. J., and Woodbury, D. M. (1967): Extracellular space of rat cerebral cortex. *Am. J. Physiol.,* 212:367–370.
93. Yajima, H., Kitagawa, K., and Segawa, T. (1973): Studies on peptides. XXXVIII. Structure-activity correlations in Substance P. *Chem. Pharm. Bull. (Tokyo),* 21:2500–2506.
94. Yanaihara, N., Yanaihara, Ch., Hirohashi, M., Sato, H., Iizuka, Y., Hashimoto, T., and Sakagami, M. (1977): Substance P analogs: Synthesis, and biological and immunological properties. In: *Substance P,* edited by U. S. von Euler and B. Pernow, pp. 27–33. Raven Press, New York.
95. Yokota, T. (1976): Two types of tooth pulp units in the bulbar lateral reticular formation. *Brain Res.,* 104:325–329.
96. Young, R. F., and Nord, S. G. (1975): Experimental modulation of medullary dental pulp units by mechanical stimulation of oro-facial fields. *Exp. Neurol.,* 49:813–821.
97. Yu, Y. J., and King, R. B. (1974): Trigeminal main sensory nucleus polymodal unit responses to noxious and non-noxious stimuli. *Brain Res.,* 72:147–152.
98. Zandberg, P., Palkovits, M., and De Jong, W. (1977): The area postrema and control of arterial blood pressure: Absence of hypertension after excision of the area postrema in rat. *Pflügers Arch.,* 372:169–173.

Neuropeptides and Neural Transmission,
edited by C. Ajmone Marsan and W. Z. Traczyk.
Raven Press, New York © 1980.

Neurotensin as a Hormone in Man

Sune Rosell, Åke Rökaeus, *M. L. Mashford, Kjell Thor, Ding
Chang, and **Karl Folkers

*Department of Pharmacology, Karolinska Institutet, S-104 01 Stockholm, Sweden; *Surgery Clinic, Ersta Hospital, Stockholm, Sweden; and **Institute for Biomedical Research, University of Texas at Austin, Texas 78712*

Neurotensin (NT) is a tridecapeptide with the sequence < Glu-Leu-Tyr-Glu-Asn-Lys-Pro-Arg-Arg-Pro-Tyr-Ile-OH (8) which was first found in the bovine hypothalamus by Carraway and Leeman (7). It is noteworthy that in the rat some 85% of the body's NT is located in the gut and particularly in the more distal part of the small bowel (9). Recently Folkers et al. (14) suggested that the acid analog (Gln⁴)-neurotensin, rather than NT, may be the naturally occurring peptide. We have found that (Gln⁴)-neurotensin and NT have the same activities in several biological systems. Immunofluorescence histochemical studies have shown glandular cells in the mucosa of the ileum which react with antibodies against NT (5,17,22,23,27).

ACTIONS OF NEUROTENSINS

Our results of pharmacological studies in dogs indicate that the most relevant dose to use in studying the actions of neurotensins in the dog seems to be in the range of 6 to 30 pmoles/kg/min administered intravenously. In this dose range discrete effects are noted in the gastrointestinal tract without any general actions on blood pressure or heart rate (Table 1). For example, the spontaneous motor activity in antral pouches of the stomach in conscious dogs is inhibited by 8 pmoles/kg/min of NT or (Gln⁴)-NT infused intravenously (Fig. 1). Furthermore, gastric acid secretion induced by pentagastrin or a test meal is inhibited to 75% by NT at an infusion rate of 30 pmoles/kg/min (1). In this dose NT and (Gln⁴)-neurotensin produce a prolonged vasoconstriction in subcutaneous adipose tissue (24) and vasodilatation in the gastrointestinal tract (Fig. 2). These vascular actions suggest that NT may redistribute blood flow from the subcutaneous fat to the gastrointestinal tract at doses that do not change cardiac output or blood pressure. To induce hypotension or hyperglycemia, higher infusion

---

* Present address: University of Melbourne, Department of Medicine, St. Vincent's Hospital, Fitzroy 3065, Australia.

TABLE 1. *Effects of NT in dogs*

Infusion i.v. (pmoles/kg/min)	Effect	Remarks
6	Inhibition of pressure motility in the antrum of the stomach.	Conscious (ref. 2)
12	Transient vasodilatation in small intestine. Delayed vasoconstriction in adipose tissue.	Pentobarbital (ref. 24)
30	Inhibition of gastric acid secretion stimulated by pentagastrin, test meal.	Conscious (ref. 1)
60	Increase in blood glucose concentration. Slight hypotension.	Pentobarbital (ref. 24)

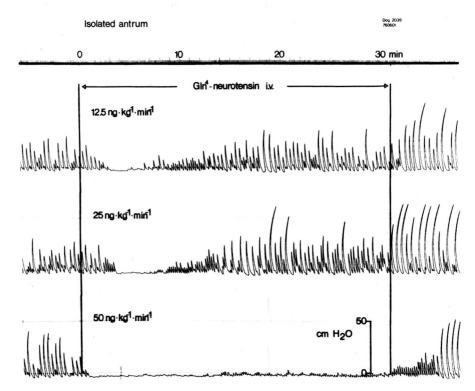

FIG. 1. Inhibitory effect of three different doses of (Gln[4])-NT on antral motility in one and the same dog. (From Andersson et al., ref. 2, with permission.)

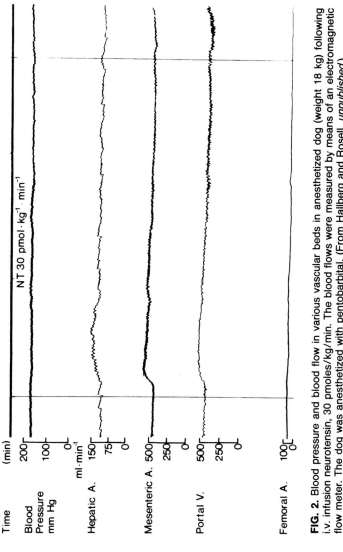

FIG. 2. Blood pressure and blood flow in various vascular beds in anesthetized dog (weight 18 kg) following i.v. infusion neurotensin, 30 pmoles/kg/min. The blood flows were measured by means of an electromagnetic flow meter. The dog was anesthetized with pentobarbital. (From Hallberg and Rosell, *unpublished*.)

rates are needed. The actions which NT exerts at low doses must be the most relevant to any endocrine function which the peptide may have. This is the reason we have focused attention primarily on the gastrointestinal action of NT.

RELEASE OF NT-LIKE IMMUNOREACTIVITY

One requirement for a circulating substance to be regarded as a hormone is that it be released from its storage site into the blood. In order to demonstrate such release, the terminal 20 cm of the ileum of anesthetized dogs were perfused *in situ* with a buffered solution and blood was collected from the carotid artery, femoral vein, and a mesenteric vein draining the terminal ileum (20). There was a positive V-A difference across the terminal ileum (Table 2). Evidently NT-like immunoreactivity (NTLI) is released into the blood by the terminal ileum, but also finds its way into the lumen of the gut.

TABLE 2. *NTLI in dogs*

Source	Concentration (pM)	V-A (pM)	Release (fmoles/min)
Carotid artery	$40 \pm 6.7(8)$		
Venous blood draining distal ileum	$91 \pm 9.7(7)$	51 ± 11^a	233 ± 46.8
Femoral vein	$46 \pm 5.9(8)$		
Perfusate, distal ileum	$521 \pm 160(7)$		

[a] $p < 0.01$.
From Mashford et al., ref 20, with permission.

It is necessary at this point to consider what the radioimmunoassay for NTLI is actually measuring. Our antibody reacts with NT, NT (1–12), (Gln[4])-NT, and (Gln[4])-NT (1–11), but not with NT (4–13) or smaller C-terminal fragments. It shows effectively no cross-reactivity with vasoactive intestinal polypeptide, (VIP), secretin, cholecystokinin-33, cholecystokinin-39, pancreatic glucagon, substance P, insulin, somatostatin, gastric inhibitory polypeptide (GIP), bovine pancreatic polypeptide (BPP), gastrin-17, gastrin-34, or trypsinized gastrin-34, which presumably contains the N-terminal heptadecapeptide. The assay can measure levels down to 5 pM. However, NTLI should not be identified unequivocally as NT since it has not been isolated and chemically characterized. Moreover, experimental data indicate that some of the actions of NT may be caused by substance(s) formed from NT (26). Since the antibody is directed towards the N-terminus of the NT molecule, shorter N-terminal sequences of NT may have been detected.

INGESTION OF FOOD AND THE PLASMA CONCENTRATION
OF NTLI

Another requirement for NT to be regarded as a hormone is that its concentration in blood vary in a reproducible way in relation to some physiologically important event. One such event is evidently food ingestion (4,19). In human volunteers the mean concentration of NTLI after an overnight fast was 65 ± 12 pM (N = 6) and continued fasting was associated with further fall in the blood concentration (Fig. 3). However, a meal consisting of an aperitif of 40 ml whisky, a white bread roll and 4 g butter, steak, fried potatoes and béarnaise sauce, 100 ml wine, and coffee produced a pronounced rise in NTLI. The mean concentration at 45 min was 233 ± 86 pM. The NTLI concentration fell thereafter but remained elevated in all subjects for the 2 hr and 45 min during which sampling continued (20). The consistent pattern of change in the blood concentration of NTLI associated with food ingestion suggested to us that the circulating NT or a NT metabolite is serving some hormonal function in relation to eating. To elucidate that possibility it is of importance to know if one or more of the principal nutrients in a mixed meal may have the major influence on the plasma NTLI. Therefore, 6 healthy male volunteers ingested on separate occasions amino acids (430 ml as Vamin N, Vitrum), glucose (30 g as 300 ml Glucose ACO), or fat (11 g as 55 ml Intralipid Vitrum 200 mg/ml) (25). Water was added to each test meal to a final volume of 500 ml. Following ingestion of Intralipid there was a significant increase in the plasma NTLI concentration from 42 ±

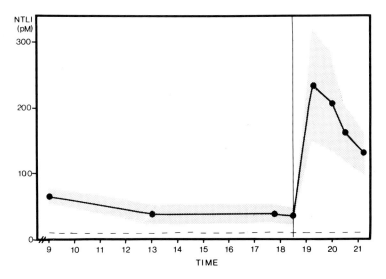

FIG. 3. NTLI levels in 6 subjects during fasting and after a meal. The *abscissa* represents the time of the day. The *shaded area* indicates the SEM. The *dotted line* indicates levels below the sensitivity of the method. (From Mashford et al., ref. 19, with permission.)

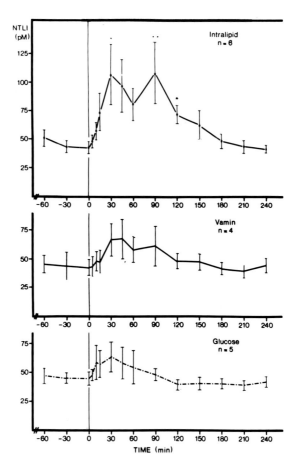

FIG. 4. Concentrations of NTLI in plasma after oral intake of Intralipid, Vamin, or glucose. *N*, number of subjects. The *vertical bars* indicate the SEM. *$p < 0.05$; **$p < 0.01$. (From Rosell et al., ref. 25, with permission.)

5.2 pM (mean $\pm$ SEM, $N = 6$) to a peak value of 109 $\pm$ 27 pM at 90 min with return of the plasma level by 180 min (Fig. 4). The isocaloric test meals comprising Vamin and glucose did not change the plasma concentration of NTLI. Therefore, it seems that ingestion of fat has a marked effect on the concentration of NTLI in plasma.

Gastric secretion and gastric motility are inhibited when ingested fat reaches the small intestine (3,13). As long as 50 years ago experimental evidence had been obtained in dogs that there is an inhibition of gastric function elicited by fat in the intestine and that this is caused by a hormone from the intestinal mucosa which Kosaka and Lim (18) named "enterogastrone." Several recent studies have dealt with the action of fat in the small intestine on gastric secretion and motility in man. Windsor et al. (27) found that instillation of fat into the duodenum and small intestine depressed a near maximal gastric acid output by approximately 50%. Similarly, Christiansen and co-workers (11) have demonstrated a pronounced inhibition of gastric acid secretion in the human small intestine following infusion of Intralipid 40 to 50 cm distal to the ligament of Treitz. Clain et al. (12) diverted the chyme from the intestine at a site 100 cm distal to the ligament of Treitz and this resulted in an increased gastric secretory response to a meal. They suggested that the distal small intestine plays an inhibitory role in postprandial gastric secretion. Thus, several groups have demonstrated in man the existence of a potent postprandial gastric acid inhibitory mechanism in the small intestine which is activated by fat.

Enterogastrone activity has been suggested for several substances including secretin, cholecystokinin, and GIP, but none of these have been established as the responsible hormone (see refs. 3,6,10,16). Our finding that ingestion of fat causes a pronounced increase in the plasma concentration of NTLI for 2 hr or more, suggest that NT or a metabolite of NT must now be considered for a causal role in the postprandial inhibition of the gastric motility and gastric acid secretion excerted from the small intestine.

ACTIONS OF NT IN MAN

Before NT or some metabolite in blood can be ascribed a physiological hormonal function as an enterogastrone, it will be necessary to show that administration of exogenous NT to produce elevation of NTLI concentrations in blood to the levels found after ingestion of fat is capable of inhibiting gastrointestinal motility or gastric acid secretion in humans.

As is evident from Fig. 5 (Gln[4])-NT infused intravenously at a rate of 6 pmoles/kg/min, inhibits the lower esophageal sphincter (LES) pressure within 3 min when the NTLI concentration in blood is about 50 pM. By comparing this concentration of NTLI with the mean value after a meal (233 pM), it is

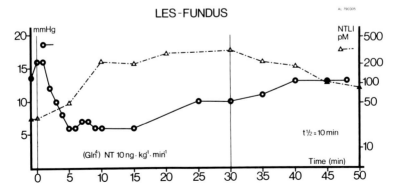

FIG. 5. The LES-fundus pressure and the concentration of NTLI in plasma following i.v. infusion of (Gln[4])-neurotensin in a healthy human volunteer (6 pmoles (10 ng)/kg/min).

quite evident that the decrease of the LES pressure occurs at physiological concentrations.

SUMMARY

Our experimental data show that NT or a NT metabolite satisfies the rather rigid physiological criteria for true hormone status. Thus, the gastrointestinal actions are produced by very small concentrations, the release into the blood is produced by a physiological stimulus (ingestion of food), and the plasma concentrations of NTLI following ingestion of food are comparable to those achieved by exogenous NT at doses that produce effects in the gastrointestinal tract. NT or a NT metabolite in blood may have a physiological role as a hormone with enterogastrone-like functions.

ACKNOWLEDGMENTS

These studies were supported by the Swedish Medical Research Council (Grant No. 3518), Julins Fond and the Robert A. Welch Foundation.

REFERENCES

1. Andersson, S., Chang, D., Folkers, K., and Rosell, S. (1976): Inhibition of gastric acid secretion in dogs by neurotensin. *Life Sci.,* 19:367–370.
2. Andersson, S., Rosell, S., Hjelmquist, U., Chang, D., and Folkers, K. (1977): Inhibition of gastric and intestinal motor activity in dogs by (Gln^4)-neurotensin. *Acta Physiol. Scand.,* 100:231–235.
3. Babkin, B. P. (1950): *Secretory Mechanism of the Digestive Glands.* Hoeber, New York, 2nd ed.
4. Besterman, H. S., Sarson, D. L., Johnston, D. I., Stewart, J. S., Guerin, S., Bloom, S. R., Blackburn, A. M., Patel, H. R., Modigliani, R., and Mallison, C. N. (1978): Gut-hormone profile in caeliac disease. *Lancet,* 1:785–788.
5. Bloom, S. R., and Polak, J. M. (1978): Gut hormones overview. In: *Gut Hormones,* edited by S. R. Bloom. Churchill Livingstone, Edinburgh.
6. Brown, J. C., Dryburgh, J. R., Ross, S. A., and Dupre, J. (1975): Identification and actions of gastric inhibitory polypeptide. *Rec. Prog. Horm. Res.,* 31:487–532.
7. Carraway, R., and Leeman, S. E. (1973): The isolation of a new hypotensive peptide. Neurotensin from bovine hypothalami. *J. Biol. Chem.,* 248:6854–6861.
8. Carraway, R., and Leeman, S. E. (1975): The amino acid sequence of a hypothalamic peptide. Neurotensin. *J. Biol. Chem.,* 250:1907–1911.
9. Carraway, R., and Leeman, S. E. (1976): Characterization of radioimmunoassayable neurotensin in the rat; its differential distribution in the central nervous system, small intestine and stomach. *J. Biol. Chem.,* 251:7045–7052.
10. Cataland, S. (1978): Physiology of GIP in man. In: *Gut Hormones,* edited by S. R. Bloom, pp. 288–293. Churchill Livingstone, Edinburgh.
11. Christiansen, J., Rehfeld, J. F., and Stadil, F. (1976): Effect of intrajejunal fat on meal-stimulated acid and gastrin secretion in man. *Scand. J. Gastroent.,* 11:673–676.
12. Clain, J. E., Liang, V., and Malagelada, J. R. (1978): Inhibitory role of the distal small intestine on the gastric secretory response to meals in man. *Gastroenterology,* 74:704–707.
13. Ewald, C. A., and Boas, J. (1886): Beiträge zur Physiologie und Pathologie der Verdaunung. *Virchows Arch.,* 104:271–305.
14. Folkers, K., Chang, D., Humphries, J., Carraway, R., Leeman, S. E., and Bowers, C. J. (1976):

Synthesis and activities of neurotensin, and its acid and amide analogs: Possible natural occurence of (Gln⁴)-neurotensin. *Proc. Natl. Acad. Sci. USA,* 73:3833–3837.

15. Frigerio, B., Ravazola, M., Ito, S., Buffa, R., Capella, C., Solcia, E., and Orci, L. (1977): Histochemical and ultrastructural identification of neurotensin cells in the dog ileum. *Histochemistry,* 54:123–131.

16. Gregory, R. A. (1967): Enterogastrone—a reappraisal of the problem. In: *Gastric Secretion. Mechanisms and Control,* edited by T. S. Shnitka, J. A. L. Gilbert, and R. C. Harrison. Pergamon, New York.

17. Helmstaedter, V., Taugner, C. H., Feurle, G. E., and Forsmann, W. G. (1977): Localisation of neurotensinimmunoreactive cells in the small intestine of man and various mammals. *Histochemistry,* 53:35–41.

18. Kosaka, T., and Lim, R. K. S. (1930): Demonstration of the humoral agent in fat inhibition of gastric secretion. *Proc. Soc. Exp. Biol. NY,* 27:890–891.

19. Mashford, M. L., Nilsson, G., Rökaeus, Å., and Rosell, S. (1978): The effect of food ingestion on circulation neurotensin-like immunoreactivity (NTLI) in the human. *Acta Physiol. Scand.,* 104:244–246.

20. Mashford, M. L., Nilsson, G., Rökaeus, Å., and Rosell, S. (1978): Release of neurotensin-like immunoreactivity (NTLI) from the gut in anaesthetized dogs. *Acta Physiol. Scand.,* 104:375–376.

21. Orci, L., Baetens, O., Rufener, C., Brown, M., Vale, W., and Guillemin, R. (1976): Evidence for immunoreactive neurotensin in dog intestinal mucosa. *Life Sci.,* 19:559–562.

22. Polak, J. M., Sullivan, S. N., Bloom, S. R., Buchan, A. M. J., Facer, P., Beown, M. R., and Pearse, A. G. E. (1977): Specific localisation of neurotensin to the N cell in human intestine by radioimmunoassay and immunocytochemistry. *Nature,* 270:183–184.

23. Rosell, S., Burcher, E., Chang, D., and Folkers, K. (1976): Cardiovascular and metabolic actions of neurotensin and (Gln⁴)-neurotensin. *Acta Physiol. Scand.,* 98:484–491.

24. Rosell, S., and Rökaeus, Å. (1979): The effect of ingestion of amino acids, glucose and fat on circulating neurotensin-like immunoreactivity (NTLI) in man. *Acta Physiol. Scand.,* 107:263–267.

25. Rosell, S., Rökaeus, Å., Chang, D., and Folkers, K. (1978): Indirect vascular actions of (Gln⁴)-neurotensin in canine adipose tissue. *Acta Physiol. Scand.,* 102:143–147.

26. Sundler, F., Håkansson, R., Hammer, R. A., Alumets, J., Carraway, R., Leeman, S. E., and Zimmerman, E. A. (1977): Immunohistochemical localization of neurotensin in endocrine cells of the gut. *Cell Tiss. Res.,* 178:313–321.

27. Windsor, C. W. O., Cockel, R., and Lee, M. J. R. (1969): Inhibition of gastric secretion in man by intestinal fat infusion. *Gut,* 10:135–142.

Neuropeptides and Neural Transmission,
edited by C. Ajmone Marsan and W. Z. Traczyk.
Raven Press, New York © 1980.

Enkephalins, Endorphins, and Their Receptors

H. W. Kosterlitz

Unit for Research on Addictive Drugs, University of Aberdeen, Aberdeen AB9 1AS, Scotland

One of the significant advances made recently in our knowledge of the role played by the enkephalins and endorphins has been the recognition that there are two independent opioid peptidergic systems in the central nervous system. The first is represented by the small peptides, Met-enkephalin (β-lipotropin$_{61-65}$) and Leu-enkephalin (12), and is spread unevenly throughout the brain, spinal cord, and peripheral autonomic nervous system (6,11,21). The second system contains the larger β-endorphin (β-lipotropin$_{61-91}$) and extends from the hypothalamic-pituitary axis into the midline regions of the diencephalon and anterior pons (3,20,24). The presence of the opioid peptides in nerve terminals suggests that they may play a role of neurotransmitters or neuromodulators. This topical issue has recently been dealt with in several symposia, and, although this presentation follows closely that given at the *Second International Congress of the International Association for the Study of Pain* (13), new data have been taken into consideration.

INTERACTION OF OPIATES AND ENDOGENOUS OPIOID PEPTIDES WITH OPIATE RECEPTORS

The question arises of whether or not the two enkephalins and β-endorphin interact with one and the same receptor. The findings obtained with the opioid peptides in four parallel assays indicate that they interact with at least two receptors, the μ-receptor and the δ-receptor (14,16). In order to make a direct comparison between these results possible, the relative agonist potencies of the opioid peptides in the guinea-pig ileum and mouse vas deferens were expressed as multiples of the potency of Met-enkephalin in the mouse vas deferens and their potencies to inhibit ^{3}H-naltrexone and ^{3}H-Leu-enkephalin as multiples of the potency of Met-enkephalin to inhibit ^{3}H-Leu-enkephalin (Table 1). In the guinea-pig ileum, the potency of Met-enkephalin is only 11% of that in the mouse vas deferens; similarly, its potency to inhibit ^{3}H-naltrexone binding is only 18% of that to inhibit ^{3}H-Leu-enkephalin binding. Compared with Met-enkephalin, the potency of Leu-enkephalin is increased in the mouse vas deferens and lowered in the guinea-pig ileum; its affinity to the ^{3}H-Leu-enkephalin binding site is lowered only a little, but the decrease in affinity to the ^{3}H-naltrexone

TABLE 1. Assessment of the relative potencies of opioid peptides and morphine

Compound	Inhibition of contractions in:			Inhibition of binding of:		
	Mouse vas deferens	Guinea-pig ileum	Gpi/Mvd	^{3}H-Leu-enkephalin	^{3}H-naltrexone	Naltrexone/ Leu-enkephalin
Met-enkephalin	1	0.11	0.11	1	0.18	0.18
Leu-enkephalin	1.6	0.04	0.025	0.76	0.05	0.066
Morphine	0.03	0.19	6.3	0.01	0.07	7.0
Tyr-D-Ala^2-Gly-MePhe-Met(O)-ol	1.1	2.0	1.8	0.03	0.40	13.3
β-Endorphin	0.32	0.38	1.2	1.31	0.66	0.5
γ-Endorphin	0.46	0.05	0.11	0.02	0.01	0.5

The binding tests were performed at 0–4°C for 150 min to reduce enzymatic degradation (14,16).
From Kosterlitz et al., ref. 13, with permission.

binding site is reduced by 70%. When morphine is compared with the two enkephalins, it is more potent in the guinea-pig ileum and much less potent in the mouse vas deferens. This finding is mirrored by the very low affinity of morphine to the ³H-Leu-enkephalin binding site, whereas the affinity to the ³H-naltrexone binding site is of the same order of magnitude as that of the enkephalins.

β-Endorphin behaves very differently in these parallel assays, although the first five amino acids are identical with the sequence of Met-enkephalin (12). It is resistant to the action of exopeptidases but is cleaved by a lysosomal endopeptidase at residues 77–78 to give γ-endorphin (9). β-Endorphin is unique amongst the natural opioid peptides in that it is almost equipotent in the two pharmacological models and in the binding tests, respectively. This characteristic property may, at least in part, explain its high antinociceptive and other activities (7,8,15). On the other hand, γ-endorphin has only 1.5% of the binding affinity of β-endorphin, although it still is active in the mouse vas deferens and, to a lesser extent, in the guinea-pig ileum. In this context, it should be remembered that the binding assays were performed at 0 to 4°C while the two tissue models were maintained at 36 to 37°C.

PHARMACOLOGICAL PATTERN OF ENKEPHALIN ANALOGUES

Since the biological half-time of the two naturally occurring enkephalins is very short (10), many stable analogues with strong antinociceptive activity have been synthesized. It is important to know which alterations in the molecule are permissible without concomitant changes in the pattern of pharmacological activity. If in position 2 of Leu-enkephalin glycine was replaced by the synthetic amino acid D-Ala, the potencies in both guinea-pig ileum and mouse vas deferens were increased by factors of 14 and 7, respectively. Since the affinities to the ³H-naltrexone and ³H-Leu-enkephalin binding sites determined at 0°C were not significantly altered, this effect was most likely due to a decrease in the enzymatic degradation of the peptide in the pharmacological models maintained at 36 to 37°C. Replacement of L-Leu by D-Leu increased activity in the mouse vas deferens (2) without a major change in the affinity to the binding sites; on the other hand, the activity in the guinea-pig ileum was somewhat reduced. The pharmacological pattern was therefore still of the type characteristic of Leu-enkephalin, perhaps even to an exaggerated extent since the peptide was much more potent in the mouse vas deferens than in the guinea-pig ileum. This peptide has antinociceptive activity after injection into the cerebral ventricles (1). When the C-terminal amino acid residue of the enkephalins was replaced by amides of proline (22), the most important changes were an increase in potency in the guinea-pig ileum and an increase in the affinity for the ³H-naltrexone binding site with a simultaneous loss in affinity for the ³H-Leu-enkephalin binding site. Székely et al. (22) found that such compounds have antinociceptive activity after intravenous and subcutaneous injection. Another peptide of great interest is the Met-enkephalin analogue Tyr-D-Ala²-Gly-MePhe-Met(O)-ol (FK 33–824, Sandoz) introduced by Roemer et al. (19). It is about as potent as the enkephalins in the mouse vas deferens, but 20 times more potent in the guinea-pig ileum (Table 1). It has a very low affinity to the ³H-Leu-enkephalin binding site, but is more potent than Met-enkephalin at the ³H-naltrexone binding site. It therefore follows that this potent analogue has lost at least some of the characteristics of methionine-enkephalin and has become rather more like morphine. In a trial on human volunteers, non-morphine-like side-effects were observed after intramuscular injections of 0.025 to 1.2 mg, which gave peak plasma concentrations of 25 to 80 nM (23).

It has been stressed (16) that the low effectiveness of naloxone against the action of the naturally occuring opioid peptides in the mouse vas deferens is strong supporting evidence for the view that the receptors of the mouse vas deferens are different from the μ-receptors with which the classic opiates interact. It is likely that the δ-receptors of the mouse vas deferens are closely related to the ³H-Leu-enkephalin binding sites in the brain. However, the fact that the opioid peptides are active in the guinea-pig ileum and that their action is antagonized by naloxone as readily as that of morphine suggests that they can interact also with μ-receptors. If the view is correct that in the mouse vas deferens the enkephalins and endorphins interact preferentially with δ-receptors less sensitive to the antagonist effect of naloxone than the μ-receptors, then naloxone should be a weaker antagonist against enkephalin analogues which retain their enkephalin-like pharmacological pattern, as for instance Try-D-Ala-Gly-Phe-D-Leu, than against enkephalin analogues which are more morphine-like, as for instance Tyr-D-Ala-Gly-NH(CH₂)₂Ph or Tyr-D-Ala-Gly-MePhe-Met(O)-ol. The results obtained with several analogues are compatible with this concept. It has been found that, in the mouse vas deferens, the equilibrium dissociation constant (K_e) of naloxone against normorphine is about 2; the corresponding values against Met-enkephalin or β-endorphin are about 22 (16). Whereas the K_e value against Tyr-D-Ala-Gly-Phe-D-Leu, which has enkephalin-like properties, is 32, the corresponding value against the morphine-like enkephalin analogue for Tyr-D-Ala-Gly-MePhe-Met(O)-ol is 4.1 (14).

SPECIFIC PROTECTION OF μ- AND δ-RECEPTORS

Phenoxybenzamine has been found to cause a long-lasting inactivation of opiate receptors in homogenates of guinea-pig brain. Both μ- and δ-receptors are affected to the same extent. Table 2 shows that this effect is selectively prevented when, before the exposure to phenoxybenzamine, the homogenate is pre-incubated with ligands of high affinity to either the μ- or the δ-receptor binding site, dihydromorphine for the former on D-Ala²-D-Leu⁵-enkephalin for the latter. With D-Ala²-L-Leu⁵-enkephalin amide, which has high affinities to both binding sites, no selective protection has been observed (18).

TABLE 2. *Specific protection from the inactivating action of phenoxybenzamine (2.4 μM) on opiate receptors of homogenates of guinea-pig brain*

Protecting cold ligand	Protection (IC$_{50}$, nM) of binding of:	
	^{3}H-dihydromorphine (0.6nM)	^{3}H-D-Ala^2-D-Leu^5-enkephalin (1.4 nM)
Dihydromorphine	13.1 ± 3.2	90.5 ± 8.1
D-Ala^2-D-Leu^5-enkephalin	73.7 ± 12.8	4.6 ± 0.4
D-Ala^2-L-Leu^5-enkephalin amide	14.4 ± 2.0	5.5 ± 1.0

The values are the means $\pm$ SEM of 3–5 observations.
Modified from Robson and Kosterlitz, ref. 18.

POSSIBLE PHYSIOLOGICAL SIGNIFICANCE

Since our knowledge of the possible physiological functions of the opioid peptides is still very limited, great care has to be taken to avoid speculation for which the experimental basis is insecure. It is likely that the peptides will mimic the actions of morphine, such as limitation of experience of pain, euphoric changes of mood, depression of respiration, changes in the extrapyramidal motor system, and constipation. Although it is not possible at present to allocate different physiological functions to the different peptides and to the receptors represented by the enkephalin and naltrexone binding sites, it is likely that the various peptides, the long-chain endorphins and short-chain enkephalins, may subserve different physiological functions. This concept may have its structural basis on the apparent independence of the enkephalin and endorphin systems (3).

The naturally occurring Met- and Leu-enkephalins are poor antinociceptive agents, even after injection into the cerebral ventricles or directly into the brain substance, because they are rapidly inactivated by peptidases. Enzyme-resistant analogues such as D-Ala^2-Met-enkephalin amide, N-CH$_3$-Tyr^1-Met-enkephalin amide, and particularly the Pro^5 analogues and FK 33–824, are potent antinociceptive peptides (7,8,17,19,22). It is not clear yet how far the antinociceptive effect is correlated with affinity to the naltrexone or enkephalin binding sites. In this context, it is of interest that, after injection into the cerebral ventricles of rats, D-Ala^2-D-Leu^5-enkephalin (Wellcome), which has a high affinity to δ-receptors and a low one to μ-receptors, has only 1% (Bläsig and Herz, *personal communication*) of the antinociceptive activity of D-Ala^2-MePhe^4-Met(O)-ol^5-enkephalin (Sandoz), whose affinity to the μ-receptors is as high as that of the Wellcome analogue to the δ-receptor. As a corollary, the affinity of the Sandoz compound to the δ-receptors is as low as that of the Wellcome compound to the μ-receptors. It is therefore possible that the μ-receptors are more important for antinociceptive effects than the δ-receptors. β-Endorphin may owe its high antinociceptive potency to the fact that it binds equally well to μ-receptors and δ-receptors. This interpretation would go a long way to explain the difficulty experienced by many observers to obtain a hyperalgesic effect in normal animals with naloxone.

Although the longer-chain peptides are resistant to the action of exopeptidases, their antinociceptive potencies vary greatly. β-Endorphin or C fragment is the most potent of these peptides; its antinociceptive effect after injection into the cerebral ventricles has been found to be greater than that of morphine (4,5,7,8, 15,17). The effect of β-endorphin is long-lasting as is that of the enzyme-resistant enkephalin analogues, in contrast to the transient effects of the naturally occurring enkephalins. Since the onset of action of the natural enkephalins is rapid and the action is readily terminated enzymatically, they are good candidates for a possible role of inhibitory neurotransmitters or neuromodulators, and thus limit the experience of excessive sudden pain rather than act as analgesics.

CONCLUSIONS

The evidence presented in this chapter indicates that the opioid peptidergic system is complex. The three agonists, Met-enkephalin, Leu-enkephalin, and β-endorphin have different pharmacological patterns. It may be of particular importance that they vary in their relative affinities to the enkephalin and naltrexone binding sites in the brain; the former are probably related to δ-receptors prevalent in the mouse vas deferens, and the latter to μ-receptors prevalent in the guinea-pig. It is possible that μ-receptors are more important for the mediation of analgesic effects than δ-receptors.

ACKNOWLEDGMENTS

Supported by grants from the Medical Research Council, the National Institute on Drug Abuse (DA 00662), and the Committee on Problems of Drug Dependence.

REFERENCES

1. Baxter, M. G., Goff, D., Miller, A. A., and Saunder, I. A. (1977): Effect of a potent synthetic opioid pentapeptide in some antinociceptive and behavioural tests in mice and rats. *Br. J. Pharmacol.,* 59:455–456P.
2. Beddell, C. R., Clark, R. B., Hardy, G. W., Lowe, L. A., Ubatuba, F. B., Vane, J. R., Wilkinson, S., Chang, K.-J., Cuatrecasas, P., and Miller, R. J. (1977): Structural requirements for opioid activity of analogues of the enkephalins. *Proc. Roy. Soc. Lond. (Biol.),* 198:249–265.
3. Bloom, F., Battenberg, E., Rossier, J., Ling, N., and Guillemin, R. (1978): Neurons containing β-endorphin in rat brain exist separately from those containing enkephalin: Immunocytochemical studies. *Proc. Natl. Acad. Sci. USA,* 75:1591–1595.
4. Bradbury, A. F., Feldberg, W., Smyth, D. G., and Snell, C. R. (1976): Lipotropin C-fragment: An endogenous peptide with potent analgesic activity. In: *Opiates and Endogenous Opioid Peptides,* edited by H. W. Kostelitz, pp. 9–17. North-Holland, Amsterdam.
5. Bradbury, A. F., Smyth, D. G., Snell, C. R., Deakin, J. F. W., and Wendlandt, S. (1977): Comparison of the analgesic properties of lipotropin C-fragment and stabilized enkephalins in the rat. *Biochem. Biophys. Res. Commun.,* 74:748–754.
6. Elde, R., Hökfelt, T., Johansson, O., and Terenius, L. (1976): Immunohistochemical studies

using antibodies to leucine-enkephalin: Initial observations on the nervous system of the rat. *Neuroscience,* 1:349–351.

7. Feldberg, W., and Smyth. D. G. (1977): Analgesia produced in cats by the C-fragment of lipotropin and by a synthetic pentapeptide. *J. Physiol. (Lond.),* 265:25–27P.
8. Feldberg, W., and Smyth, D. G. (1977): C-fragment of lipotropin—an endogenous potent analgesic peptide. *Br. J. Pharmacol.,* 60:445–453.
9. Gráf, L., and Kenessey, A. (1976): Specific cleavage of a single peptide bond (residues 77–78) in β-lipotropin by a pituitary endopeptidase. *FEBS Lett.,* 69:255–260.
10. Hambrook, J. M., Morgan, B. A., Rance, M. J., and Smith, C. F. C. (1976): Mode of deactivation of the enkephalins by rat and human plasma and rat brain homogenates. *Nature,* 262:782–783.
11. Hughes, J., Kosterlitz, H. W., and Smith, T. W. (1977): The distribution of methionine-enkephalin and leucine-enkephalin in the brain and peripheral tissues. *Br. J. Pharmacol.,* 61:639–647.
12. Hughes, J., Smith, T. W., Kosterlitz, H. W., Fothergill, L. A., Morgan, B. A., and Morris, H. R. (1975): Identification of two related pentapeptides from the brain with potent opiate agonist activity. *Nature,* 258:577–579.
13. Kosterlitz, H. W. (1979): Interaction of endogenous opioid peptides and their analogs with opiate receptors. In: *Advances in Pain Research and Therapy, Vol. 3,* edited by J. J. Bonica J. C. Liebeskind, and D. G. Albe-Fessard, pp. 377–384. Raven Press, New York.
14. Kosterlitz, H. W., Lord, J. A. H., Paterson, S. J., and Waterfield, A. A. (1980): Effects of changes in the structure of enkephalins and narcotic analgesic drugs on their interactions with μ-receptors and δ-receptors. *Br. J. Pharmacol.,* 68:333–342.
15. Loh, H. H., Tseng, L. F., Wei, E., and Li, C. H. (1976): β-Endorphin as a potent analgesic agent. *Proc. Natl. Acad. Sci. USA,* 73:2895–2898.
16. Lord, J. A. H., Waterfield, A. A., Hughes, J., and Kosterlitz, H. W. (1977): Endogenous opioid peptides: Multiple agonists and receptors. *Nature,* 267:495–499.
17. Pert, A. (1976): Behavioural pharmacology of D-alanine²-methionine-enkephalin amide and other long-lasting opiate peptides. In:*Opiates and Endogenous Opioid Peptides,* edited by H. W. Kosterlitz, pp. 87–94. North-Holland, Amsterdam.
18. Robson, L. E., and Kosterlitz, H. W. (1979): Specific protection of the binding sites of D-Ala²-D-Leu⁵-enkephalin (δ-receptors) and dihydromorphine (μ-receptors). *Proc. Roy. Soc. Lond. (Biol.),* 205:425–432.
19. Roemer, D., Buescher, H. H., Hill, R. C., Pless, J., Bauer, W., Cardinaux, F., Closse, A., Hauser, D., and Huguenin, R. (1977): A synthetic enkephalin with prolonged parenteral and oral analgesic activity. *Nature,* 268:547–549.
20. Rossier, J., Vargo, T. M., Minick, S., Ling, N., Bloom, F. E., and Guillemin, R. (1977): Regional dissociation of β-endorphin and enkephalin contents in rat brain and pituitary. *Proc. Natl. Acad. Sci. USA,* 74:5162–5165.
21. Simantov, R., Kuhar, M. J., Uhl, G. R., and Snyder, S. H. (1977): Opioid peptide enkephalins: Immunohistochemical mapping in the rat central nervous system. *Proc. Natl. Acad. Sci. USA,* 74:2167–2171.
22. Székely, J. I., Rónai, A. Z., Dunai-Kovács, Z., Miglécz, E., Bertzétri, I., Bajusz, S., and Gráf, L. (1977): (D-Met²,Pro⁵)-Enkephalin amide: A potent morphine-like analgesic. *Eur. J. Pharmacol.,* 43:293–294.
23. Von Graffenried, B., del Pozo, E., Roubicek, J., Krebs, E., Pöldinger, W., Burmeister, P., and Kerp, L. (1978): Effects of the synthetic enkephalin analogue FK 33–824 in Man. *Nature,* 272:729–730.
24. Watson, S. J. and Barchas, J. D. (1979): Anatomy of the endogenous opioid peptides and related substances: the enkephalins, β-endorphin, β-lipotropin and ACTH. In: *Mechanisms of Pain and Analgesic Compounds,* edited by R. F. Beers and E. G. Bassett, pp. 227–237. Raven Press, New York.

Neuropeptides and Neural Transmission,
edited by C. Ajmone Marsan and W. Z. Traczyk.
Raven Press, New York © 1980.

Opioid Peptides as Inhibitory Neurotransmitters Acting on Sensory Neurones in the Rat Medulla

R. G. Hill

*Department of Pharmacology, University of Bristol Medical School,
Bristol BS8 1TD, United Kingdom*

It is well established that electrical stimulation of specific sites in the brain, electroacupuncture, and transcutaneous nerve stimulation can all produce analgesia in man and cause antinociception in animals (17,19). The mechanisms underlying these observations are still only partially understood in spite of the large number of experimental studies that have been performed in the last decade; but it is reasonable to suppose, where central mechanisms are involved, that the end result in each case is either to prevent the excitation or to cause the inhibition of those relay neurones that are normally excited after a noxious stimulus. The observation that stimulus-evoked analgesia is usually attenuated by administration of naloxone (1,17) leads to the assumption that endorphins are involved in the type of process described above, and there is now a great deal of biochemical and histochemical evidence (8,13,20,23) for the presence of enkephalin-containing neurones and nerve terminals in sensory nuclei of the rat brain. However, there is little objective evidence for a specific inhibitory transmitter function for these substances. This problem has been investigated by searching for synaptic inhibitions of neurones in the rat caudal medulla that are reversed by the specific opiate antagonist naloxone.

METHODS

All experiments were performed in adult albino rats anaesthetized with halothane (1–1.5%) or urethane (0.5 ml/25% wt/vol solution per 100 g body weight) and prepared for recording from the caudal medulla as previously described (17). Single or multibarrelled micropipettes, for extracellular action potential recording and application of drugs, were inserted perpendicular to the surface of the medulla, caudal to the obex, using a motor driven hydraulic micromanipulator. Penetrations were made between 0.5 and 1.5 mm lateral to the midline in order to locate neurones in the dorsal column (cuneate and gracile) nuclei and nucleus reticularis ventralis (NRV), and were made between 1.5 mm lateral and the lateral borders of the exposed medulla to locate trigeminal caudalis neurones. When neurones were encountered, they were identified by their responses to natural adequate stimuli applied to appropriate locations on the body surface. Anatomical positions of the neurones, from which recordings were made, were obtained from reconstruction of electrode tracks in transverse sections of the formalin-fixed medulla, and this procedure was facilitated by making dye spots during the experiment with pontamine sky blue expelled from the micropipette by iontophoresis.

Conventional five- or six-barrelled micropipettes were constructed from borosilicate glass tubing with an integral fibre, as previously described (12). Recording barrels of all pipettes were filled with 4 M NaCl solution, or in some experiments 2.5% pontamine sky blue (G. T. Gurr Ltd.) in 0.2 M sodium acetate buffer at pH 5.6. One peripheral barrel of multibarrelled pipettes always contained 1 M NaCl for automatic current neutralization and to provide a return path for the iontophoresis currents. Drug barrels of the pipettes contained combinations of glutamic acid (Sigma, 0.5 M, pH 8.5), gamma-aminobutyric acid (GABA) (Sigma, 0.5 M, pH 3.5), morphine sulphate (Macfarlan Smith, 50 mM), met-enkephalin hydrochloride (Burroughs Wellcome, 8 mM), and naloxone hydrochloride (Endo, 50 mM).

Solutions of the GABA antagonists picrotoxin and bicuculline (12) and of naloxone were prepared in normal saline and used for systemic injection.

Natural stimuli classed as noxious included immersion of the tail in water at 50 to 55°C (18), pinching folds of skin with toothed forceps, and firm pressure with a needle (4). Non-noxious stimuli included deflection of vibrissae and hairs with an oscillating air jet, stroking, and tapping.

Attempts were made in some experiments to duplicate the peripheral electrical stimulation conditions used in studies on behavioral analgesia (23) when rectangular pulses were delivered from an isolated stimulator to pairs of needle electrodes inserted subcutaneously.

RESULTS

Direct Effects of Exogenous Opioids

Met-enkephalin (20–100 nA) depressed the spontaneous and glutamate-evoked firing of all neurones to which it was applied (10 in the cuneate and gracile nuclei, 20 in trigeminal nucleus caudalis, and 17 in NRV). Morphine was not applied to any cuneate or gracile neurones, but when applied with currents of 10 to 75 nA, depressed 17 of 18 trigeminal nucleus caudalis neurones and excited the remaining one. In NRV, morphine (10–50 nA) was applied to 8 neurones, exciting 5 and depressing 3. Similar excitant effects of morphine have been reported for other reticular formation neurones. Depressant effects of the opioids were reversed by naloxone (10–40 nA), although direct depressant effects of the antagonist predominated on some neurones in all three areas.

As reported earlier (10), met-enkephalin had no effect on the synaptic excitation of cuneate neurones and had a similar lack of effect on that of most low-threshold trigeminal neurones. Met-enkephalin or morphine did, however, reduce the synaptic excitation of polymodal and high-threshold trigeminal neurones, as described by other workers in the cat trigeminal (2). In NRV, met-enkephalin reduced the excitatory effects of noxious peripheral stimuli, and this effect was reversible with naloxone. These results will be reported in detail elsewhere, but it is noteworthy that neurones in all three areas were depressed by met-enkephalin for although the trigeminal nucleus caudalis contains dense fibre and terminal immunofluorescence for this peptide and there are smaller amounts in NRV, the dorsal column nuclei do not appear to contain any (20,22). It is therefore not possible to use sensitivity to opioids as a criterion in order to determine which neurones are likely to be inhibited by synaptically released endorphins. Accordingly, synaptic inhibition of neurones in all three areas was challenged with naloxone, applied iontophoretically or injected systemically.

Synaptic Inhibition in Dorsal Column Nuclei

Seven neurones were studied, four in the cuneate nucleus and three in the gracile, and all were excited by air jet hair deflection or brushing within a restricted receptive field on the ipsilateral fore or hind limbs, respectively. Electrical stimulation within the receptive field, using subcutaneous needle electrodes produced a burst of action potentials at a short latency, followed by inhibition lasting between 50 and 100 msec. Five neurones showed no response to noxious stimuli applied inside or outside their receptive fields, the remaining two being inhibited by such stimuli. All inhibitions studied were resistant to intravenously administered naloxone in doses up to 10 mg/kg, but in three neurones subsequent administration of bicuculline (0.2 mg/kg) or picrotoxin (1.5–3.0 mg/kg) clearly reduced the inhibition.

Synaptic Inhibition in Trigeminal Nucleus Caudalis and Associated Reticular Nuclei

Nine polymodal neurones (2,4) with receptive fields on the face and located within the main body of the trigeminal nucleus or within the closely adjacent reticular formation (nucleus reticularis dorsalis or parvocellularis) (4) were studied. Inhibitions were evoked either by electrical stimulation via subcutaneous electrodes or by noxious stimulation outside the excitatory receptive field. The neurone illustrated in Fig. 1 represents an example of this latter group. Pressure with a needle or pinching with toothed forceps within quite a small area of the face produced a marked inhibition of the firing of this neurone. Intravenous naloxone in a dose of 1 mg/kg failed to modify this inhibitory response, even though repeated administration up to a total dose of 5 mg/kg was made.

Figure 2 shows the responses of a second cell, this time having a very wide inhibitory receptive field encompassing the entire ipsilateral face. Electrical stimulation of the tooth pulp of one upper incisor also inhibited this neurone and

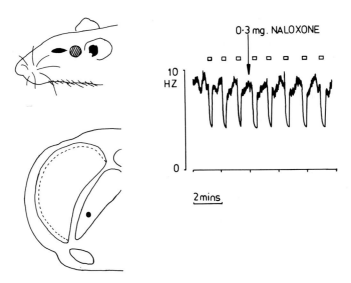

FIG. 1. Responses of a polymodal trigeminal neurone that was excited by both noxious and non-noxious stimulation applied to the mysticial pad. Pressure on, or pinching of, the *hatched area* shown in the outline of the rat's face strongly inhibited the firing of this neurone. The neurone was shown, from subsequent histology, to be located within the nucleus reticularis parvocellularis (indicated by the *filled circle* on the diagram of the medulla), but its characteristics were identical with those of neurones located within the main trigeminal nucleus caudalis. The analogue rate meter trace on the right of the figure shows the response of this neurone to pressure with a needle on the inhibitory receptive field, the stimulus being applied for the duration of the open bars above the record. Intravenous injection of naloxone 0.3 mg (1 mg/kg) failed to modify this inhibitory response as did subsequent doses (not illustrated) up to a total of 5 mg/kg.

this can be readily seen in the post-stimulus time histograms. Following the intravenous injection of 3 mg/kg naloxone, the inhibitory response of this neurone was unchanged. Subsequent injection of picrotoxin (1.5 mg/kg) halved the duration of the inhibitory response, however.

These results were typical and antagonism of inhibition by naloxone was not seen on any of these trigeminal neurones; but on the three neurones tested with picrotoxin (1.5–2.0 mg/kg) and the two tested with bicuculline (0.2–0.3 mg/kg), attenuation of the inhibition was always apparent.

Synaptic Inhibition in NRV

The properties of neurones in this nucleus were recently described (5,18) and subsequent investigation of a total of 230 neurones confirms the conclusions of this report. Our observation that some neurones in this nucleus were inhibited by noxious peripheral stimulation and that these inhibitions were reversed by intravenous naloxone, has now been confirmed in a detailed study of 20 neurones that showed strong and reproducible inhibition following noxious peripheral

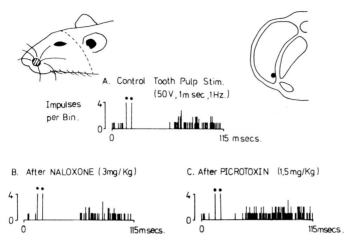

FIG. 2. Responses of a second polymodal trigeminal neurone (located within the main nucleus caudalis), that was excited by noxious pressure applied within the *hatched area* on the diagram of the rat's face and was also excited by displacement of the vibrissae with an air jet. Noxious stimulation over a large area of the face (shown by the *dotted line*) inhibited the firing of this neurone as did electrical stimulation of the pulp of one upper incisor. The inhibition produced by tooth pulp stimulation is displayed in post-stimulus time histograms **(A–C)** constructed over 32 sweeps, and in these records the stimulus artifacts are shown by dots above the histograms. **A** shows the control response and **B** the unchanged response 10 min after the intravenous injection of naloxone (3 mg/kg). **C** shows that following the injection of picrotoxin, a GABA antagonist (1.5 mg/kg), the inhibition was much reduced.

stimulation. Of the 20 neurones studied, 17 showed either attenuation or complete antagonism of the inhibition with doses of naloxone between 0.5 and 10 mg/kg, the responses of one neurone are illustrated in Fig. 3. No excitatory receptive field was detected for this neurone, but a variety of intense stimuli applied to a wide area of the body surface strongly inhibited its firing. The responses shown indicate the inhibitory responses to pressure with a needle to the ipsilateral face, pinching of the ipsilateral hind paw, and distention of the vagina with a blunt probe. Following the intraperitoneal administration of 0.5 mg/kg naloxone, these responses were all attenuated.

On five further NRV neurones inhibited by noxious peripheral stimulation, microiontophoretic application of naloxone (10–40 nA) was used in an attempt to block the inhibition, and a reduction in the size of the inhibitory response was seen in three neurones, although the effects were less marked than with systemic naloxone.

Four neurones were found on which a different type of inhibitory response occurred. These neurones all showed strong excitatory responses to noxious stimulation, but repetitive electrical stimulation outside the excitatory receptive field reduced the size of this response without causing a depression of the background firing rate of the neurone. Electrical stimulation was effective when stimulus parameters similar to those used to produce behavioural analgesia were

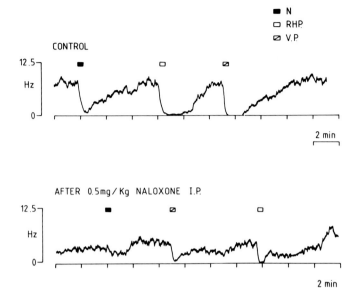

FIG. 3. Analogue rate meter records of the firing of a neurone located within NRV. No excitatory receptive field could be identified for this neurone, but noxious stimuli applied to a wide area of the body produced a long-lasting inhibition. The responses illustrated were produced by pressure with a needle to the ipsilateral face (N), pinching of the ipsilateral hind paw (RHP), and distention of the vagina with a blunt probe (VP); the duration of the stimuli is indicated by the *bars* above the record. Following the injection of naloxone (0.5 mg/kg i.p.) 15 min previously, these inhibitory responses were much reduced and this was more evident on the duration of the response than on the maximum depression achieved.

used (23), and stimulation had to be applied for 5 to 30 min before it reduced the size of the nociceptive response. Figure 4 illustrates the responses of a neurone that was excited by a noxious pinch applied to the ipsilateral hind paw, but showed a reduction in the size of this nociceptive response after 25 min electrical stimulation of the contralateral hindpaw. Some 10 to 12 min after discontinuing the electrical stimulation the nociceptive responses returned to their original size. Figure 5 shows the effect of iontophoretic naloxone on the responses of this neurone. The electrical stimulation was commenced 10 min before the start of the record illustrated and produced a reduction in the size of the nociceptive response. Iontophoretic application of naloxone 20 nA reversed the effects of the electrical stimulation and, on removal of the stimulus, some enhancement of the nociceptive response was seen. On removal of the naloxone current the control response returned to its initial size. Two of the four neurones of this type studied so far showed a reduction in the conditioning effect of repetitive electrical stimulation with currents of naloxone of between 10 and 40 nA, the others being unaffected.

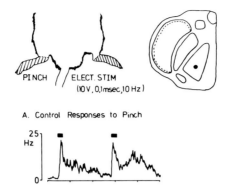

A. Control Responses to Pinch

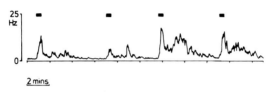

B. Responses after 25 mins Electrical Stim. to Contralateral Paw.

2 mins

FIG. 4. Analogue rate meter records of another neurone located in NRV. The position of this neurone within the nucleus is shown on the diagram of a transverse section of caudal medulla. Pinching the ipsilateral hind paw (indicated by the *filled bars* above the record) produced a long duration excitation of this neurone (record **A**), and when repetitive electrical stimulation of the contralateral hind paw was maintained for about 25 min, a reduction in the size of the response was seen (the stimulus being discontinued just before the start of record **B**). The inhibitory effect was maintained for about 10 min after the end of the stimulus and then responses returned to their control amplitude.

DISCUSSION

The lack of response of synaptic inhibition in the dorsal column nuclei to naloxone is not unexpected, as there is no evidence for the presence of enkephalin-containing terminals or cell bodies in this area (20,22). These negative responses do serve, however, to confirm that, in the doses used, naloxone is not producing a non-specific blockade of synaptic inhibition operated by other neurotransmitters such as GABA (6).

It is surprising, however, that evidence for naloxone-sensitive synaptic inhibition could not be obtained in the trigeminal nucleus caudalis where met-enkephalin containing terminals and perikarya are abundant (20,22), but it should be noted that other workers have failed to demonstrate naloxone-sensitive inhibition (7) in the dorsal horn of the spinal cord where a similar distribution of met-enkephalin and opiate receptors is found (3,20). One possibility not tested in our experiments is that the met-enkephalin neurones in the trigeminal complex may only be able to be activated by central stimulation, but evidence in the

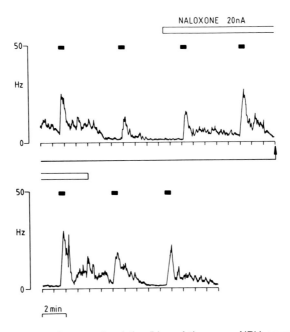

FIG. 5. Analogue rate meter records of the firing of the same NRV neurone illustrated in Fig. 4. Pinching of the ipsilateral hind paw is indicated by the *filled bars* above the record, and electrical stimulation (10 V, 0.1 msec, 10 Hz) of the contralateral hind paw, which was commenced 10 min. before the start of the record, is indicated by the *continuous line* below the trace. A clear reduction in the size of the response to pinching was obtained and then naloxone, 20 nA *(open bar)*, was applied to the neurone. This antagonized the effects of the electrical stimulation and on discontinuing the stimulation an enhanced nociceptive response was evident. Control responses were recovered when the naloxone application was ended.

literature suggests that descending inhibition in the dorsal horn seems more likely to operate by monoamine pathways than by endorphins (9,17,20). The type of experiment described in this chapter would not detect inhibitions that were exclusively presynaptic, and it may be that in the rat trigeminal nucleus caudalis the physiological role of met-enkephalin is at this site. This suggestion is supported by the observations that the release of substance P, the putative neurotransmitter in unmyelinated nociceptive fibres, from trigeminal nucleus slices is blocked by met-enkephalin (14), and that opiate receptors are concentrated on primary afferent terminals (15).

In NRV, although met-enkephalin concentrations are patchy (20,22) and precise details of distribution of the peptide vary slightly from one research group to another, it is clear that fibres containing the peptide are present particularly on the lateral border of the nucleus. The demonstration of naloxone-sensitive synaptic inhibition in this area provides a functional role for these fibres, but the physiological significance of this nucleus is still not clear and can only be explored when more details of its input pathways and projections are obtained.

It is noteworthy that the inhibitory effects seen on the majority of these neurones needed stimuli of noxious intensity to evoke them; this is consistent with clinical findings that the endorphin systems only produce a level of analgesia when a certain basal level of noxious stimulus is present (16).

Those inhibitions in NRV that produce a pronounced depression in the background firing rate of the neurone seem likely to be postsynaptic (24,25) and may reflect the action of endogenous opioid at the receptors where iontophoretic met-enkephalin acts to depress these neurones. The neurones that show conditioning of their nociceptive responses by repetitive electrical stimulation may reflect a presynaptic action of opioids in this area (21) as background firing rates are not affected.

The finding that, on some neurones in NRV, inhibitions could be reduced by iontophoretic application of naloxone suggests that synaptically released endorphins are acting locally within NRV, but the possibility that systemic naloxone may not be acting within NRV, but remotely, is still present and it should be noted that the effects of iontophoretic naloxone were short of complete block of the inhibition.

In conclusion, this examination of synaptic inhibitory processes in the sensory nuclei of the rat caudal medulla has shown that the inhibition of dorsal column nuclei and trigeminal nucleus caudalis neurones by peripheral stimuli was not sensitive to blockade by the opiate antagonist naloxone, but was reduced by the GABA antagonists picrotoxin and bicuculline. The significance of the abundant met-enkephalin present within the trigeminal nucleus caudalis therefore remains to be explained. Naloxone-sensitive inhibitions were located, however, within the ventral reticular nucleus of the medulla, and provide a role for the met-enkephalin containing fibres present within parts of this nucleus. The physiological significance of the wide receptive field neurones within this nucleus will remain obscure until more information on its synaptic connections with other areas is obtained.

ACKNOWLEDGMENTS

I am grateful to Susan Ayliffe and M. L. Mayer for allowing me to use results obtained in our collaborative experiments. Thanks are due to S. Stoter and A. Duncan for skilled technical assistance, and to Endo Laboratories for the gift of naloxone and to Wellcome Research Laboratories for the gift of met-enkephalin. This research was supported by grants from the Wellcome Trust and Royal Society.

REFERENCES

1. Akil, H., Mayer, D. J., and Liebeskind, J. S. (1976): Reduction of stimulation-produced analgesia by the narcotic antagonist naloxone. *Science,* 191:961–962.
2. Andersen, R. K., Lund, J. P., and Puil, E. (1977): The effects of iontophoretic applications of morphine and putative neurotransmitters on neurons of the trigeminal nuclei oralis and

caudalis. In: *Pain in the Trigeminal Region,* edited by B. Anderson and D. Matthews, pp. 271–284. Elsevier/North Holland, Amsterdam.

3. Atweh, S. F., and Kuhar, M. J. (1977): Autoradiographic localization of opiate receptors in rat brain. I. Spinal cord and lower medulla. *Brain Res.,* 124:53–67.
4. Ayliffe, S. J., and Hill, R. G. (1979): Responses of cells in the trigeminal subnucleus caudalis of the rat to noxious stimuli. *J. Physiol.* (Lond.), 287:18–19P.
5. Benjamin, R. M. (1970): Single neurones in the rat medulla responsive to nociceptive stimulation. *Brain Res.,* 24:525–529.
6. Dingledine, R. (1977): Naloxone as a GABA antagonist. In: *Iontophoresis and Transmitter Mechanisms in the Mammalian CNS,* edited by R. W. Ryall and J. S. Kelly, pp. 314–316. Elsevier, Amsterdam.
7. Duggan, A. W., and Griersmith, B. T. (1979): Inhibition of the spinal transmission of nociceptive information by supraspinal stimulation in the cat. *Pain,* 6:149–161.
8. Elde, R., Hökfelt, T., Johnsson, O., and Terenius, L. (1976): Immunohistochemical studies using antibodies to leucine-enkephalin, initial observations on the nervous system of the rat. *Neuroscience,* 1:349–361.
9. Headley, P. M., Duggan, A. W., and Griersmith, B. T. (1978): Selective reduction by noradrenaline and 5-hydroxytryptamine of nociceptive responses of cat dorsal horn neurones. *Brain Res.,* 145:185–189.
10. Hill, R. G., and Pepper, C. M. (1978): Selective effects of morphine on the nociceptive responses of thalamic neurones in the rat. *Br. J. Pharmacol.,* 64:137–143.
11. Hill, R. G., Pepper, C. M., and Mitchell, J. F. (1976): The depressant action of iontophoretically applied met-enkephalin on single neurones in rat brain. In: *Opiates and Endogenous Opioid Peptides,* edited by H. W. Kosterlitz, pp. 225–230. Elsevier/North Holland, Amsterdam.
12. Hill, R. G., Simmonds, M. A., and Straughan, D. W. (1976): Antagonism of γ-aminobutyric acid and glycine by convulsants in the cuneate nucleus of cat. *Br. J. Pharmacol.,* 56:9–19.
13. Hökfelt, T., Ljungdahl, A., Terenius, L., Elde, R., and Nilsson, G. (1977): Immunohistochemical analysis of peptide pathways possibly related to pain and analgesia: Enkephalin and substance P. *Proc. Natl. Acad. Sci. USA,* 74:3081–3085.
14. Jessel, T. M., and Iversen, L. L. (1977): Opiate analgesics inhibit substance P release from rat trigeminal nucleus. *Nature,* 268:549–551.
15. La Motte, C., Pert, C. B., and Snyder, S. H. (1976): Opiate receptor binding in primate spinal cord; distribution and changes after dorsal root section. *Brain Res.,* 112:407–412.
16. Levine, J. D., Gordon, N. C., and Fields, H. L. (1979): Naloxone dose dependently produces analgesia and hyperalgesia in post-operative pain. *Nature,* 278:740–741.
17. Mayer, D. L., and Price, D. D. (1977): Central nervous system mechanisms and analgesia. *Pain,* 2:379–404.
18. Mayer, M. L, and Hill, R. G. (1978): The effects of intravenous fentanyl, morphine and naloxone on nociceptive responses of neurones in the rat caudal medulla. *Neuropharmacology,* 17:533–539.
19. Reynolds, D. V. (1969): Surgery in the rat during electrical analgesia induced by focal brain stimulation. *Science,* 164:444–445.
20. Sar, M., Stumpf, W. E., Miller, R. J., Chang, K.-J., and Cuatrecasas, P. (1978): Immunohistochemical localization of enkephalin in rat brain and spinal cord. *J. Comp. Neurol.,* 182:17–38.
21. Sastry, B. R. (1979): Presynaptic effects of morphine and methionine-enkephalin in feline spinal cord. *Neuropharmacology,* 18:367:375.
22. Uhl, G. R., Goodman, R. R., Kuhar, M. J., Childers, S. R., and Snyder, S. H. (1979): Immunohistochemical mapping of enkephalin containing cell bodies, fibres and nerve terminals in the brain stem of the rat. *Brain Res.,* 166:75–94.
23. Woolf, C. J., Barrett, G. D., Mitchell, D., and Myers, R. A. (1977): Naloxone-reversible peripheral electroanalgesia in intact and spinal rats. *Eur. J. Pharmacol.,* 45:311–314.
24. Zieglgänsberger, W., and Bayerl, H. (1976): The mechanism of inhibition of neuronal activity by opiates in the spinal cord of cat. *Brain Res.,* 115:111–128.
25. Zieglgänsberger, W., and Tulloch, I. F. (1979): The effects of methionine-and leucine-enkephalin on spinal neurones of the cat. *Brain Res.,* 167:53–64.

Neuropeptides and Neural Transmission,
edited by C. Ajmone Marsan and W. Z. Traczyk.
Raven Press, New York © 1980.

Metabolism of Enkephalins and Endorphins

Tadeusz Lesław Chruściel

Institute for Drug Research and Control, Chełmska Strasse, PL-00725 Warszawa, Poland

The endogenous peptide structure responsible for morphine-like activity is Tyr-Gly-Gly-Phe-(X), where X is a hydrophobic amino acid such as methionine (in Met-enkephalin) or leucine (in Leu-enkephalin). This amino acid sequence occurs also in β-lipoprotein (LPH) as sequence LPH_{61-65}. All fragments of LPH commencing with residues 61-65 have opioid activity to some extent: However, peak activity is seen with the C-terminal fragment of β-LPH, β-endorphin (LPH_{61-91}).

There is now evidence that a family of related lipotropin/corticotropin hypophysis intermediate lobe peptides are derived from a common glycoprotein precursor pro-opiocortin, a glycosylated peptide of molecular weight 30,000. Thus, pro-opiocortin contains a number of potentially active molecules and the knowledge of its cleavage mechanisms is of considerable importance (20). Relatively little is yet known of the controlling and inactivating mechanisms and of the enzymes responsible for pro-opiocortin sequence cleavage. Much more is known about the enkephalins.

A weak and transient analgesia upon intracerebroventricular administration and the relative lack of analgesic activity following systemic injection of natural enkephalins (3,5,17) has been attributed to their rapid metabolism.

Hughes (19) observed a complete loss of inhibition of neurally evoked contractions of the mouse vas deferens and guinea-pig mesenteric plexus when 5 μg equivalents of the purified brain extract, containing natural enkephalins, were incubated with carboxypeptidase A for 10 min, or leucine aminopeptidase for 20 min. It was found that a 50% inactivation occurred in 70 ± 10 sec with carboxypeptidase (2 units/ml) and in 190 ± 20 sec with leucine aminopeptidase (20 μg/ml). The boiled enzymes had no effect on the brain extract and the inactivation was completely prevented at 0°C. Supernatant preparations from guinea-pig myenteric plexus and mouse vas deferens homogenates exhibited marked inactivating activity. Hughes (19) has also shown that direct addition of carboxypeptidase (4 units/ml) or leucine aminopeptidase (30 μg/ml) to the organ bath reversed the inhibitory action of morphine or normorphine.

Similarly, Hambrook et al. (18) have shown, using the depressant effect of the enkephalins on the electrically evoked contractions of the mouse vas deferens as a bioassay, that the half-life of both Met-enkephalin and Leu-enkephalin in rat plasma was very short. The breakdown of the enkephalins takes place also very rapidly in the presence of rat brain homogenates: ^{3}H-Tyr-Leu^5-enkephalin (10^{-7} M) was completely destroyed within 1 min at 37°C in a homogenate of whole rat brain containing approximately 3 mg protein/ml. The mode of deactivation seems to be identical with that observed in plasma for both enkephalins. Enkephalins are indeed rapidly metabolized *in vitro* in plasma (18) and in brain membrane preparations (24,27). Half-lives of 2 min or more have been calculated for Met^5-enkephalin (18,24,27). The primary step in the breakdown of Met-enkephalin in rat plasma is assigned as cleavage of the Tyr-Gly-amide bond. Experiments carried out using human plasma showed that an essentially identical pattern of breakdown was taking place, though the rate of cleavage seemed to be somewhat slower.

On the basis of similar experiments with labelled Leu-enkephalin, Hambrook et al. (18) conclude that Leu-enkephalin is degraded in rat and human plasma in a way that is identical with Met-enkephalin, which is by cleavage of the Tyr-Gly-amide bond. Guinea-pig ileum tissue preparations contain enkephalin-hydrolysing activity (8). Similar activity is also found in the bath fluid surrounding ileum preparations.

Puig et al. (28) studied the inactivation in the guinea-pig ileum and in the rat brain membrane preparations of Met-enkephalin, Leu-enkephalin, Met-enkephalin amide, S-benzyl sulphonium analogue of Met-enkephalin, and 3-benzyl-tyrosine analogues of both Leu- and Met-enkephalin. Met-enkephalin amide was relatively more resistant to the ileum peptidases than were the other peptides, but was destroyed at the same rate by brain membranes; this variation in inactivation of Met-enkephalin amide probably indicates the presence of different peptidases in each tissue preparation.

Amino acid analyzer (AAA) was used for the determination of ratio of amino acids in different enkephalins and their analogues following an acid hydrolysis of the examined compounds. Puig et al. (28) hydrolyzed peptides for analysis by heating in sealed tubes for 22 hr at 110°C with 6 N HCl containing 1 mg/ml each of 2-mercaptoethanol and phenol. Amino acid ratios were determined in the hydrolysates; the results are shown in Table 1.

In the Department of Hormonal Drugs of the Institute for Drug Research and Control in Warsaw, Dr. Grochulski, Mrs. Tyska, Dr. Wilk, Dr. Szczygieł, and myself have elaborated a nonradiochemical assay of enkephalin-hydrolysing

TABLE 1. *Amino acid analysis of peptides*

Peptide	Amino acid ratios found				
	Gly	Phe	Tyr	Met	Leu
Leu-enk.	2.05	1.00	1.02	—	0.93
Met-enk.	2.03	1.05	0.97	0.97	—

Data from Puig et al., ref. 28.

activity of tissue homogenates (14). In control assays both Leu-enkephalin and Met-enkephalin solutions in phosphate buffer (pH 7.2) did not produce peaks, indicating a good stability of peptides. A mixture of 2.7 ml of freshly prepared enkephalin solution containing a known amount of the compound (usually 1 mg) in 0.025 M phosphate buffer (pH 7.2) and 0.3 ml of the rat brain homogenate supernatant, prepared as above, was used for the AAA assay. This mixture was incubated for 20 min in room temperature, deproteinized, and run for 5 hr against a standard amino acid set in the AAA. The same supernatant, appropriately diluted and deproteinized was used as blank. The amounts of amino acid present in the supernatant, calculated from the blank run, were subtracted from those obtained in the experimental run, and enkephalin-hydrolysing activity was expressed as a percentage of the theoretically calculated amounts of the four constituent **respective** amino acids of the intact pentapeptide. When inhibitors were used in the AAA assay, 0.9 ml of supernatant was incubated for 5 min with 0.1 ml of solution of inhibitor; 0.3 ml of this mixture was used for AAA assay.

We have found that the brain homogenate supernatant, after being mixed with approximately μmole/ml solution of enkephalins in room temperature, produced tyrosine, the amino-terminal amino acid, in large amounts (Table 2). In one experiment the release of tyrosine reached 64% of its content in peptapeptide; in other experiments it was approximately 33%. The carboxy-terminal amino acid, either methionine or leucine, appeared in smaller amounts. Free glycine and phenylalanine were also released but in much smaller amounts. Addition of either bacitracine or inhitrypsin [a peptide (Biomed, Krakow) extracted from urine] to the incubation mixture in room temperature did not, however, inhibit the enkephalin-hydrolysing activity of the supernatant, although a decrease of this activity was observed. The results of one of our experiments are presented in Table 3.

In our experiments free tyrosine was the main degradation product of both enkephalins; indicating that the brain supernatant is primarily attacking the tyrosine-glycine bond. This further confirms the supposition that the aminopeptidase seems to be the main enzyme involved in the biological disposition of enkephalins, although we expect that there is more than one aminopeptidase involved.

Simantov et al. (30) studied the effect of the proteolytic enzymes trypsin, chymotrypsin, carboxypeptidase A, and leucine aminopeptidase on the activity of enkephalins of natural origin from rhesus monkey and other laboratory animal brains. The natural enkephalins have been extracted from the brain and partially purified by ion-exchange chromatography. The enkephalin-hydrolysing activity of monkey brain extracts was not appreciably diminished by trypsin; it was somewhat reduced by chymotrypsin, and markedly degraded by carboxypeptidase A and leucine aminopeptidase, thus resembling the sensitivity of calf, rat, and pig brain enkephalins to proteolytic enzymes.

Simantov et al. (30) measured the effect of various ions on the enkephalin

TABLE 2. *Amino acids released from enkephalins by rat brain homogenate supernatant*

Enkephalin	Amino acid	Exp. no.	AA content in substrate[a]	
			mg/cm^3	% Released
Met-enkephalin	Tyrosine	1	0.093	64.1
		2	0.050	34.9
		3	0.040	27.6
	Glycine	1	0.002	1.7
		2	0.001	0.7
		3	0.001	0.9
	Phenylalanine	1	0.0075	5.8
		2	0.007	3.0
		3	0.003	2.2
	Methionine	1	0.013	11.1
		2	0.003	2.3
		3	0.002	1.7
	Total AA	1	0.115	22.7
		2	0.058	11.4
		3	0.045	8.8
Leu-enkephalin	Tyrosine	2	0.043	29.2
		3	0.057	38.7
	Glycine	2	0.001	0.8
		3	0.001	0.8
	Phenylalanine	2	0.002	1.5
		3	0.002	1.5
	Leucine	2	0.002	1.9
		3	0.002	1.9
	Total AA	2	0.048	9.4
		3	0.062	12.2

[a] AA, aminoacid. % Released is the percentage of AA released in relation to its content in enkephalin contained in substrate.

activity of a monkey brain extracts. Sodium chloride (15 mM) markedly reduced enkephalin activity; potassium chloride (15 mM) and calcium chloride (1 mM) had no effect, while manganese chloride (1 mM) increased the activity.

Pasternak et al. (26) have found in mammals that enkephalin activity is degraded by carboxypeptidase A and leucine aminopeptidase, but is resistant to trypsin and neuraminidase.

Peptidyl-dipeptidase from vascular endothelial cells also metabolizes enkephalins *in vitro* and *in vivo* (10).

Knight and Klee (22) stated that enkephalins are rapidly inactivated by a membrane-associated aminopeptidase present in the brain. They suggest that enkephalin binding to opiate receptors is coupled to subsequent aminopeptidase degradation. Enkephalin degradation at concentrations four orders of magnitude below the K_m, proceeds at essentially the same rate whether or not the peptide is bound to receptors, and opiates and enkephalins have no direct effect upon the rate of aminopeptidase action at the concentrations used in experiments. Thus, Knight and Klee (22) conclude that receptor binding may serve as a

TABLE 3. *Amino acids released from Met-enkephalin by rat brain homogenate supernatant in the presence of inhitrypsin (100 U) or bacitracine (500 (μg/cm³)*

| Amino acid released | Amino acid content in substrate | | | |
| | Without inhib. | | With inhitrypsin | |
	mg/cm³	% Released	mg/cm³	% Released
Tyrosine	0.054	38.1	0.050	35.9
Glycine	0.004	2.1	0.003	1.4
Phenylalanine	0.010	7.8	0.008	5.7
Methionine	0.009	7.8	0.007	5.7
Total AA	0.077	15.2	0.067	13.1
			With bacitracine	
Tyrosine	0.045	31.6	0.041	28.7
Glycine	0.003	2.8	0.002	1.8
Phenylalanine	0.007	5.1	0.004	3.1
Methionine	0.006	5.4	0.004	3.1
Total AA	0.061	12.0	0.051	9.94

concentration mechanism which ensures the efficient inactivation of enkephalin by a nearby peptidase after it has interacted with the receptor.

The aminopeptidase functions optimally at neutral pH and obeys Michaelis-Menten kinetics over at least five orders of magnitude of substrate concentration (K for Met-enkephalin is 4.5×10^{-5} M). Bacitracin enhances enkephalin-mediated effects on cyclic guanosine monophosphate accumulation in slices of rat neostriatum (25). This enhancement may well be due to inhibition of peptidase activity by the antibiotic. Many peptides, such as angiotensin, bacitracin, bradykinin, somatostatin, and substance P are inhibitors of the enzyme. Chelating agents such as 1,10-phenanthroline and 8-OH-quinoline are effective inhibitors of enkephalin destruction by peptidases, indicating that these might be metalloenzymes (8). However, the most effective inhibitor ($K_I = 2 \times 10^{-7}$ M) is the peptide analogue puromycin (22).

Meek et al. (24) examined the metabolism of enkephalins using high pressure liquid chromatography. They have found that the "opiate receptor" fraction of brain commonly used to measure enkephalin contains a large amount of aminopeptidase activity capable of metabolizing enkephalin but not β-endorphin. The release of tyrosine from enkephalin was at least 20 times faster than glycine or leucine. When carrier-free ³H-enkephalin was injected intraventricularly, more than 90% was broken down within 1 min.

In vivo studies (20) have indicated that after radioactive Met⁵-enkephalin or D-Ala³-Met⁵-enkephalin amide intravenous injection, radioactivity is lost from the plasma rapidly (half-life less than 1 min for both compounds), and that the radioactivity from both compounds entered the brain within 5 sec.

Dupont et al. (9) have separated ³H-Met⁵-enkephalin from its metabolites and have demonstrated an extremely short plasma half-life (2–4 sec) for this intact peptapeptide. Only a small amount (6% of the total radioactivity) of the peptide remained in the brain 2 min after injection.

Von Voigtlander and Lewis (31) confirmed that both Met[5]-enkephalin and D-Ala[2]-Met[5]-enkephalin amide rapidly enter the brain of mice. The $t_{1/2}$ for D-Ala[2]-Met[5]-enkephalin amide in the brain was calculated as 0.7 min.

Craves et al. (7) confirmed and extended previous observations demonstrating susceptibility of enkephalins to rapid metabolism by brain tissues. The enzymatic activity was ubiquitous, but non-membranous fractions were most active. Acidic pH (4.0) and lowering the temperature (0°C) inhibited, but did not prevent, metabolism nor did concentrations of bacitracine which enhance the activity of metenkephalin in *in vitro* opiate assays.

In order to determine the rate of metabolism *in vivo,* Craves et al. (7) administered ^{3}H-Met-enkephalin either as bolus into the right lateral ventricle of rats or perfused through the rat ventricular system. The perfusate in both cases was collected from the cisterna magna and the radiolabelled peptide was analyzed. In contrast to the *in vitro* studies, *in situ* the initial enzymatic attack is at the Gly-Gly or Gly-Phe bond rather than at the terminal Tyr-Gly.

Lane et al. (23) have found a heterogeneous distribution of enkephalin-hydrolysing activity in rat brain subfractions and considered this as evidence for enzyme heterogenicity. Their study has shown that substantial enkephalin-hydrolysing activity is present in intact synaptosomes.

β-Endorphin, unlike the enkephalins, has a high potency in its central action (2,4,11,21) and is relatively stable to brain peptidases (1,5,22). NH$_2$-terminal tyrosine of β-endorphin resists the action of aminopeptidases (1), and the COOH-terminal sequence is highly resistant to attack by carboxypeptidases (14).

Austen and Smyth (2) have shown that four soluble endopeptidases catalyze the cleavage of C-fragment of LPH (Fig. 1). Renin, chymotrypsin, Armillaria mellea protease, and trypsin catalysed cleavage of β-endorphin at positions 77–78, 78–79, 78–79, and 79–80, respectively.

Gráf and Kenessey (13) showed that a crude homogenate of porcine hypophysis contains an endopeptidase capable of cleaving β-lipoprotein (LPH$_{1-91}$) specifically between residues Leu[77] and Phe[78] yielding LPH$_{1-77}$ and LPH$_{78-91}$ at an optimum pH of 6.5. At pH 8, three other media fragments could be identified, namely LPH$_{1-46}$, LPH$_{1-60}$, and LPH$_{1-79}$.

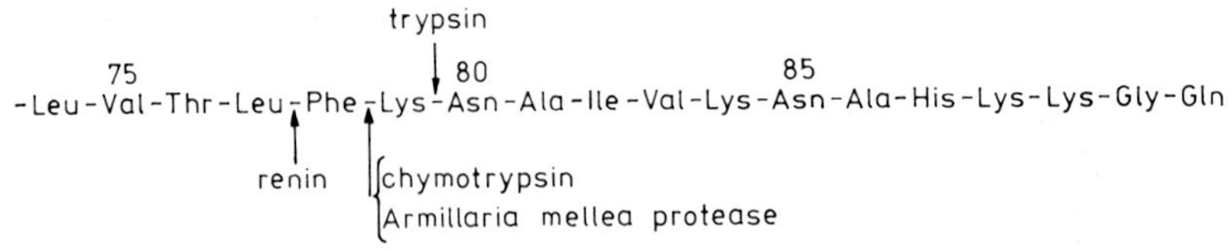

```
                                trypsin
       75                         │ 80                        85
  -Leu-Val-Thr-Leu┬Phe┬Lys┬Asn-Ala-Ile-Val-Lys-Asn-Ala-His-Lys-Lys-Gly-Gln
                   │    ↑
                   ↓    │
                 renin ││chymotrypsin
                       │Armillaria mellea protease
```

FIG. 1. Sites of cleavage of C-fragment under mild conditions of endopeptidase digestion (Data from Austen and Smyth, ref. 2.)

Seidah et al (29) found that tonin (a rat enzyme) cleaves β-lipotropin into sequences 1–50, 1–51, 51–60, 52–60, 61–78, and 79–91, thereby selectively releasing the opiate-like acting segment 61–78, containing Met-enkephalin.

The long peptides seem to possess preferred conformations which protect the NH_2-terminal region from the degradative enzyme (1,15,18). The COOH-terminal residues of β-endorphin, Lys-Lys-Gly-Glu, are highly resistant to the action of carboxypeptidases in brain (13,14). The COOH-terminal region of C-fragment of lipotropin confers stability on the peptide against proteolysis. Thus, β-endorphin seems more suited to a hormone role, but what this role is remains yet obscure.

REFERENCES

1. Austen, B. M., and Smyth, D. G. (1977): The NH_2-terminus of C-fragment is resistant to the action of aminopeptidases. *Biochem. Biophys. Res. Commun.,* 76:477–482.
2. Austen, B. M., and Smyth, D. G. (1977): Specific cleavage of lipotropin C-fragment by endopeptidases; evidence for a preferred conformation. *Biochem. Biophys. Res. Commun.,* 77:86–94.
3. Belluzzi, J. D., Grant, N., Garsky, V., Sarantakis, D., Wise, C. D., and Stein, L. (1976): Analgesia induced in vivo by central administration of enkephalin in rat. *Nature,* 260:625–626.
4. Bradbury, A. F., Smyth, D. G., Snell, C. R., Deakin, J. F. W., and Wendlandt, S. (1977): Comparison of the analgesic properties of lipoprotein C-fragment and stabilized enkephalins in the rat. *Biochem. Biophys. Res. Commun.,* 74:748–754.
5. Buescher, H. H., Hill, R. C., Roemer, D., Carinaux, F., Closse, A., Hauser, D., and Pless, J. (1976): Evidence for analgesic activity of enkephalin in the mouse. *Nature,* 261:423–425.
6. Chruściel, T. L., Grochulski, A., Tyska, J., Wilk, M., and Szyzygieł, M. (1980): Non-radiochemical assay of enkephalin hydrolysing activity of rat brain and liver tissue homogenates *(in preparation).*
7. Craves, F. B., Law, P. Y., Hunt, C. A., and Loh, H. H. (1978): The metabolic disposition of radiolabelled enkephalins in vitro and in situ. *J. Pharmacol. Exp. Ther.,* 206:492–506.
8. Craviso, G. L., and Musacchio, J. M. (1978): Inhibition of enkephalin degradation in the guinea-pig ileum. *Life Sci.,* 23:2019–2020.
9. Dupont, A., Cusan, L., Gavon, M., Alvaredo-Urbino, G., and Labrie, F. (1977): *Life Sci.,* 21:907–914.
10. Erdös, E. G., Johnson, A. R., and Boyden, N. T. (1978): Hydrolysis of enkephalin by cultured human endothelial cells and by purified peptidyl dipeptidase. *Biochem. Pharmacol.,* 27:843–846.
11. Feldberg, W. S., and Smyth, D. G. (1976): The C-fragment of lipotropin—a potent analgesic. *J. Physiol. (Lond.),* 260:30P–31P.
12. Feldberg, W. S., and Smyth, D. G. (1977): Analgesia produced in cats by the C-fragment of lipotropin and by a synthetic pentapeptide. *J. Physiol., (Lond.)* 265:25P–27P.
13. Gráf, L., and Kenessey, A. (1976): Specific cleavage of a single peptide bond (residues 77–78) in beta-lipotropin by a pituitary endopeptidase. *FEBS Lett.,* 69:255–260.
14. Graf, L., Szekely, J. I., Rónai, A. Z., Dunai-Kovàcs, Z., and Bajusz, S. (1976): Comparative study on analgesic effects of met⁵-enkephalin and related lipotropin fragments. *Nature,* 263:240–242.
15. Geisow, M. J., Deakin, J. F. W., Dostrovsky, J. O., and Smyth, D. G. (1977): Analgesic activity of lipotropin C-fragment depends on carboxyl terminal tetrapeptide. *Nature,* 269:167–168.
16. Geisow, M. J., and Smyth, D. G. (1977): Lipotropin C-fragment has a terminal COOH-sequence with high intrinsic resistance to the action of exopeptidases. *Biochem. Biophys. Res. Commun.,* 75:625–629.
17. Goldstein, A. (1978): Endorphins: Physiology and clinical implications. *Ann. NY Acad. Sci.,* 331:49–55.

18. Hambrook, J. M., Morgan, B. A., Rance, M. J., and Smith, C. F. C. (1976): Mode of deactivation of the enkephalins by rat and human plasma and rat brain homogenates. *Nature,* 262:782–783.
19. Hughes, J. (1975): Isolation of an endogenous compound from the brain with pharmacological properties similar to morphine. *Brain Res.,* 88:295–308.
20. Hughes, J. (1979): Opioid peptides and their relatives. *Nature,* 278:394–395.
21. Kastin, A. J., Nissen, C., Schally, A. V., and Coy, D. H. (1978): Blood-brain barrier, half-time disappearance and brain disappearance for labelled enkephalins and a potent analog. *Brain Res. Bull.,* 1:538–589.
22. Knight, M., and Klee, W. A. (1978): The relationship between enkephalin degradation and opiate receptor occupancy. *J. Biol. Chem.,* 253:3843–3847.
23. Lane, A. C., Rance, M. J., and Walter, D. S. (1977): Subcellular localisation of leucine-enkephalin-hydrolysing activity in rat brain. *Nature,* 269:75–76.
24. Meek, J. L., Yang, H. Y. T., and Costa, E. (1977): Enkephalin catabolism in vitro and in vivo. *Neuropharmacology,* 16:151–154.
25. Minneman, K. P., and Iversen, L. I. (1976): Enkephalin and opiate narcotics increase cyclic GMP acccumulation in slices of rat neostriatum. *Nature,* 262:313–314.
26. Pasternack, G. W., Simantov, R., and Snyder, S. H. (1976): Characterization of an endogenous morphine-like factor (enkephalin) in mammalian brain. *Mol. Pharmacol.,* 12:504–513.
27. Pert, C., Bowie, D. L., Fong, B. T. W., and Chang, J. K. (1976): Synthetic analogues of met-enkephalin which resists enzymatic destruction. In: *Opiates and Endogenous Opioid Peptides,* edited by H. W. Kosterlitz, pp. 79–86. North-Holland, Amsterdam.
28. Puig, M. M., Gascon, P., Craviso, G. L., Bjur, R. A., Matsueda, G., Stewart, J. M., and Musacchio, J. N. (1977): The effect of enkephalin and enkephalin analogues on the guinea-pig ileum and rat brain opiate receptor. *Arch. Int. Pharmacodyn.,* 226:69–80.
29. Seidah, N. G., Chan, J. S. D., Mardini, G., Benjannet, S., Chretien, M., Boucher, R., and Genest, J. (1979): Specific cleavage of β-LPH and ACTH by tonin: Release of an opiate-like peptide β-LPH (61–78). *Biochem. Biophys. Res. Commun.,* 86:1002–1013.
30. Simantov, R., Snowman, A. M., and Snyder, S. H. (1976): *Brain Res.,* 107:650–657.
31. Von Voigtlander, P. F., and Lewis, R. A. (1978): In vitro disposition and metabolism of enkephalin: Relationship to analgesic properties. *Res. Commun. Chem. Pathol. Pharmacol.,* 20:265–274.

Neuropeptides and Neural Transmission,
edited by C. Ajmone Marsan and W. Z. Traczyk.
Raven Press, New York © 1980.

Behavioral Effects of Neuropeptides Related to ACTH and β-LPH

D. de Wied

*Rudolf Magnus Institute for Pharmacology, Medical Faculty, University of Utrecht,
Utrecht, The Netherlands*

The implication of adrenocorticotropic hormone (ACTH), α-melanocyte-stimulating hormone (α-MSH), and the neurohypophyseal hormones on adaptive behavior was first suggested by classic endocrine methods, i.e., by the removal of the endocrine gland (in this case, the pituitary), the subsequent demonstration of a deficiency, and finally the correction of the deficient function by treatment with hormones produced by the extirpated gland. Removal of the anterior lobe of the pituitary (68) or the whole gland (2,67,71) in rats impairs acquisition of shuttle box avoidance behavior. Removal of the posterior pituitary does not materially affect acquisition, but interferes with the maintenance of shuttle box avoidance behavior (69). These behavioral impairments could be corrected with ACTH, but also with α-MSH and fragments of ACTH/MSH which are devoid of corticotropic effects. In addition, these impairments could be removed by treatment with [Lys⁸]-vasopressin (LVP) and [des-Gly⁹-Lys⁸]vasopressin (DG-LVP), the latter being virtually devoid of the classic endocrine effects of vasopressin (8,41,71). These results suggested that the behavioral effects of pituitary hormones are not mediated through an influence on their endocrine target tissues. Pituitary hormones may therefore be regarded as precursor molecules for neuropeptides involved in acquisition and maintenance of adaptive behavior.

ACTH and related peptides delay extinction of one-way and two-way active avoidance behavior in intact animals (70,71). The effect of the peptides is of a relatively short-term nature and lasts for a few hours (70). A plausible explanation for the short-term effect of ACTH seems to be a temporary increase in motivation. Several studies support this hypothesis. Facilitation of acquisition of shuttle box avoidance behavior at a low footshock level (58), facilitation of acquisition of food-rewarded behavior in a multiple T-maze (33), and improvement of maze performance (20) suggest a motivational effect. Furthermore, ACTH and related peptides facilitate passive-avoidance behavior (20,37,38,43,44,72), delay extinction of food motivated behavior in hungry rats (20,22,29,42,56), delay extinction of sexually motivated approach behavior (9), and delay extinction of conditioned taste aversion (53). Memory processes may be affected as well. ACTH fragments alleviate amnesia produced by CO_2 inhalation or electroconvulsive shock (54,55) by intracerebral administration of the protein synthesis inhibitor puromycin (19) or anisomycin (20,52). Rigter et al. (52) demonstrated that amnesia induced by CO_2 can be reversed by $ACTH_{4-10}$ only when given 1 hr prior to the retention test, but not when administered before the induction of amnesia suggesting an influence on retrieval processes. Observations in man revealed that $ACTH_{4-10}$ facilitates selective visual attention (38) and influences memory retrieval (12), but evidence for a motivational hypothesis has been provided as well (21).

Cardiovascular changes, particularly heart rate alteration might be regarded as a measure of psychological processes underlying behavior, such as motivation, attention, and arousal. Classic conditioning, involving an unavoidable footshock as the conditioned stimulus, results in development of conditioned bradycardia which gradually disappears during extinction. $ACTH_{4-10}$ delays extinction of this conditioned bradycardia (6). Thus, $ACTH_{4-10}$ not only affects instrumental learning but also acquired autonomic responding. Bradycardia is also found during retention of passive-avoidance behavior. The rate of bradycardia depends on the intensity and the duration of the shock experience during the learning trial. $ACTH_{4-10}$ facilitates passive-avoidance behavior but the effect of the peptide is accompanied by tachycardia. This tachycardia suggests that $ACTH_{4-10}$ increases the state of arousal (7). This is corroborated by electrophysiological observations. $ACTH_{4-10}$ induces a frequency shift in theta activity in hippocampus and thalamic structures evoked by stimulation of the reticular formation in freely moving rats (64). Similar shifts can be obtained by increasing the stimulus intensity, indicating that $ACTH_{4-10}$ increases the arousal state in limbic midbrain structures.

In conclusion, behavioral and electrophysiological observations suggest that ACTH and related peptides temporarily enhance the motivational influence of specific environmental cues. This increases the probability that stimulus specific behavioral responses occur. To accomplish such responses memory components are involved as well as goal-directed aspects of perception and attention, as a result of a temporary increase in the arousal state of limbic midbrain structures.

The behavioral activity of ACTH fragments can be completely dissociated from endocrine and peripheral metabolic activities by modification of the molecule. Substitution of Met^4 by methionine sulfoxide, Arg^8 by D-Lys, and Trp^9 by Phe yields a peptide $(4-Met(O_2)8-D-Lys, 9-Phe\ ACTH_{4-9})$ (Org 2766) which is behaviorally a thousand times more active than $ACTH_{4-10}$ (30) and activity is retained even after oral administration. It possesses, however, a thousand times less MSH activity and its steroidogenic action is markedly reduced. It has no fat mobilizing activity nor opiate-like effects (62,77). Structure activity studies designed to determine the essential elements required for the behavioral effect of ACTH revealed that $ACTH_{4-7}$ is as effective as the whole ACTH molecule in delaying extinction of pole-jumping avoidance behavior (30,77). More activity sites are present in ACTH since $ACTH_{7-10}$ and $ACTH_{11-24}$ also delay extinction of pole-jumping avoidance behavior but at a much higher dose level than $ACTH_{4-7}$. Similar observations have been made for other pituitary hormone activities. Eberle and Schwyzer (17) also identified two active sites in α-MSH, i.e., MSH_{4-10} and MSH_{11-13}, which have melanocyte-stimulating activity. The residual potency of $ACTH_{7-10}$ can be increased to the same level of $ACTH_{4-7}$ by extending the carboxyl terminus with $ACTH_{11-16}$ to $ACTH_{7-16}$ (77). The tripeptide H-Phe-D-Lys-Phe-OH, which is the major breakdown product of the highly potent hexapeptide Org 2766, in itself has only minor behavioral effects (80). Again, chain elongation with $ACTH_{10-16}$ restores the potency. Substitution of Lys^{11} by the D-enantiomer augments the effect on avoidance behavior and extension of the NH_2-terminus with $Met(O)^4$-Glu^5-His^6 further potentiates the behavioral effect to yield a peptide that is three hundred thousand more active than $ACTH_{4-10}$ (73) (Org 5041). The potency of this peptide depends on the residues Gly^{10} and Lys^{16}. Removal of either of these amino acids markedly reduces the effect on extinction of pole-jumping avoidance behavior (73). Chain elongation and structure modification result in increased metabolic stability (80). However, the marked increase in potency may also indicate a much greater affinity/or intrinsic activity for presumptive receptor sites (74).

These structural modifications provided peptides with a similar behavioral profile as the parent $ACTH_{4-10}$ fragment. The only exception is replacement of the amino acid residue phenylalanine in position 7. Replacement of this amino acid by the D-enantiomer in $ACTH_{1-10}$, $ACTH_{4-10}$, or $ACTH_{4-7}$ causes an effect on extinction of avoidance behavior opposite to that found with nonsubstituted ACTH fragments. Such (D-Phe^7) ACTH analogs facilitate extinction of active avoidance behavior or approach behavior motivated by food (10,22, 30,71). However, D-Phe^7 $ACTH_{4-10}$ like $ACTH_{4-10}$ facilitates passive-avoidance behavior when given prior to the retention test (72), but in relatively high doses attenuates passive-avoidance behavior when administered immediately following the learning trial (20) and delays extinction of conditioned taste aversion (53). In view of the specific activity of D-Phe^7 analogs of ACTH and the highly potent derivatives, one might assume that the pituitary contains other possibly more specific and potent neuropeptides involved in motivational, learning, and memory processes.

Peptides related to ACTH, MSH, and β-lipotropic hormone (β-LPH) induce a stretching and yawning syndrome following intracerebral administration only (18,23). In rodents, the onset of the syndrome is preceded by a display of excessive grooming (18,27,34,51). In rats $ACTH_{1-24}$ and α- and β-MSH possess equipotent excessive grooming activity (27). $ACTH_{4-10}$ is less active in rabbits (3) and inactive in rats (27) and mice (51) but [D-Phe^7] $ACTH_{4-10}$ has appreciable activity. $ACTH_{4-10}$ could be activated by C-terminal chain elongation but also by shortening to $ACTH_{4-7}$. This peptide is as active as [D-Phe^7] $ACTH_{4-10}$ (78). $ACTH_{4-7}$ is also the shortest sequence that exerts full activity in the pole-jumping avoidance test (30). Excessive grooming induced by ACTH analogs can be completely suppressed by pretreatment with specific opiate antagonists, while morphine itself induces this syndrome. This suggests an interaction with opiate receptors in the brain (25). In addition, Terenius (59) found that $ACTH_{1-28}$

and $ACTH_{4-10}$ had affinity for opiate receptors. Subsequent structure activity studies pointed to an active site within $ACTH_{4-10}$ with some indication for a second site distal to the C-terminus of this heptapeptide (62). Analysis of the binding revealed low selectivity of these peptides for agonist and antagonist binding sites, comparable to that of the partial agonist nalorphine (60). In addition, ACTH and related peptides exert affinity for an intrinsic activity on opioid receptors in the mouse vas deferens preparation and bind to morphine antiserum (47). In view of the relatively low affinity for the opiate receptor (IC_{50} of the order of 10^{-6}–10^{-5} M), $ACTH_{4-10}$ cannot be regarded as a physiological ligand for opiate receptors in the brain in contrast to C-terminal β-LPH fragments which exhibit high affinity for brain opiate receptors (11). But the fact that ACTH interacts with opiate receptors in the brain may explain the interaction of these peptides with the analgesic effect of morphine (26). Morphine-induced spinal reflex activity is reduced by ACTH in preparations *in vivo* and *in vitro* (81) and ACTH counteracts the analgesic effect of morphine in rodents (79). Gispen et al. (24) found that ACTH and ACTH fragments reduce the analgesic response of morphine by 50 to 60% as measured in the hot plate test. The peptides themselves had no effect on the response of the rats on the hot plate. Interestingly, this *in vivo* effect corresponds rather well with the affinity to brain opiate receptor sites *in vitro*. Excessive grooming probably is mediated by opiate receptors in the brain. In fact, the endorphins are more potent than ACTH since intraventricular administration of doses as low as 10 ng β-endorphin elicits excessive grooming (24). α-Endorphin is much less active while Met-enkephalin is virtually inactive. The grooming effect of β-endorphin is like that of ACTH readily blocked by naloxone (24).

The observation that β-endorphin injected intraventricularly or intracerebrally in rats at rather high dose levels causes, as does morphine, a catatonic- or cataleptic-like syndrome, led to the suggestion that β-endorphin might be associated with mental disorders (5,35). Furthermore, the endorphins have been implicated in schizophrenia. The first evidence came from the observation that the level of opioid-like substances was increased in the cerebrospinal fluid of schizophrenic patients (63). Clinical studies supported these assumptions. Opiate antagonists temporarily decreased the psychotic symptoms in about 30% of the patients (61) and β-endorphin had some beneficial effects in a number of psychotic patients (39).

Acquisition and extinction of conditioned avoidance behavior in rats are sensitive parameters for neuroleptic activity and are impaired even by low dose levels of neuroleptics (14,36,40). Neuropeptides modulate extinction of conditioned avoidance behavior. Relatively low doses of ACTH, β-endorphin, and several fragments of these peptides delay extinction of the avoidance response (73,75). However, a particular fragment of β-endorphin, γ-endorphin (β-LPH_{61-77}), appeared to facilitate extinction of avoidance behavior. These effects are independent of interaction with opiate receptor sites in the brain.

Des-tyrosine-γ-endorphin (DTγE, β-LPH$_{62-77}$), which has no opiate-like activity, is even more potent than γ-endorphin in facilitating extinction of avoidance behavior (76). The pharmacological profile of DTγE indicated neuroleptic-like activity. DTγE and haloperidol both facilitated extinction of pole-jumping avoidance behavior, attenuated passive-avoidance behavior (40,76), decreased the response rate for electrical self-stimulating behavior elicited via electrodes implanted in the ventral tegmental-medial substantia nigra area (16), decreased heroin self-administration (Van Ree, *unpublished observations*), and were active in various grip tests (76). However, DTγE did not cause the typical locomotor and sedative effects of haloperidol. Because of these findings it was postulated that β-endorphin and its fragments play an important role in brain homeostatic mechanisms and that derangements in the fragmentation of β-endorphin may be a factor in the etiology of schizophrenia. The balance between α- and β-type endorphins on the one hand and γ-type endorphins on the other, may be of special importance in the manifestation of psychotic symptoms and, in addition, may explain the variability with which the schizophrenic syndrome manifests itself (49,74). An imbalance between β-endorphin fragments may lead, at least in some cases, to the accumulation of β-endorphin, a peptide which induces a catatonia-like syndrome in experimental animals (35,57) and which would be responsible for the catatonic symptomatology of schizophrenic patients. An excess of α-type endorphin might give rise to aggressive or paranoid forms of the schizophrenic syndrome, since α-endorphin and related peptides induce effects which in some respects resemble those of amphetamine (16,40,74). Drugs such as amphetamines are known to exacerbate the psychotic symptoms in patients and to induce schizophrenic (paranoid) psychosis in normal individuals (15,46). An eventual increase in the level of α- or β-type endorphins could explain the temporary relief of psychotic symptoms subsequent to naloxone administration (1,31,61). The possibility that this hypothetical balance between endorphins operates physiologically in the brain is supported by the fact that the enzymatic breakdown of β-endorphin occurs *in vitro* in the presence of brain membranes. Enzyme activity with an optimum of pH 5 in brain and pituitary has been found which metabolizes β-endorphin as well as β-LPH at the Leu[77]-Phe[78] bond (28), thus generating γ-endorphin. Subsequent carboxypeptidase activity would give α-endorphin (45). Burbach et al. (13) found that β-endorphin incubated at pH 7.4 was converted so as to yield γ-endorphin and DTγE, while γ-endorphin and α-endorphin were the main products at a lower pH.

The neuroleptic-like activity of DTγE seen in animal experiments was also found in humans since the psychotic symptoms of a number of chronic schizophrenic patients markedly diminished during DTγE treatment. In some of the patients the improvement appeared to be long-lasting (49,65). Although DTγE mimics the action of neuroleptics in some respects, its mode of action may be quite different from that of these drugs. Accordingly, DTγE does not displace radioactive haloperidol or spiperone from dopaminergic or serotonergic brain binding sites *in vitro* (50). Moreover, DTγE reduced substantia nigra self-stimulation at currents just above the threshold for eliciting the behavior, while haloperidol had the same effect at both threshold and high current intensities (16). This suggests that DTγE acts more as a neuromodulator than as a blocker of neurotransmitter activity, as do classic neuroleptics. The influence of DTγE on substantia nigra self-stimulation and its interference with dopaminergic transmission in restricted brain areas (66) may link the DTγE hypothesis of schizophrenia (74) to the involvement of noradrenaline and/or dopamine in this mental disorder (4,15,48).

Evidence was provided for an interaction of endorphins with catecholaminergic neuronal systems after intraventricular administration of various endorphin fragments in doses as low as 100 ng. This is at least one hundred times below those needed to elicit opiate-like effects and in the range of doses needed to modify avoidance behavior (66). The effects of α-endorphin were observed to be widespread in the brain and without exception the peptide caused a decrease in (α-MPT)-induced catecholamine disappearance. Dopamine turnover was decreased in caudate nucleus, globus pallidus, medial septal nucleus, the nucleus interstitialis striae terminalis, paraventricular nucleus, zona incerta, and medial amygdaloid nucleus. The effects of DYγE and β-endorphin were more limited and increases as well as decreases in catecholamine turnover were noted after synthesis inhibition. In contrast to α-endorphin, in some regions (paraventricular nucleus and zona incerta), DTγE caused an enhanced dopamine turnover. Most regions where effects were observed were in close association with fibers and terminal regions of the endorphin neuronal systems (66). DTγE did not cause changes in dopamine disappearance in the nigrostriatal system. It may be, therefore, that the neuroleptic-like effects of this neuropeptide are the result of an interaction with other dopaminergic systems. However, DTγE, like haloperidol, inhibits excessive grooming of rats induced by intracerebroventricular ACTH following local application in the nigrostriatal area (Gispen et al., *unpublished observations*) and it decreases intracranial self-stimulation of rats elicited via electrodes in the same area (16). The exact influence of DTγE on dopamine transmission, therefore, remains to be elucidated. Schizophrenia, according to our hypothesis, is the result of a relative excess of α-type endorphins in the brain (74). If this were true, an excess of α-type endorphins would be associated with a decreased catecholamine metabolism in various limbic midbrain regions. Versteeg et al. (66) found an increased concentration of noradrenaline following synthesis inhibition by α-MPT in rats in the medial septal nucleus, dorsomedial nucleus, central amygdaloid nucleus, subiculum, the ventral part of the nucleus reticularis medullae oblongatae, and the A_1-regions. In this respect it is noteworthy that Hornykiewicz et al. (32) reported a significant increase in noradrenaline levels in a few limbic regions (ventral septum, bed nucleus of the stria terminalis and nucleus accumbens, and possibly the mammilary body) in 4 postmortem brains of patients with chronic paranoid schizophrenia.

REFERENCES

1. Akil, H., Watson, S. J., Berger, P. A., and Barchas, J. D. (1978): Endorphins, β-LPH and ACTH: Biochemical, pharmacological and anatomical studies. In: *Advances in Biochemical Psychopharmacology, Vol. 18: The Endorphins,* edited by E. Costa and M. Trabucchi, pp. 125–139. Raven Press, New York.
2. Applezweig, M. H., and Baudry, F. D. (1955): The pituitary-adrenocortical system in avoidance learning. *Psychol. Rep.,* 1:417–420.
3. Baldwin, D. M., Haun, Ch. K., and Sawyer, Ch. H. (1974): Effects of intraventricular infusions of $ACTH_{1-24}$ and $ACTH_{4-10}$ on LH release, ovulation and behaviour in the rabbit. *Brain Res.,* 80:291–301.
4. Berger, P. A. (1978): Medical treatment of mental illness. *Science,* 200:974–981.
5. Bloom, F., Segal, D., Ling, N., and Guillemin, R. (1976): Endorphins: Profound behavioral effects in rats suggest new etiological factors in mental illness. *Science,* 194:630–632.
6. Bohus, B. (1973): Pituitary-adrenal influences on avoidance and approach behavior of the rat. In: *Progress in Brain Res., Vol. 39: Drug Effects on Neuroendocrine Regulation,* edited by E. Zimmermann, W. H. Gispen, B. H. Marks, and D. de Wied, pp. 407–420. Elsevier, Amsterdam.
7. Bohus, B. (1975): Pituitary peptides and adaptive autonomic responses. In: *Progress in Brain Res., Vol. 42: Hormones, Homeostasis and the Brain,* edited by W. H. Gispen, Tj. B. van Wimersma Greidanus, B. Bohus, and D. de Wied, pp. 275–283. Elsevier, Amsterdam.
8. Bohus, B., Gispen, W. H., and Wied, D. de (1973): Effect of lysine vasopressin and $ACTH_{4-10}$ on conditioned avoidance behavior of hypophysectomized rats. *Neuroendocrinology,* 11:137–143.
9. Bohus, B., Hendrickx, H. H. L., Kolfschoten, A. A. van, and Krediet, T. G. (1975): Effect of $ACTH_{4-10}$ on copulatory and sexually motivated approach behavior in the male rat. In: *Sexual Behavior: Pharmacology and Biochemistry,* edited by M. Sandler and G. L. Gessa, pp. 269–275. Raven Press, New York.
10. Bohus, B., and Wied, D. de (1966): Inhibitory and facilitatory effect of two related peptides on extinction of avoidance behavior. *Science,* 153:318–320.
11. Bradbury, A. F., Smyth, D. G., Snell, C. R., Birdsall, N. J. M., and Hulme, E. C. (1976): C-fragment of lipotropin has a high affinity for brain opiate receptors. *Nature,* 260:793–795.
12. Branconnier, R. J., Cole, J. O., and Cardos, G. (1979): $ACTH_{4-10}$ in the amelioration of neuropsychological symptomatology associated with senile organic brain syndrome. *Psychopharmacology,* 61:161–165.
13. Burbach, J. P. H., Loeber, J. G., Verhoef, J., Kloet, E. R. de, and Wied, D. de (1979): Biotransformation of endorphins by a synaptosomal plasma membrane preparation of rat brain and by human serum. *Biochem. Biophys. Res. Commun.,* 86:1296–1303.
14. Courvoisier, S., Fournel, J., Ducrot, R., Kolsky, M., and Koetschet, P. (1952): Propriétés pharmacodynamiques du chlorhydrate de chloro-3 (diméthylamino-3-propyl)-10 phénothiazine (4.560 RP). *Arch. Int. Pharmacodyn. Ther.,* 92:305–361.
15. Crow, T. J., Johnstone, E. C., Longden, A., and Owen, F. (1978): Dopamine and schizophrenia. In: *Advances in Biochemical Psychopharmacology, Vol. 19: Dopamine,* edited by P. J. Roberts, G. N. Woodruff, and L. L. Iversen, pp. 301–309. Raven Press, New York.
16. Dorsa, D. M., van Ree, J. M., and Wied, D. de (1979): Effects of [Des-Tyr^1]-γ-endorphin and α-endorphin on substantia nigra self-stimulation. *Pharmacol. Biochem. Behav.,* 10:599–905.
17. Eberle, A., and Schwyzer, R. (1975): Hormone-receptor interaction: Demonstration of two message sequences (active sites) in α-melanotropin. *Helv. Chim. Acta,* 58:1528-1535.
18. Ferrari, W., Gessa, G. L., and Vargiu, L. (1963): Behavioral effects induced by intracysternally injected ACTH and MSH. *Ann. NY Acad. Sci.,* 104:330–345.
19. Flexner, J. B., and Flexner, L. B. (1971): Pituitary peptides and the suppression of memory by puromycin. *Proc. Natl. Acad. Sci. USA,* 68:2519–2521.
20. Flood, J. F., Jarvik, M. E., Bennett, E. L., and Orme, A. E. (1976): Effects of ACTH peptide fragments on memory formation. *Pharmacol. Biochem. Behav.,* 5(Suppl. 1):41–51.
21. Gaillard, A. W. K., and Sanders, A. F. (1975): Some effects of $ACTH_{4-10}$ on performance during a serial reaction task. *Psychopharmacologia,* 42:201–208.
22. Garrud, P., Gray, J. A., and Wied, D. de (1974): Pituitary-adrenal hormones and extinction of rewarded behavior in the rat. *Physiol. Behav.,* 12:109–119.

23. Gessa, G. L., Pisano, M., Vargiu, L., Crabai, F., and Ferrari, W. (1967): Stretching and yawning movements after intracerebral injections of ACTH. *Rev. Can. Biol.,* 26:229–236.
24. Gispen, W. H., Buitelaar, J., Wiegant, V. M., Terenius, L., and Wied, D. de (1976): Interaction between ACTH fragments, brain opiate receptors and morphine-induced analgesia. *Eur. J. Pharmacol.,* 39:393–397.
25. Gispen, W. H., and Wiegant, V. M. (1976): Opiate antagonists suppress ACTH$_{1-24}$-induced excessive grooming in the rat. *Neurosci. Lett.,* 2:159–164.
26. Gispen, W. H., Wiegant, V. M., Bradbury, A. F., Hulme, E. C., Smyth, D. G., Snell, C. R., and Wied, D. de (1975): Induction of excessive grooming in the rat by fragments of lipotropin. *Nature,* 264:794–795.
27. Gispen, W. H., Wiegant, V. M., Greven, H. M., and Wied, D. de (1975): The induction of excessive grooming in the rat by intraventricular application of peptides derived from ACTH/structure activity studies. *Life Sci.,* 17:645–652.
28. Gráf, L., and Kenessey, A. (1976): Specific cleavage of a single peptide bond (residues 77–78) in β-lipotropin by a pituitary endopeptidase. *FEBS Lett.,* 69:255–260.
29. Gray, J. A. (1971): Effect of ACTH on extinction of rewarded behavior is blocked by previous administration of ACTH. *Nature,* 229:52–54.
30. Greven, H. M., and Wied, D. de (1973): The influence of peptides derived from corticotropin (ACTH) on performance. Structure activity studies. In: *Progress in Brain Research, Vol. 39: Drug Effects on Neuroendocrine Regulation,* edited by E. Zimmermann, W. H. Gispen, B. H. Marks, and D. de Wied, pp. 429–442. Elsevier, Amsterdam.
31. Herz, A., Bläsig, J., Emrich, H. M., Cording, C., Pirée, S., Kölling, A., and Zerssen, D. von (1978): Is there some indication from behavioral effects of endorphins for their involvement in psychiatric disorders? In: *Advances in Biochemical Psychopharmacology, Vol. 18: The Endorphins,* edited by E. Costa and M. Trabucchi, pp. 333–339. Raven Press, New York.
32. Hornykiewicz, O., Farley, I. J., and Shannak, K. S. (1979): Brain monoamine changes in paranoid schizophrenia. *Abstract First International Colloquium on Receptors, Neurotransmitters and Peptide Hormones.* Capri, May 13–18, 1979, p. 56.
33. Isaacson, R. L., Dunn, A. J., Rees, H. D., and Waldock, B. (1976): ACTH$_{4-10}$ and improved use of information in rats. *Physiol. Psychol.,* 4:159–162.
34. Izumi, K., Donaldson, J., and Barbeau, A. (1973): Yawning and stretching in rats induced by intraventricularly administered zinc. *Life Sci.,* 12:203–210.
35. Jacquet, Y. F., and Marks, N. (1976): The C-fragment of β-lipotropin: An endogenous neuroleptic or antipsychotogen? *Science,* 194:632–634.
36. Janssen, P. A. J., and Niemegeers, C. J. E. (1961): Analysis of the influence of haloperidol and pharmacologically related drugs on learned avoidance-escape habits of the Wistar rat in a "jumping box" situation. *Arzneim. Forsch.,* 11:1037–1043.
37. Kastin, A. J., Plotnikoff, N. P., Schally, A. V., and Sandman, C. A. (1976): Endocrine and CNS effects of hypothalamic peptides and MSH. In: *Reviews of Neuroscience, Vol. 2,* edited by S. Ehrenpreis and I. J. Kopin, pp. 111–148. Raven Press, New York.
38. Kastin, A. J., Sandman, C. A., Stratton, L. O., Schally, A. V., and Miller, L. H. (1975): Behavioral and electrographic changes in rat and man after MSH. In: *Progress in Brain Research, Vol. 42: Hormones, Homeostasis and the Brain,* edited by W. H. Gispen, Tj. B. van Wimersma Greidanus, B. Bohus, and D. de Wied, pp. 143–150. Elsevier, Amsterdam.
39. Kline, N. S., Li, C. H., Lehman, H. E., Lajtha, A., Laski, E., and Cooper, T. (1977): β-Endorphin-induced changes in schizophrenic and depressed patients. *Arch. Gen. Psychiatr.,* 34:1111–1113.
40. Kovács, G. L., and de Wied, D. (1978): Effects of amphetamine and haloperidol on avoidance behavior and exploratory activity. *Eur. J. Pharmacol.,* 53:103–107.
41. Lande, S., Witter, A., and Wied, D. de (1971): Pituitary peptides. An octapeptide that stimulates conditioned avoidance acquisition in hypophysectomized rats. *J. Biol. Chem.,* 246:2058–2062.
42. Leonard, B. E. (1969): The effect of sodium-barbitone alone and together with ACTH and amphetamine on the behavior of the rat in the multiple "T" maze. *Int. J. Neuropharmacol.,* 8:427–435.
43. Levine, S., and Jones, L. E. (1965): Adrenocorticotropic hormone (ACTH) and passive avoidance learning. *J. Comp. Physiol. Psychol.,* 59:357–360.
44. Lissák, K., and Bohus, B. (1972): Pituitary hormones and avoidance behavior of the rat. *Int. J. Psychobiol.,* 2:103–115.

45. Marks, N. (1978): Biotransformation and degradation of corticotrophins, lipotropins and hypothalamic peptides. In: *Frontiers in Neuroendocrinology, Vol. 5,* edited by L. Martini and W. F. Ganong, pp. 329–377. Raven Press, New York.
46. Meltzer, H. I. Y., and Stahl, S. M. (1976): Dopamine hypothesis of schizophrenia, a review. *Schizophrenia Bull.,* 2:19–75.
47. Plomp, G. J. J., and Ree, J. M. van (1978): Adrenocorticotropic hormone fragments mimic the effect of morphine *in vitro. Br. J. Pharmacol.,* 64:223–227.
48. Praag, H. M. van. (1977): *Depression and Schizophrenia.* Spectrum, New York.
49. Ree, J. M. van, Verhoeven, W. M. A., Praag, H. M. van, and Wied, D. de (1978): Antipsychotic action of [des-Tyr^1]-γ-endorphin (β-LPH$_{62-77}$). In: *Characteristics and Function of Opioids,* edited by J. M. van Ree and L. Terenius, pp. 181–184. Elsevier/North-Holland Biomedical Press, Amsterdam.
50. Ree, J. M. van, Witter, A., and Leysen, J. E. (1978): Interaction of destyrosine-γ-endorphin (DTγE, β-LPH$_{62-77}$) with neuroleptic binding sites in various areas of rat brain. *Eur. J. Pharmacol.,* 52:411–413.
51. Rees, H. D., Dunn, A. J., and Juvone, P. M. (1976): Behavioral and biochemical responses of mice to the intraventricular administration of ACTH analogs and lysine vasopressin. *Life Sci.,* 18:1333–1340.
52. Rigter, H., Elbertse, R., and Riezen, H. van (1975): Time-dependent antiamnesic effect of ACTH$_{4-10}$ and desglycinamide-lysine vasopressin. In: *Progress in Brain Research, Vol. 42: Hormones, Homeostasis and the Brain,* edited by W. H. Gispen, Tj. B. van Wimersma Greidanus, B. Bohus, and D. de Wied, pp. 163–171. Elsevier, Amsterdam.
53. Rigter, H., and Popping, A. (1976): Hormonal influences on the extinction of conditioned taste aversion. *Psychopharmacologia,* 46:255–261.
54. Rigter, H., and Riezen, H. van (1975): Anti-amnesic effect of ACTH$_{4-10}$: Its dependence of the nature of the amnesic agent and the behavioral test. *Physiol. Behav.,* 14:563–566.
55. Rigter, H., Riezen H. van, and Wied, D. de (1974): The effects of ACTH and vasopressin analogues on CO$_2$-induced retrograde amnesia in rats. *Physiol. Behav.,* 13:381–388.
56. Sandman, C. A., Kastin, A. J., and Schally, A. V. (1969): Melanocyte-stimulating hormones and learned appetitive behavior. *Experientia,* 25:1001–1002.
57. Segal, D. S., Browne, R. G., Bloom, F., Ling, N., and Guillemin, R. (1977): β-Endorphin: Endogenous opiate or neuroleptic? *Science,* 198:411–414.
58. Stratton, L. O., and Kastin, A. J. (1974): Avoidance learning at two levels of motivation in rats receiving MSH. *Horm. Behav.,* 5:149–155.
59. Terenius, L. (1975): Effect of peptides and aminoacids on dihydromorphine binding to the opiate receptor. *J. Pharm. Pharmacol.,* 27:450–452.
60. Terenius, L. (1976): Somatostatin and ACTH are peptides with partial agonist-like selectivity for opiate receptors. *Eur. J. Pharmacol.,* 38:211–213.
61. Terenius, L. (1978): The implications of endorphins in pathological states. In: *Characteristics and Function of Opioids,* edited by J. M. van Ree and L. Terenius, pp. 143–158. Elsevier/North-Holland Biomedical Press, Amsterdam.
62. Terenius, L., Gispen, W. H., and Wied, D. de (1975): ACTH-like peptides and opiate receptors in the rat brain: Structure-activity studies. *Eur. J. Pharmacol.,* 33:395–399.
63. Terenius, L., Wåhlstrom, A., Lindstrom, C., and Widerlöo, E. (1975): Increased CSF levels of endorphins in chronic psychosis. *Neurosci. Lett.,* 3:157–162.
64. Urban, I., and Wied, D. de (1976): Changes in excitability of the theta activity generating substrate by ACTH$_{4-10}$ in the rat. *Exp. Brain Res.,* 24:325–344.
65. Verhoeven, W. M. A., Praag, H. M. van, Ree, J. M. van, and Wied, D. de (1979): Improvement of schizophrenic patients treated with [Des-Tyr^1]-γ-endorphin (DTγE). *Arch. Gen. Psychiatry,* 36:294–298.
66. Versteeg, D. H. G., Kloet, E. R. de, and Wied, D. de (1979): Effects of α-endorphin, β-endorphin and [des-try^1]-γ-endorphin on α-MPT-induced catecholamine disappearance in discrete regions of the rat brain. *Brain Res.,* 179:5–92.
67. Weiss, J. M., McEwen, B. S., Silva, M., and Kalkut, M. (1970): Pituitary-adrenal alterations and fear responding. *Am. J. Physiol.,* 218:864–868.
68. Wied, D. de (1964): Influence of anterior pituitary on avoidance learning and escape behavior. *Am. J. Physiol.,* 207:255–259.
69. Wied, D. de (1965): The influence of the posterior and intermediate lobe of the pituitary and

pituitary peptides on the maintenance of a conditioned avoidance response in rats. *Int. J. Neuropharmacol.,* 4:157–167.

70. Wied, D. de (1966): Inhibitory effect of ACTH and related peptides on extinction of conditioned avoidance behavior in rats. *Proc. Soc. Exp. Biol. Med.,* 122:28–32.
71. Wied, D. de (1969): Effects of peptide hormones on behavior. In: *Frontiers in Neuroendocrinology 1969,* edited by W. F. Ganong and L. Martini, pp. 97–140. Oxford University Press, London/ New York.
72. Wied, D. de (1974): Pituitary-adrenal system hormones and behavior. In: *The Neurosciences, Third Study Program,* edited by F. O. Schmitt and F. G. Worden, pp. 653–666. MIT Press, Cambridge.
73. Wied, D. de (1977): Behavioral effects of neuropeptides related to ACTH, MSH and β-LPH. *Ann. NY Acad. Sci.,* 297:263–274.
74. Wied, D. de (1978): Psychopathology as a neuropeptide dysfunction. In: *Characteristics and Function of Opioids,* edited by J. M. van Ree, and L. Terenius, pp. 113–122. Elsevier/North-Holland Biomedical Press, Amsterdam.
75. Wied, D. de, Bohus, B., Ree, J. M. van, and Urban, I. (1978): Behavioral and electrophysiological effects of peptides related to lipotropin (β-LPH). *J. Pharmacol. Exp. Ther.,* 204:570–580.
76. Wied, D. de, Kovács, G. L., Bohus, B., Ree, J. M. van, and Greven, H. M. (1978): Neuroleptic activity of the neuropeptide β-LPH$_{62-77}$ ([des-Tyr^1]-γ-endorphin; DTγE). *Eur. J. Pharmacol.,* 49:427–436.
77. Wied, D. de, Witter, A., and Greven, H. M. (1975): Behaviorally active ACTH analogues. *Biochem. Pharmacol.,* 24:1463–1468.
78. Wiegant, V. M., Gispen, W. H., Terenius, L., and Wied, D. de (1977): ACTH-like peptides and morphine: Interaction at the level of the CNS. *Psychoneuroendocrinology,* 2:63–69.
79. Winter, C. A., and Flataker, L. (1951): The effect of antihistaminic drugs upon the performance of trained rats. *J. Pharmacol. Exp. Ther.,* 101:156–162.
80. Witter, A., Greven, H. M., and Wied, D. de (1975): Correlation between structure, behavioral activity and rate of biotransformation of some ACTH$_{4-9}$ analogs. *J. Pharmacol. Exp. Ther.,* 193:853–860.
81. Zimmermann, E., and Krivoy, W. A. (1973): Antagonism between morphine and the polypeptides ACTH, ACTH$_{1-24}$, and β-MSH in the nervous system. In: *Progress in Brain Research, Vol. 39: Drug Effects on Neuroendocrine Regulation,* edited by E. Zimmermann, W. H. Gispen, B. H. Marks, and D. de Wied, pp. 383–394. Elsevier, Amsterdam.

Neuropeptides and Neural Transmission,
edited by C. Ajmone Marsan and W. Z. Traczyk.
Raven Press, New York © 1980.

Opioid Peptides as Brain Neurotransmitters with Therapeutic Potential: Basic and Clinical Studies

Robert C. A. Frederickson, Edward L. Smithwick,
and David P. Henry

Lilly Research Laboratories, Eli Lilly and Company, Indianapolis, Indiana 46285

The demonstration of stereospecific receptors for opiates in brain (16,18,21) followed by the discovery of their endogenous peptide ligands (11,24) has provided a major advance in our understanding of the receptor concept and of drug activity. This work, furthermore, promises to stimulate major advances in the development of chemical therapeutics. The family of putative endogenous ligands includes the various endorphins such as β-endorphin, α-endorphin, γ-endorphin, Met-enkephalin and Leu-enkephalin, and possibly other peptide and nonpeptide materials as well (8,9,12).

The enkephalins are the most widely studied of these and apparently function in brain as neurotransmitters mediating various physiological functions including reaction to pain (3,22). Much of the most promising drug development to date has focused on these pentapeptides. The potential rewards for such effort are obvious. In addition to the role in modulation of recognition and/or response to noxious stimuli, these peptides probably also have a role in the hypothalamic control of pituitary function (5,17) and may play a part in sexual maturation and function (1,14,15) and dysfunction in these systems; furthermore, they may be related to various forms of psychiatric illness (23).

The pentapeptides seem to have significant advantages over the larger endorphins from the point of view of drug development since pharmacological activity resides in the smaller fragment which is easier and more economical to synthesize. Because the natural enkephalins are too labile to have therapeutic utility, the research challenge has been to provide structural modification which would infer enzymatic protection without destroying affinity and efficacy at the desired receptors.

Our approach to this problem was to first determine the structure-activity relationships for Met-enkephalin, *in vitro* to bypass pharmacokinetic problems, and then, having deduced the essential structural requirements for receptor activation, to make minimal modifications to provide enzymatic protection and increase blood-brain barrier permeation. pA_2[1] values for naloxone versus interest-

---

[1] Negative logarithm of the molar concentration of an antagonist that reduces the effect of a double dose of an agonist to that of a single dose.

ing enkephalin analogs were determined to facilitate a judgement of whether these analogs were interacting with the same receptors (δ-receptors) as were the natural peptides. Peptides were prepared so that when injected intraventricularly, they were as much as 100,000 times more potent than were the natural materials as analgesics. Many of the compounds proved to be analgesics even after systemic administration. One compound in particular, LY 127623, was of similar potency to morphine and meperidine in rodent tests for analgesia and had less tendency to produce respiratory depression or tolerance and physical dependence. It is presently undergoing initial clinical trials in man.

METHODS

Synthesis and Characterizaton of Peptides

Peptides were prepared by classic solution methodology. The general approach involved the dicyclohexylcarbodiimide-hydroxybenzotriazole mediated coupling of an $N\alpha$-Boc-protected N-terminal tripeptide with the desired C-terminal dipeptide amide or ester. All intermediates were crystalized or preparatively chromatographed on silica-gel to give pure compounds with correct ($\pm$ 3%) amino acid analysis, elemental analysis ($\pm 0.3\%$), and thin-layer homogeneity in several solvent systems. All final peptide products were purified when necessary by chromatography on DEAE-Sephadex A-25 in 1% pyridine: 0.05% acetic acid aqueous buffer. Characterization included, in addition to the methods used for blocked intermediates, high-performance liquid chromatography on C_{18} reverse-phase silica (effluent monitoring at 210 and 280 nm) in an appropriate aqueous acetonitrile-salt buffered eluting solution.

Mouse Vas Deferens

Single vas deferens from mature mice (Cox, 30–40 g) were suspended in 3 ml modified Kreb's solution (10) aerated with 95% O_2-5% CO_2 and maintained at 37°C. The twitch induced by field stimulation (0.15 Hz, 1 msec, 40 V) was recorded on a polygraph (Grass Model 78) via an isometric transducer (Grass FTO3C). Drugs were added to the bath in 20- to 30-μl aliquots with Hamilton syringes. Dose-response curves were constructed by cumulative addition of appropriate amounts of drug to the bath. Comparison of relative agonist potency was made on the basis of IC_{50} values (concentration causing a depression of 50% of the electrically evoked contraction). The peptides were compared with normorphine as a standard of reference.

Analgesic Tests

The hot plate test utilized an apparatus with an electrically heated, thermostatically controlled metal plate (Technilab Instruments, Model 475). A plexiglass cylinder, 12 inches (30 cm) high and 4.75 inches (12 cm) inner diameter, was used to confine the animals to a defined surface of the hot plate. The hot plate was maintained at 52°C for the studies reported here. The time in seconds from contact with the plate until a hind paw lick occurred was recorded as the response latency. The latency until an escape jump occurred was also recorded. Each mouse was used only once. Rat tail heat and mouse writhing tests were also used to test analgesia. These tests are described elsewhere (7,19). Drugs were administered either subcutaneously, intravenously, or intraventricularly. Hamilton microsyringes bearing 27-gauge needles with stops at 2.5 mm from the needle tip were utilized for intraventricular administration (4).

Physical Dependence

Male Sprague-Dawley rats (90–100 g at start of experiment, Harlan Industries) were used to assess primary dependence liability of opioids. The rats were injected subcutaneously four times daily for 14 days with either saline or an opioid drug (morphine, meperidine, pentazocine, codeine, or enkephalin analog) with doses increasing gradually from 10 to 160 mg/kg per injection. The degree of dependence development was assessed at days 4, 7, 10, and 14 by challenge with naloxone and scoring of the resulting withdrawal signs. This withdrawal scoring technique has been previously described (2,7).

Similar studies were also done with mice using the naloxone-induced jumping response to measure withdrawal severity. Mice were treated four times daily with saline or opioid drug for either 3 days or 5 days. Jumps were counted after challenge with subcutaneous naloxone at 100 mg/kg.

RESULTS

Mouse Vas Deferens Data

The mouse vas deferens preparation was utilized to develop structure-activity relationships without interference from pharmacokinetic factors. Some of these data have been already published (3,5). A comparison of LY 127623 (D-Ala^2-N(Me)Met^5-enkephalin amide) with normorphine and natural Met-enkephalin on the mouse vas deferens is shown in Fig. 1. The replacement of Gly^2 with D-Ala^2 provided protection from cleavage by peptidases from the N-terminal, while amidation and N-methylation at the peptide link at position 5 provided protection at the C-terminal. These modifications did not interfere with binding to the receptor but, in fact, resulted in increased receptor activity. LY 127623 was approximately 50 times more potent, while Met-enkephalin was approximately 20 times more potent, than normorphine on this preparation. Analysis of pA$_2$ revealed that normorphine used one receptor type in this tissue (pA$_2$ for naloxone = 8.2) while Met-enkephalin and LY 127623 shared a second type of receptor (pA$_2$ for naloxone = 7.6).

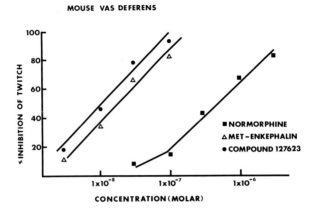

FIG. 1. Comparative dose-response curves of the inhibition of the electrically induced twitch of the mouse vas deferens by normorphine, Met-enkephalin, and compound LY 127623.

Analgesic Data

Intraventricular Injection

The mouse hot plate test for analgesia was utilized to assess the activity of synthetic peptides compared with morphine. In initial studies the compounds were administered directly into the lateral ventricles in order to bypass the blood-brain barrier. The activity of LY 127623 compared with morphine is shown in Fig. 2. LY 127623 was more than 100 times more potent than morphine and at least 30,000 times more potent than Met-enkephalin when administered directly into the ventricles. This analgesic activity could be antagonized by naloxone, although this required 3 to 10 times as much naloxone as required to comparatively antagonize morphine.

Systemic Injection

LY 127623 was active after subcutaneous or intravenous administration in the mouse hot plate, mouse writhing, and rat tail heat tests for analgesia. The comparative intravenous ED_{50} values of LY 127623 and meperidine on the hind paw lick and jump responses in the mouse hot plate test are shown in Table 1. Further analgesic data are published elsewhere (5,6). By the subcutaneous route of administration the duration of action of LY 127623 is intermediate between that of meperidine and morphine, while after intravenous administration it is of faster onset and shorter than meperidine.

Physical Dependence

The relative capacity of LY 127623 to substitute in morphine-dependent mice, rats, and monkeys was compared with that of morphine, meperidine, pentazocine,

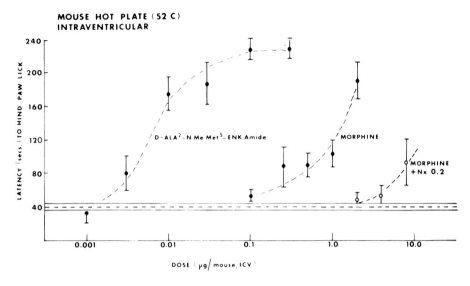

FIG. 2. Comparative dose-response curves of morphine and D-Ala²-*N*(Me)Met⁵-enkephalin amide (LY 127623) in the mouse hot plate test. The drugs were administered into the lateral ventricles. The ordinate is the latency in seconds to the hind paw lick response. The horizontal lines give the mean control (saline-treated mice) latency (± SE). Latencies were determined at 30 min after injection of morphine and 15 min after D-Ala²-*N*(Me)Met⁵-enkephalin amide. Nx 0.2 = Naloxone, 0.2 mg/kg s.c., given 15 min before testing.

and codeine. LY 127623 was the least effective of all the agents tested. The ability of LY 127623 to produce physical dependence after chronic treatment of mice and rats was also compared with the standard analgesics mentioned above. Rats were treated chronically with each of the drugs for 14 days as described in Methods and the withdrawal scores obtained on each of the test days after injection of naloxone are shown in Fig. 3. Morphine produced a high level of dependence and meperidine and pentazocine produced an intermediate level of dependence. LY 127623 produced only slightly more dependence than did saline in this test. Similar results were obtained in the mouse withdrawal jumping test. LY 127623 was also found to have less respiratory depressant activity than morphine in rodent tests.

TABLE 1. *Intravenous ED₅₀ values (mg/kg) in mouse hot plate test[a]*

	Hind paw lick	Jump
LY 127623	0.28	0.15
Meperidine	0.49	0.91

[a] Values were determined at the time of peak effect which was 2 min.

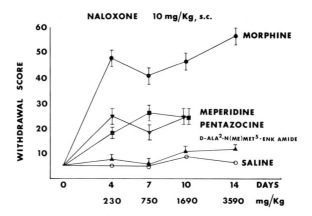

FIG. 3. Naloxone precipitated withdrawal scores after chronic treatment of rats with morphine, meperidine, pentazocine, D-Ala^2-N(Me)Met^5-enkephalin amide or saline as described in Methods. Withdrawal was precipitated at day 4, 7, 10, and 14 by the injection of naloxone at 10 mg/kg s.c. Withdrawal signs were scored for 15 min after injection of naloxone. The numbers below the abscissa give the total dose of compound in mg/kg administered by each time of testing. There is no data for meperidine or pentazocine after day 10 since the rats died after further treatment with these drugs.

Clinical Data

LY 127623 was administered intramuscularly as a single weekly injection to each of 4 normal male volunteers in doses increasing gradually from 0.5 to 90 mg. A characteristic pharmacologic pattern was apparent at doses of 12.5 mg or greater, but showed only slight increases in intensity and duration with increase of dose from 25.0 to 90 mg.

No adverse effects were seen as monitored by routine clinical chemistry, electrolytes, urinalysis, hemograms, or EKG. No clinically relevant effects were

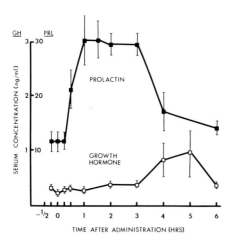

FIG. 4. Effect of LY 127623 on serum prolactin (PRL) and growth hormone (GH) in man. The points represent the mean values ($\pm$ S.E.) determined from 4 subjects given an intramuscular injection of 75 mg of LY 127623 at time zero. There are no significant effects on growth hormone.

observed on blood pressure or heart rate, even at the dose of 90 mg. All subjects, however, at doses greater than 12.5 mg reported a mild retroorbital burning sensation which began 1 to 3 min after administration of the drug and subsequently progressed to nasal congestion and dry mouth which were of 3 to 4 hr duration. The subjects reported a heavy sensation in the extremities which lasted about 1 hr. Emotional detachment and conjunctival injection were also observed. No flushing or changes in bowel sounds were noted. Flare or wheal formation did not occur after intradermal administration. The above pharmacologic profile was also observed in these subjects when they received 75 mg LY 127623 in a single-blinded placebo-controlled study.

A prompt and significant increase in serum prolactin concentration occurred after the administration of 75 mg LY 127623 (Fig. 4). No significant change in growth hormone was observed however (Fig. 4).

DISCUSSION

There is substantial evidence that Met-enkephalin is a neurotransmitter in brain and there is evidence, furthermore, for tonic activity in endogenous opioid systems modulating pain perception and neuroendocrine release (3,5,22). We undertook to develop the therapeutic potential for this opioid pentapeptide. After extensive structure-activity studies on the mouse vas deferens preparation, we attempted minimal structural modification of the Met-enkephalin molecule to provide enzymatic protection and increase bioavailability to the central nervous system after systemic administration. One result of these studies was the preparation of LY 127623 (D-Ala^2-N(Me)Met^5-enkephalin amide) whose pharmacology we have described here.

LY 127623 proved to be more active on the mouse vas deferens than Met-enkephalin which itself is 20 to 30 times more potent than normorphine on this preparation. The observation that naloxone had the same pA$_2$ value versus LY 127623 as versus Met-enkephalin provided further evidence that we had not altered receptor selectivity by our modifications.

Indeed, the compound also acted on the appropriate receptors in brain since it was at least 100 times as potent an analgesic as morphine after direct injection into the lateral ventricles. LY 127623 was active in several analgesic tests after systemic administration as well. It was 5 to 15 times more potent on a molar basis than meperidine in the mouse hot plate test when given intravenously. By the subcutaneous route it was of similar potency to morphine or meperidine in the mouse hot plate and mouse writhing tests, but it was of somewhat lesser potency in rats. The duration of its analgesic activity was similar to that of meperidine or pentazocine.

LY 127623 produced very little primary dependence after chronic treatment (3–14 days) in mice and rats, and appeared to have much less dependence liability in these tests than any of the analgesic standards to which it was compared, such as morphine, meperidine, codeine, or pentazocine. It was also less potent than these drugs in suppressing withdrawal phenomena in morphine-dependent mouse, rat, and monkey, and had reduced capacity to produce respiratory depression when compared with morphine. The pharmacological profile of LY 127623 suggested that it would have advantages over existing drugs as a parenteral analgesic and has been chosen for clinical trials.

Little is known about the pharmacology of enkephalins in man. The only previous studies are those with FK 33-824 (13,20,25), another synthetic enkephalin analog. In this chapter we have described the results of the first administration to humans of LY 127623. The results with FK 33824 and LY 127623 suggest that the opioid peptide agonists have a distinct pharmacology which differs from that of conventional opiates. These two synthetic peptides share some pharmacological effects, but more importantly there appear to be differences in the pharmacologic and neuroendocrinologic profiles of these two compounds in man. Both induce a subjective sensation of heaviness of the extremities, conjunctival injection, nasal stuffiness, and dry mouth and both increase serum prolactin. FK 33-824, however, stimulated the release of growth hormone while LY 127623 did not. FK 33-824, furthermore, produced facial and whole body flushing, an impressive increase in bowel sounds, a transient increase in pulse rate, and a flare reaction after intradermal injection, none of which were observed with LY 127623. None of the pharmacology generally seen with opioids was seen with either compound.

Caution must be exercised in interpreting these preliminary findings since FK 33-824 and LY 127623 have not been compared side-by-side after the same doses by the same routes of administration. The existing data, nevertheless, suggest differences in the pharmacologic profile between these opioid peptides and conventional narcotic analgesics and differences between these two peptide analogs themselves. These observations provide support for the concept of multiple opioid receptors and raises hope for the development of pharmacologic agents with specificity for the various physiological functions apparently mediated by the endogenous opioids.

ACKNOWLEDGMENTS

We thank Robert Shuman, Carolyn E. Harrell, Vigo Burgis, and J. David Edwards for technical assistance, J. David Edwards for preparation of the figures, and Arline Scott for typing the manuscript.

REFERENCES

1. Blank, M. S., Panerai, A. E., and Friesen, H. G. (1979): Opioid peptides modulate luteinizing hormone secretion during sexual maturation. *Science,* 203:1129–1131.
2. Frederickson, R. C. A. (1975): Morpine withdrawal response and central cholinergic activity. *Nature,* 257:131–132.
3. Frederickson, R. C. A. (1977): Enkephalin pentapeptides: A review of current evidence for a role in vertebrate neurotransmission. *Life Sci.,* 21:23–42.

4. Frederickson, R. C. A., Burgis, V., and Edwards, J. D. (1978): Dual actions of substance P on nociception: Possible role of endogenous opioids. *Science,* 199:1359–1362.
5. Frederickson, R. C. A., and Smithwick, E. L. (1979): Evidence for tonic activity of enkephalins in brain and development of systemically active analogues with clinical potential. In: *Endorphins in Mental Research,* edited by E. Usdin, W. E. Bunney, Jr., and N. S. Kline. MacMillan, London.
6. Frederickson, R. C. A., Smithwick, E. L., and Shuman, R. (1978): Opioid peptides: Structure activity studies and development of analogues with clinical potential. In: *Characteristics and Function of Opioids,* edited by J. van Ree and L. Terenius. Elsevier, Amsterdam.
7. Frederickson, R. C. A., and Smits, S. E. (1973): Time course of dependence and tolerance development in rats treated with "slow release" morphine suspensions. *Res. Commun. Chem. Pathol. Pharmacol.,* 5:867–870.
8. Gintzler, A. R., Gershon, M. D., and Spector, S. (1978): A nonpeptide morphine-like compound: Immunocytochemical localization in the mouse brain. *Science,* 199:447–448.
9. Goldstein, A. (1976): Opioid peptides (endorphins) in pituitary and brain. *Science,* 193:1081–1086.
10. Henderson, G., Hughes, J., and Kosterlitz, H. W. (1972): A new example of a morphine-sensitive neuro-effector junction: Adrenergic transmission in the mouse vas deferens. *Br. J. Pharmacol.,* 46:764–766.
11. Hughes, J. (1975): Isolation of an endogenous compound from the brain with pharmacological properties similar to morphine. *Brain Res.,* 88:295–308.
12. Hughes, J., Smith, T. W., Kosterlitz, H. W., Fothergill, L. A., Morgan, B. A., and Morris, H. R. (1975): Identification of two related pentapeptides from the brain with potent opiate agonist activity. *Nature,* 258:577–579.
13. Leslie, R. D. G., Pyke, D. A., and Stubbs, W. A. (1979): Sensitivity to enkephalin as a cause of non-insulin dependent diabetes. *Lancet,* Feb. 17:341–343.
14. Meyerson, B. J., and Terenius, L. (1977): β-Endorphin and male sexual behavior. *Eur. J. Pharmacol.,* 42:191–192.
15. Pellegrini-Quarantotti, B., Corda, M. G., Paglietti, E., Biggio, G., and Gessa, G. L. (1978): Inhibition of copulatory behavior in male rats by D-ala²–met-enkephalin amide. *Life Sci.,* 23:673–678.
16. Pert, C. B., and Snyder, S. H. (1973): Opiate receptor: Demonstration in nervous tissue. *Science,* 179:1011–1014.
17. Shaar, C. J., Frederickson, R. C. A., Dininger, N. B., and Jackson, L. (1977): Enkephalin analogues and naloxone modulate the release of growth hormone and prolactin—evidence for regulation by an endogenous opioid peptide in brain. *Life Sci.,* 21:853–860.
18. Simon, E. J., Hiller, J. M., and Edelman, I. (1973): Stereospecific binding of the potent narcotic analgesic ³H-etorphine to rat brain homogenate. *Proc. Natl. Acad. Sci. USA,* 70:1947–1949.
19. Smits, S. E., and Myers, M. B. (1974): Some comparative effects of racemic methadone and its optical isomers in rodents. *Res. Commun. Chem. Pathol. Pharmacol.,* 7:651–662.
20. Stubbs, W. A., Delitala, G., Jones, A., Jeffcoate, W. J., Edwards, C. R. W., Ratter, S. J., Besser, G. M., Bloom, S. R., and Alberti, K. G. M. (1978): Hormonal and metabolic responses to an enkephalin analogue in normal man. *Lancet,* Dec. 9:1225–1227.
21. Terenius, L. (1973): Characteristics of the "receptor" for narcotic analgesics in synaptic plasma membrane fraction from rat brain. *Acta. Pharmacol. Toxicol.,* 33:377–384.
22. Terenius, L. (1978): Endogenous peptides and analgesia. *Annu. Rev. Pharmacol. Toxicol.,* 18:189–204.
23. Terenius, L. (1978): The implications of endorphins in pathological states. In: *Characteristics and Function of Opioids,* edited by J. van Ree and L. Terenius. Elsevier, Amsterdam.
24. Terenius, L., and Wahlstrom, A. (1975): Search for an endogenous ligand for the opiate receptor. *Acta Physiol. Scand.,* 94:74–81.
25. von Graffenried, B., del Pozo, E., Roubicek, J., Krebs, E., Poldinger, W., Burmeister, P., and Kerp, L. (1978): Effects of the synthetic enkephalin analogue FK33–824 in man. *Nature,* 272:729–730.

Neuropeptides and Neural Transmission,
edited by C. Ajmone Marsan and W. Z. Traczyk.
Raven Press, New York © 1980.

The Inhibition of the Development of Tolerance to and Physical Dependence on Morphine by Peptides

R. F. Ritzmann, Roderich Walter, *Hemendra N. Bhargava,
and **William Krivoy

*Department of Physiology and Biophysics, and *Department of Pharmacognosy and Pharmacology, University of Illinois at the Medical Center, Chicago, Illinois 60612; and **Department of Health, Education and Welfare, National Institute on Drug Abuse, Addiction Research Center, Lexington, Kentucky 40583*

The tolerance to and physical dependence on opiates which occurs after chronic drug administration has been suggested to be a form of central nervous system (CNS) adaption (6), which may be similar in some aspects to learning and memory (8). In support of this concept, there are a number of procedures that have been shown to interfere with the development of tolerance, dependence, and memory processes. Among these procedures are cortical ablations (5,9), inhibition of protein synthesis (3,13,14), the depletion of neurotransmitters such as serotonin (4,10) and norepinephrine (12,16), and electroconvulsive shock (7,15). Recently, a considerable interest has been generated in the role of neurohypophyseal peptides and fragments both in acute response to opiates and in the development of tolerance to these drugs. Reports have implied that oxytocin (OXT) and, to a lesser extent, arginine vasopressin (AVP) facilitate the development of tolerance to and physical dependence on morphine (17).

These two peptides have also been shown to alter certain aspects of memory processes (2). Studies from our laboratory have shown the C-terminal tripeptide of OXT, Pro-Leu-Gly-NH$_2$ [melanocyte release-inhibiting factor (MIF); also known as melanocyte-stimulating hormone–release-inhibiting factor (MSH-RIF)] was more potent that OXT in attenuating the amnesia caused by puromycin in mice (18). Various fragments and analogs of MIF were also active in these tests. A recent report has indicated that OXT may actually produce amnesia (1). Initial studies have indicated that MIF and several other small peptides related to MIF, may also have the opposite effect as OXT on morphine tolerance and physical dependence (19); that is, these peptides appear to block or inhibit the development of morphine tolerance and physical dependence.

Because of the potential clinical, as well as the theoretical importance of this finding, the present series of experiments were designed to investigate a selected number of peptides [MIF, cyclo(leu-Gly), and Z-Pro-D-Leu] in order to evaluate their relative ability in altering the acute response to morphine, the development of tolerance to the analgesic properties of the opiate, as well as the development of physical dependence on morphine. We also performed a structure activity analysis of a wide range of tri- and dipeptides in order to compare the potency of these compounds in altering the response to morphine with their ability to alter learning and memory.

MATERIALS AND METHODS

A double-blind procedure was used for all experiments, and each peptide was tested in at least two independent experiments. Male Swiss Webster mice (Scientific Small Animal Farm Inc., Melrose Park, Ill.) weighing 24 ± 2g (mean ± SD) were used. The mice were housed 5 or 6 per cage in temperature (23 ± 1°C) and light (light 6 A.M.–6 P.M.) controlled rooms and were kept in our laboratory for a minimum of 7 days prior to the initiation of experiments. Food (Purina Laboratory Chow) and water were available *ad lib.*

Mice were randomly divided into two groups. One group received subcutaneous injections of 0.1 ml of water (vehicle). The other group received peptide dissolved in 0.1 ml of water; in the case of the structure–activity studies, a single dose of 50 μg of peptide per mouse was given on day 1, and in the dose response studies 50, 5, 0.5, or 0.005 μg of peptide was administered to the respective groups of mice. Two hours later the mice were implanted with either morphine or placebo pellets. Morphine pellets, containing 75 mg of morphine (free base), were implanted subcutaneously between 10 A.M. and 11 A.M. and were removed 3 days later at the same time of day (19). The injections of vehicle and respective peptides were repeated 24 and 48 hr after the first injection in their respective groups. Controls were as described (20). To evaluate the effect of the various peptides on the acute response to morphine, the peptides were injected for 3 days; 24 hr after the last peptide injection the analgesic effect of morphine (40 mg/kg i.p.) was tested. The analgesic response was determined by measuring the jump threshold to an increasing electric current on an electrified grid attached to a BRS/LVE shock generator/scrambler. The level of analgesia was determined by comparing the change in threshold prior to, and 30 min after, the injection of morphine (20).

To determine the effects of peptide treatment on development of physical dependence, the abstinence syndrome was precipitated using the morphine antagonist naloxone (Endo Laboratories Inc., N.Y.) (0.1 mg/kg) injected intraperitoneally 1 hr following removal of morphine and placebo pellets. Pellet removal was performed 24 hr after the last peptide injection. These mice were monitored for changes in body temperature, by using a lubricated rectal probe (inserted 2.5 cm into the rectum) and telethermometer (model 43TA, Yellow Springs Instrument); the first measurement was made just prior to naloxone administration and the rest were at 15, 30, and 60 min. postinjection. The results are expressed in the tables as the difference between the 0- and 30-min readings.

Effects of removing the pellets (withdrawing morphine) was also assessed by utilizing body temperature as dependent variable, however, these measurements were made at 2 hr intervals for 10 hr after the removal of the pellets. Placebo-implanted mice were treated in the same manner as the morphine pellet-implanted mice (20).

Tolerance to hypothermic and analgesic effects of morphine injected intracerebroventricularly was assessed 24 hr after the removal of the pellets in mice not injected with naloxone. The intracerebroventricular injection was 40 μg of morphine sulfate solution in 10 μl volume (20). Body temperature was recorded prior to, and 10 and 15 min after, injection of morphine. Analgesia was determined 1 hr after the intracerebroventricular injection.

Tolerance to the analgesic effects of morphine was also measured by injecting morphine (40 mg/kg) intraperitoneally 24 hr after the removal of the pellets in separate groups of mice (20). The analgesic response was determined as described above.

Brain levels of morphine were measured in mice that had received either vehicle or peptide injections. These mice were decapitated 72 hr after the morphine pellets had been implanted. Brains were rapidly removed, frozen on dry ice, and stored at $-80°$C until assayed for morphine content. Morphine concentrations were quantified fluorometrically (20).

RESULTS

The naturally occurring peptide MIF (19) was found to be very effective in blocking the development of physical dependence on morphine when injected daily at a dose of 50 μg per mouse. The addition of a N-benzyloxycarbonyl (Z) group apparently did not alter the activity of the peptide in this testing situation, but additions of Z-Gly or substitution of pyro-Glu([Glu) for the NH$_2$-terminal proline gave derivatives with reduced activity. Replacement of the proline residue by 3,4-dehydroproline (Δ^3Pro), deletion of the proline moiety, dimethylation of the primary carboxamide group, or replacement of the glycinamide moiety by glycine resulted in inactive derivatives of MIF. However, the free dipeptide Pro-Leu exhibited activity; and, as in our previous study (20), Z-Pro-D-Leu was active under the present test conditions as well. Reminiscent of another investigation (18) of ours, in which we found the C-terminal dipeptide of oxytocin, Leu-Gly-NH$_2$, and its optical isomer, D-Leu-Gly-NH$_2$, to be very effective in attenuating puromycin-induced amnesia in mice, is the finding that all of the four possible optical isomers—i.e., Z-Pro-Leu, Z-D-Pro-Leu, Z-Pro-D-Leu, and Z-D-Pro-D-Leu—were able to block physical dependence on morphine. Likewise, the substitution of Gln, Met, or Tyr for Leu in Z-Pro-Leu gave potent derivatives, but the substitution by either Ser or ΔPhe gave peptides of reduced activity. All of the above peptides may be considered to be analogs of MIF.

Another group of peptides that can yield active derivatives are the cyclic

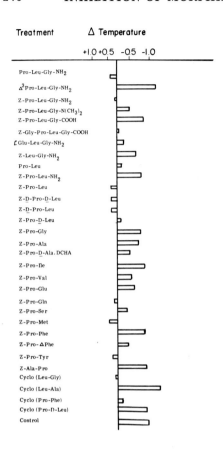

FIG. 1. Structure–activity relationship for MIF in blocking the development of physical dependence in mice. Morphine pellets were removed 72 hr after implantation; 1 hr after removal, mice were injected (i.p.) with naloxone (0.1 mg/kg). Body temperature was recorded just prior to and 30 min after naloxone injection. The data are expressed as the difference between the two temperatures.

dipeptides. Among the few tested, cyclo(Leu-Gly) and cyclo(Pro-Phe) showed activity. (See Fig. 1).

The 3-day treatment with MIF, cyclo(Leu-Gly), or Z-Pro-D-Leu did not alter the acute analgesic response to morphine; the difference between pre- and post-morphine jump thresholds was 1.0, 1.2, and 1.25, respectively, as compared with a difference of 1.26 found for vehicle-injected mice. In each case the difference between pre- and postjump threshold was significantly different ($p < 0.05$ t-test).

There was no difference in brain morphine levels 72 hr after pellets were implanted (ng/g ± SEM): vehicle 277 ± 32, MIF 291 ± 52, cyclo(Leu-Gly) 265 ± 29. The daily injection of 50 µg MIF, cyclo (Leu-Gly), or Z-Pro-D-Leu prevented the hypothermic response which occurs during either abrupt or naloxone-induced withdrawal. During abrupt withdrawal the peptide-treated mice which had been implanted with morphine pellets did not differ from either peptide- or vehicle-injected mice which had been implanted with placebo pellets at any of the time points. Vehicle-injected mice which had received the chronic morphine treatment exhibited a significant hypothermia (−1.5°C) 8 hr after

TABLE 1. *Dose-response effects of MIF and derivatives on naloxone-precipitated withdrawal*

Treatment	Dose (μg)	N	Δt (°C)[a]	p[b]
MIF	50	8	+0.25 ± 0.24	0.001
	5	4	+0.08 ± 0.28	0.001
	0.5	5	+0.18 ± 0.39	0.001
	0.05	4	−1.50 ± 0.14	ns
	0.005	4	−1.05 ± 0.17	ns
Z-Pro-D-Leu	50	11	−0.09 ± 0.58	0.001
	5	4	−0.05 ± 0.37	0.01
	0.5	6	−1.47 ± 0.12	ns
Cyclo(Leu-Gly)	50	15	−0.19 ± 0.58	0.001
	5	5	+0.47 ± 0.32	0.001
	0.5	10	+0.30 ± 0.29	0.001
	0.05	10	+0.27 ± 0.70	0.01
Vehicle	0	33	−1.18 ± 0.43	—

[a] Difference in body temperature of mice determined just prior to naloxone injection (0.1 mg/kg) and 30 min thereafter; values are expressed as mean ± SD.
[b] Means compared by Student's test, $p > 0.05$ was considered to be not significant (ns).

pellet removal. A similar relationship was found during naloxone-induced withdrawal. Vehicle-injected mice which had received morphine lost −1.8°C, while the peptide-treated mice did not demonstrate any alteration in body temperature following the injection of naloxone (Table 1).

Dose-response experiments revealed cyclo(Leu-Gly) to be the most potent peptides tested to date in blocking physical dependence on morphine (Table 1). MIF at a dose of less than 0.5 μg per mouse failed to produce any alterations in the withdrawal response, while cyclo(Leu-Gly) was still effective in blocking physical dependence at a dose as low as 0.05 μg per mouse. Z-Pro-D-Leu exhibited significant activity until a dose of less than 5 μg per mouse was administered.

Morphine-treated mice given vehicle were tolerant to the hypothermic ($p < 0.01$) and analgesic ($p < 0.01$) effects of the intracerebroventricular injection of morphine (40 μg/mouse) when compared with the vehicle-injected placebo group (Table 2). This tolerance was evident 24 hr after the removal of the pellets. Mice which had been given Z-Pro-D-Leu during chronic morphine treatment responded to the intracerebroventricular injection of morphine in a manner that was not significantly different from morphine-naive mice, but differed significantly from vehicle/morphine-treated mice ($p < 0.01$).

Administration of MIF or cyclo(Leu-Gly) inhibited the development of tolerance to morphine (40 mg/kg). In placebo pellet-implanted mice, the administration of morphine increased jump threshold significantly ($p < 0.05$) (Table 2). Morphine (40 mg/kg) administration did not alter the jump threshold in morphine-dependent mice which were injected with vehicle, MIF, or cyclo(Leu-Gly) after the tolerance had already developed. However, no tolerance to morphine developed in chronic morphine-treated mice, which were injected with

TABLE 2. *Effects of peptides on the development of tolerance to morphine*

Group	Morphine injection[a]	Δt (°C)[b]	Jump threshold[c]
Vehicle/morphine	40 μg/s i.c.v.	−0.58 ± 0.24[d]	2.66 ± 0.36[d]
Z-Pro-D-Leu/morphine	40 μg/s i.c.v.	−1.32 ± 0.34	4.33 ± 0.54
Vehicle/placebo	40 μg/s i.c.v.	−1.30 ± 0.48	4.25 ± 0.63
Z-Pro-D-Leu/placebo	40 μg/s i.c.v.	−1.48 ± 0.46	4.18 ± 0.41
Vehicle/morphine	40 mg/kg i.p.	—	4.31 ± 0.33[e]
MIF/morphine	40 mg/kg i.p.	—	6.16 ± 0.41
Cyclo(Leu-Gly)/morphine	40 mg/kg i.p.	—	6.59 ± 0.32
Vehicle/placebo	40 mg/kg i.p.	—	6.15 ± 0.23
MIF/placebo	40 mg/kg i.p.	—	5.80 ± 0.17
Cyclo(Leu-Gly)/placebo	40 mg/kg i.p.	—	5.80 ± 0.23

[a] See text for details of morphine injection.
[b] Δt is the difference between pre- and post (15 min)-morphine injection temperature.
[c] See text for method of determining jump threshold.
[d] $p < 0.01$ means ± SD (Student's t-test).
[e] $p < 0.05$ means ± SD (Student's t-test).

MIF or cyclo(Leu-Gly) during morphine treatment, as evidenced by an increase in the jump threshold following an injection of morphine which was not different from morphine-naive mice (Table 2). There were no differences among the vehicle- or peptide-injected mice in brain morphine levels.

DISCUSSION

The three peptides [(MIF, cyclo(Leu-Gly), and Z-Pro-D-Leu)] tested prevented the development of physical dependence as determined by the loss of body temperature during both abrupt or naloxone-induced withdrawal. Cyclo(Leu-Gly) appears to be the most potent peptide tested under these conditions. There was also no apparent development of tolerance to morphine. These effects were produced without altering the acute analgesic response to morphine, nor did they directly effect either body temperature or pain sensitivity at any of the doses tested. The injection of the peptides after physical dependence and tolerance had already developed, i.e., after 3 days of morphine treatment, did not alter the display of either the symptoms of withdrawal or the degree of tolerance exhibited. These data would indicate that these peptides interfere with the development of morphine tolerance and physical dependence without altering the acute response to the drug. The mechanism by which this interference is produced is not certain. Since there is no change in the acute response to morphine, it would not seem likely that the peptides are altering the ability of morphine to interact with opiate receptors. In addition, there does not appear to be any change in brain morphine levels among the various peptide-treated mice during chronic morphine treatment. The failure to observe any tolerance to an intracerebroventricular injection of morphine in peptide-treated mice which had received chronic morphine administration would also argue against the concept that these effects are a result of peripheral alterations. Similarly, the failure of these peptides to alter the display of dependence or tolerance once they had already developed indicates that these effects are not due to a blockage of efferent pathways. A recent report has indicated that the amount of cyclo(Leu-Gly) localized in the synaptosomal fraction, but not in other subcellular fractions, was highly correlated with the peptides' effect on puromycin-induced amnesia (11). It would therefore appear that these peptides are altering the genesis of morphine tolerance and physical dependence via some CNS action, possibly by a modification of some synaptic change which occurs during chronic drug exposure. Since the synpase is the most plastic element in the CNS, it has been proposed that alterations in synaptic function underlie learning and memory processes. The present findings are therefore consistent with the hypothesis that the development of tolerance and dependence as well as learning and memory may be forms of general CNS adaption to novel stimuli.

ACKNOWLEDGMENT

This work was supported by U. S. Public Health Service Grant AM-18399, by National Science Foundation Grant GB-42758, and by the Illinois Department of Mental Health and Development Disabilities Grant 904–02.

REFERENCES

1. Bohus, B., Kovacs, G. L., and de Wied, D. (1978): Oxytocin, vasopressin and memory: Opposite effects on consolidation and retrieval processes. *Brain Res., 157*:414–417.
2. de Wied, D. (1965): The influence of the posterior and intermediate lobe of the pituitary and pituitary peptide on the maintenance of a conditioned avoidance response in rats. *Int. J. Neuropharmacol., 4*:157–167.
3. Flood, J. F., Bennett, E. L., Orme, A. E., and Rosengweig, M. R. (1975): Relation of memory formation to controlled animals of brain protein synthesis. *Physiol. Behav., 15*:97–102.
4. Frankel, D., Khanna, J. M., LeBlanc, A. E., and Kalant, H. (1975): Effect of *p*-chlorophenylalanine on acquisition of tolerance to ethanol and pentobarbital. *Psychopharmacology, 44*:247–252.
5. Grossman, S. P. (1967): *A Textbook of Physiological Psychology.* Wiley, New York.
6. Hoffman, P. L., Ritzmann, R. F., Walter, R., and Tabakoff, B. (1978): Arginine vasopressin maintains ethanol tolerance. *Nature, 276*:614–616.
7. Kesner, R. P., Priano, D. J., and de Witt, J. R. (1976): Time-dependent disruption of morphine tolerance by electroconvulsive shock and frontal cortical stimulation. *Science, 194*:1079–1081.
8. LeBlanc, A. E., and Cappell, H. (1977): Tolerance as adaptation: Interactions with behavior and parallels to other adaptive processes. In: *Alcohol and Opiates, Neurochemical and Behavioral Mechanisms,* edited by K. Blume, pp. 65–77. Academic, New York.
9. LeBlanc, A. E., Matsunaga, M., and Kalant, H. (1976): Effects of frontal polar cortical ablation and cycloheximide on ethanol tolerance in rats. *Pharmacol. Biochem. Behav., 4*:175–179.
10. Ogren, S. O., Ross, S. B., and Baumann, L. (1975): 5-Hydroxtryptamine and learning: Long term effects of *p*-chloroamphetamine on acquisition. *Med. Biol., 53*:165–168.
11. Rainbow, T. C., Flexner, J. B., Flexner, L. B., Hoffman, P. L. and Walter, R. (1979): Distribution, survival and biological effects in mice of a behaviorally active, enzymatically stable peptide: Pharmacokinetics of cyclo(Leu-Gly) and puromycin-induced amnesia. *Pharmacol. Biochem. Behav., 7*:787–793.

12. Ritzmann, R. F., and Tabakoff, B. (1976): Dissociation of alcohol tolerance and dependence. *Nature,* 263:418–420.
13. Segal, D. S., Squire, L. R., and Barondes, S. H. (1971): Cycloheximide: Its effects on activity are dissociatable from its effects on memory. *Science,* 172:82–84.
14. Squire, L. R., and Barondes, S. H. (1973): Memory impairment during prolonged training in mice given inhibitors of cerebral protein synthesis. *Brain Res.,* 56:215–225.
15. Stolerman, I. P., Bunker, P., Johnson, C. A., Jarvik, M. E., Krivoy, W., and Zimmerman, E. (1976): Attenuation of morphine tolerance development of electroconvulsive shock to mice. *Neuropharmacology,* 15:309–313.
16. Tabakoff, B., Yanai, J., and Ritzmann, R. F., (1978): Brain noradrenergic systems as a prerequisite for developing tolerance to barbiturates. *Science,* 200:449–451.
17. Van Ree, J. M., and de Wied, D., (1976): Prolyl-leucyl-glycinamide (PLG) facilitates morphine dependence. *Life Sci.,* 19:1331–1340.
18. Walter, R., Hoffman, P. L., Flexner, J. B., and Flexner, L. B. (1975): Neurohypophyseal hormones, analogs, and fragments: Their effect on puromycin-induced amnesia. *Proc. Natl. Acad. Sci., USA,* 72:4180–4184.
19. Walter, P., Ritzmann, R. F., Bhargava, H. N., and Flexner, L. B., (1979): Prolyl-leucyl-glycinamide, cyclo(leucyl-glycine), and derivatives block development of physical dependence on morphine in mice. *Proc. Natl. Acad. Sci. USA,* 76:518–520.
20. Walter, R., Ritzmann, R. F., Bhargava, H. N., Rainbow, T. C., Flexner, L., and Krivoy, W. A. (1978): Inhibition by Z-Pro-D-Leu of development of tolerance to and physical dependence on morphine in mice. *Proc. Natl. Acad. Sci. USA,* 75:4573–4576.

Neuropeptides and Neural Transmission,
edited by C. Ajmone Marsan and W. Z. Traczyk.
Raven Press, New York © 1980.

The Distribution and Release of β-Endorphin in Relation to Certain Possible Functions

* R. Przewłocki, Ch. Gramsch, V. Höllt, M. J. Millan, H. Osborne, and A. Herz

Department of Neuropharmacology, Max-Planck-Institut für Psychiatrie, D–8000 München 40, Federal Republic of Germany

The isolation and synthesis of endogenous opiate-like peptides has generated a considerable interest in, and a plethora of studies directed towards the elucidation of, their localization, mechanism and regulation of release, and physiological function.

β-Endorphin, a peptide identical to the amino acid sequence 61–91 of β-lipotropin (β-LPH), is found at a high concentration in the pituitary gland of rats and other species (6,8,12,24). β-Endorphin, β-LPH, and adrenocorticotropic hormone (ACTH), which have been localized in the same pituitary cells, and even in the same granules within these cells (6,40), have been found by Mains et al. (27) to possess a common 31 K precursor. Recently, immunocytochemical studies have demonstrated β-endorphin containing cell bodies in the basal hypothalamus (5).

β-Endorphin has been implicated, both experimentally and conceptually in a number of biological processes. For example, in the processes of thermoregulation (4,28) and as a component of the closely interrelated systems of response to stress and pain (9,11,16,19,22,26,36).

The distribution in, and release of this peptide from the brain and pituitary constitutes the major part of this chapter, but since such data can be illuminatory as to at least the possible function(s) of β-endorphin, a brief discussion of this central aspect of β-endorphin physiology will be attempted.

DISTRIBUTION OF β-ENDORPHIN IN THE BRAIN

β-Endorphin immunoreactivity (β-EI) is at a maximal concentration in the hypothalamus, septum, and midbrain of the rat, whereas it is undetectable in both the striatum and pons/medulla of this species (31,37). The development of an antiserum highly avid for human β-endorphin, with a detection limit of

---

* Permanent address: Institute of Pharmacology, Polish Academy of Sciences, Cracow, Smetna 12, Poland.

less than 2 fmoles/tube, has enabled us to likewise determine the pattern of distribution of β-EI in human brain (13,14). The anterior and posterior hypothalamus, periaqueductal gray matter, mamillary bodies, and pineal gland displayed a high concentration of β-EI, it being below the detection limit in the cerebellum and cortex. Intermediate levels were consistently found in several other structures, e.g., the amygdaloid complex, septum, olfactory bulb, thalamus, midbrain, and pons/medulla. It is worthy of emphasis that the contrasting distribution of Met-enkephalin and β-endorphin in human brain, analogous to the situation in the rat, is suggestive that these endorphins exist in anatomically independent neurones in both species (5,13,39).

Bloom and his colleagues have investigated the organization of β-endorphinergic pathways in the rat CNS via an immunocytochemical approach (5). Thus, β-EI is localized in a diffuse cluster of cell bodies in the basal hypothalamus, from which varicose fibres project throughout the midline nuclear area of the diencephalon and anterior pons. The neurones are apparently dispersed in two discrete groups: one within and beyond the dorsolateral portion of the middle to posterior thirds of the arcuate nucleus; and the second, continuous with the first, extends anterolaterally almost to the lateral border of the hypothalamus. In our laboratory, however, using a highly purified anti-β-endorphin serum, only one group of neurones has been identified in the perikarya of neurones scattered throughout the arcuate nucleus of the hypothalamus.

Although our antiserum recognises neither Met- or Leu-enkephalin, nor α- or γ-endorphin, it displays about 50% cross-reactivity to β-LPH. Differentiation of the β-endorphin and β-LPH components of β-EI is naturally desirable, so β-immunoreactive material obtained was characterized by gel-filtration using a Sephadex G–50 superfine column, according to a procedure previously described by Przewłocki et al. (34).

Column chromatographic studies have revealed that in both rat and human brains, β-endorphin constitutes the majority of β-EI measured (97 and 90%, respectively) (Table 1). Further, it has been recently established that brain ACTH and alpha-melanocyte stimulating hormone (α-MSH) possess a comparable concentration ratio to that for β-endorphin and β-LPH (Kleber and Gramsch, *unpublished*). It is not unreasonable to assume that these relative proportions genuinely reflect those of *in vivo* conditions and, thus, one is tempted to speculate that α-MSH and β-endorphin, as the predominant peptides, may correspond to the actual neurotransmitter and/or modulators in the brain, whereas ACTH and β-LPH may merely represent their respective synthetic precursors.

DISTRIBUTION OF β-ENDORPHIN IN THE PITUITARY GLAND

High amounts of immunoreactive β-endorphin are found in both the anterior and intermediate lobes of pituitaries of various species (6,8,10,12,23,24). Immunocytochemical examination of the pituitary has demonstrated that intermediate

TABLE 1. *Regional distribution of β-endorphin and β-LPH in rat and human brain*

Region	Human brain[a]			Rat brain[a]	
	β-LPH	β-E		β-LPH	β-E
Hypothalamus anterior	4	40	Hypothalamus	0.5	20
Hypothalamus posterior	8	30			
Periaqueductal gray	0.2	3	Midbrain	0.2	5.2
Septum pellicidum	0	0.7	Septum	0.8	17
Olfactory bulb	0	0.2	Olfactory bulb	0.2	0.4
Pineal gland	0	0.1	Pineal gland	1.3	1.38
Medial amygdaloid nucleus	0.05	0.5	Brainstem	0.2	2.0
Substantia nigra	0.15	0.6	Striatum	0	0.9
Nucleus ruber	0.2	0.5	Hippocampus	0	0.2
Colliculus inferior	0.4	1.41	Cortex	0	0.05
Dorsal pons (including locus coeruleus)	0	0.82	Cerebellum	0	0.05

[a] β-E, β-endorphin. Values in pmoles/g tissue.

lobe cells and adenohypophyseal corticotrophs contain β-EI (6), whereas the posterior lobe (neurohypophysis) is conspicuous in being completely irresponsive to β-endorphin antiserum, but has been shown, however, to possess a high concentration of Met- and Leu-enkephalin (10,35).

Gel-filtration of extracts from the intermediate/posterior lobe of rat pituitaries has revealed that almost all the β-EI consists of β-endorphin with only a negligible contribution being made by β-LPH (31,32). In the anterior lobe, however, β-LPH constitutes about 50% of total immunoreactivity (31,32). Gel-filtration has also shown that the neurointermediate lobe contains mainly α-MSH, whereas in the anterior lobe, ACTH predominates (32). In the human anterior lobe, gel-filtration, in combination with radioimmunoassay (RIA), has shown β-LPH at a high concentration of 134 nmoles/g and β-endorphin at 45 nmoles/g. The neurohypophysis, which possibly contains rudimentary intermediate lobe tissue, contains much lower amounts of both, with β-LPH at 0.213 and β-endorphin at 0.11 nmoles/g.

To summarize, then, both human and rat anterior lobes contain high quantities of ACTH and β-LPH but lower amounts of α-MSH and β-endorphin. It has been maintained that β-EI in the anterior lobe is exclusively due to β-LPH and that any β-endorphin in this lobe may merely be generated by the extraction procedure (25). Notwithstanding the fact that a variety of such procedures have revealed a β-endorphin component in our laboratory, the relative proportions of β-endorphin and β-LPH may reflect differences in type and activity of degradative enzymes etc. And with respect to such processes, the close similarity between the β-LPH/β-endorphin and ACTH/α-MSH ratios in rat brain and intermediate lobe is suggestive of a similarity between these areas in the enzymatic processes governing their formation and breakdown.

RELEASE OF β-ENDORPHIN FROM THE BRAIN

The localization of β-endorphin in a discrete neuronal pathway corresponds to the satisfaction of one criterion necessary for the acceptance of a substance as a neurotransmitter. Recently, we have fulfilled a further important condition, in demonstrating a Ca^{2+}-dependent, three- to fourfold increase in β-EI outflow from rat hypothalamic slices, in response to a depolarizing elevated potassium ion concentration (29) (Fig. 1). Gel-filtration analysis of this effluent yielded about 70% β-endorphin, with the remaining 30% consisting of β-LPH and the 31 K precursor molecule common to both β-LPH and β-endorphin (27).

It is clearly critical, however, to determine if release can occur *in vivo*. One conventional approach to the resolution of this problem is to expose the animal to a particular stimulus in order to compare pre- and post-stimulation levels of the putative neurotransmitter, assuming a decrease in levels to be indicative of the release and subsequent degradation of the neurotransmitter in question. Rossier et al. originally reported a slight decrease in the β-EI content of the

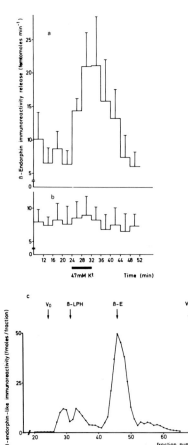

FIG. 1. Release of β-endorphin immuno-reactivity from rat hypothalamus slices **(a)** in Krebs-bicarbonate medium and **(b)** in calcium-free Krebs-bicarbonate medium. Each point represents the mean ± SD of 6–8 determinations. **(c)** Gel-filtration (Sephadex G-50 superfine column) of β-EI material released during potassium stimulation. The position of human β-LPH and synthetic human β-endorphin (β-E) are shown above.

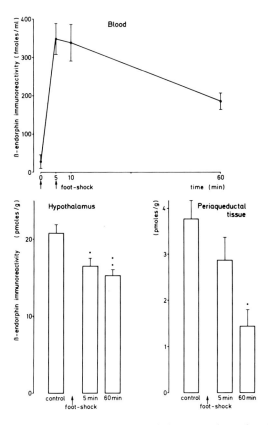

FIG. 2. The influence of foot-shock stress on hypothalamus, periaqueductal tissue and blood levels of β-EI. *$p < 0.02$, **$p < 0.01$, Student's *t*-test.

hypothalami of rats subjected to foot-shock stress (36). Using a similar procedure, we have observed not only such a depression in hypothalamic levels, but also, and perhaps more significantly, a large reduction in the β-EI content of periaqueductal tissue (Fig. 2), wherein β-endorphin is known to exist exclusively in nerve fibres and terminals (5).

RELEASE OF β-ENDORPHIN FROM THE PITUITARY

In vitro Release from the Anterior Lobe

The release of β-EI from isolated lobes of rat pituitary was achieved by Przewłocki et al. (32–34) and from anterior pituitary cells in culture by Vale et al. (38). These experiments clearly showed that the β-endorphin pools in the anterior and intermediate lobes differ both in their mechanism of release and in the regulation of this process. The application of a 50 mM solution of

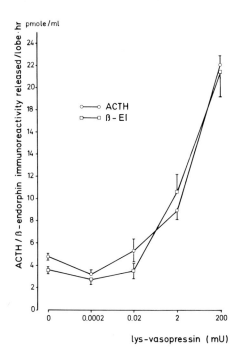

FIG. 3. Release of β-EI or ACTH from the anterior lobe of rat pituitary by Lys-vasopressin. Points represent means ± SEM of 4–5 experiments.

K$^+$-ions instigated a marked Ca^{2+}-dependent release of β-EI from the anterior lobe (32). Lys-vasopressin, hypothalamic extract (NIAMD-Rat HE-RP-1), and noradrenaline further elicited a large corticosterone-inhibitable increase in anterior lobe secretion. Propranolol, a β-adrenergic blocker, was ineffective, but dibenamine, the α-adrenergic blocker, was potent in antagonizing the noradrenaline-initiated increase, demonstrating that its action is mediated by an α-adrenergic receptor.

These results are essentially in agreement with those of Vale et al. (38), working with a tissue culture preparation of anterior lobe cells. The singular disparity between the inability of Vale et al. to release large quantities of β-endorphin dose-dependently by Arg-vasopressin and our observation that Lys-vasopressin is a powerful dose-dependently acting releaser of β-endorphin and ACTH (Fig. 3) is presumably a consequence of differences in cellular and tissue properties between the respective systems. Thus, this chapter re-asserts the importance of vasopressin as a releasing factor. In conclusion, β-endorphin is released from the anterior lobe by a corticotropin-releasing factor of hypothalamic origin (probably at least partially vasopressin), and noradrenaline possibly facilitates this release, perhaps by acting as a cofactor.

In vitro Release from the Intermediate/Posterior Lobe

The intermediate lobe proved refractory to all the above manouvres in displaying no such stimulated release. Its spontaneous release output was, however, higher than that from the anterior lobe, and this release could be inhibited by both dopamine and the ergot alkaloid ergonovine (33). A dopaminergic pathway running to the intermediate lobe is well known (2,3), and irreversible interruption of this network by a variety of means—chemical (6-hydroxydopamine) and electrolytic lesions of the basal hypothalamus, and chronic treatment with chlorpromazine, spiroperidol, and haloperidol—causes a substantial increase in the β-endorphin content of the intermediate lobe. Thus, evidence has accumulated which suggests that release from the intermediate lobe is regulated in an opposite direction to that from the anterior, with a graded activation of a tonic dopaminergic inhibitory input responsible for control of both release and cellular content.

Gel-filtration of Released β-EI from Anterior and Intermediate/Posterior Lobes

Gel-filtration of incubation fluids has allowed for the biochemical analysis of the β-EI material released, of which about 60% from the anterior lobe corresponds to (i.e., coelutes with) human β-LPH and about 30% to human β-endorphin (Fig. 4). The intermediate lobe incubation medium, being primarily composed of β-endorphin, is again clearly distinguishable from its anterior relative.

Thus, these *in vitro* studies have established that the anatomical separation of the anterior and intermediate pools of β-endorphin is accompanied by notable

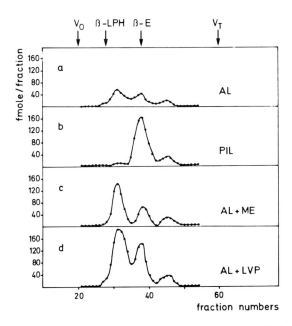

FIG. 4. Gel-filtration of incubation fluids from the anterior lobe of rat pituitary (AL) with **(a)** medium only, **(c)** hypothalamic extract (ME), and **(d)** lys-vasopressin, and of the intermediate/posterior lobe (PIL) with medium **(b)**. Elution volumes of human β-LPH and human β-endorphin (β-E) are shown. Each point represents the mean of two runs.

differences in the mechanism of release, in the regulation of this process, and in the nature of β-EI stored and secreted.

In vivo Studies

In vitro studies are largely inappropriate when considering which system the material is actually released into, and are also irrelevant to their site of action. In fact, that the anterior lobe corticotrophs release directly into the bloodstream is a cornerstone of the concept of a hypophyseal-anterior pituitary-adrenal axis responsive to stress. Most *in vivo* investigations have exploited this fact and concentrated upon various manipulations of the ACTH axis, in order to demonstrate communalities of ACTH and β-endorphin release *in vivo,* and have shown that ACTH and β-endorphin are released concurrently (16) in response to common stimuli. Thus, elimination of adrenal feedback by adrenalectomy or metyrapone results in elevated basal blood levels of β-EI, whilst dexamethasone administration depresses both basal and stimulated release of β-EI in the blood (16). It should also be added, in support of the above contention that vasopressin is a corticotropin-releasing hormone entity, that this substance also releases β-endorphin and raises its level in the blood *in vivo* (18).

In contrast, the situation of the intermediate lobe is still far from clear, and, as yet, release of either ACTH or β-endorphin into the blood from this lobe has not been unambiguously demonstrated *in vivo.* Greer et al. (15) have claimed that, in stressed adenohypophysectomized rats, insufficient ACTH is released to support the stress response, not surprising in view of the fact that ACTH is normally present at only a low concentration in this lobe. In the respect that the intermediate lobe contains vastly greater quantities of β-endorphin than any other structure, the timing of the release, and the function of this β-endorphin is, perhaps, of more pressing concern. One intriguing possibility is that the intermediate pool determines the basal level of β-endorphin in the blood or is released into the brain. Supportive of this conjecture are data from rats chronically treated with morphine: this engenders a parallel 60% decrease in intermediate lobe levels of β-endorphin (34) and depression of basal blood levels of this peptide, whilst leaving intact the large stress-evoked increase in blood β-endorphin, for which the anterior lobe is responsible.

FUNCTIONAL ASPECTS

As mentioned in the introductory remarks, release studies, in particular those performed *in vivo,* can provide certain information germane to a consideration of the potential function(s) of the released substance. Here, attention is focused primarily upon stress and associated phenomena, since it is the imposition of foot-shock stress which has achieved a decrease (probably reflecting release) in β-endorphin levels in hypothalamic and periaqueductal tissue and stress is known to be the major type of circumstances eliciting release of β-endorphin and ACTH from the adenohypophysis (16). Further, behavioral studies have frequently investigated the role of β-endorphin under condition of a reproducible stress. That certain types of stress-induced analgesia are partially blocked by the specific opiate antagonist naloxone, e.g., foot-shock (1) or cold-water immersion (7) has been forwarded as suggestive of an endorphinergic component of this analgesia. But such experiments, to obtain significant effects, have used perhaps unacceptably high doses of naloxone and contradictory to such results, we, in our laboratory, and Hayes et al. (17) have been unable to inhibit this analgesia using the more reasonable dose of 1 mg/kg, sufficient to precipitate full withdrawal in morphine-tolerant animals and, according to *in vivo* binding studies (21), saturate the opiate receptors.

The complementary technique of surgical disruption or inactivation of selective β-endorphin pools has been used in our laboratory and, in agreement with the data from naloxone effects, we have found that specific radiofrequency lesion of the β-endorphin containing arcuate nucleus in the brain only very slightly reduce foot-shock induced analgesia, whilst dexamethasone abolition of ACTH and β-endorphin release from the pituitary was likewise ineffective in reducing this analgesia. Our related observation that both hypo- and adenohypophysectomy both strongly antagonize foot-shock induced analgesia seems to demand an alternative, probably non-endorphinergic explanation.

Thus, an involvement of β-endorphin in the analgesia produced by stress is not, as yet, established, and the discovery that intracerebroventricular injection of β-endorphin into the brain induces analgesia in animals (11,19,26), and that electrical stimulation of the periaqueductal gray increases ventricular concentrations of β-EI and diminishes pain in humans (20) awaits a physiological correlate.

A second pertinent effect of microinjection of β-endorphin into the brain, in this case, of low doses into the preoptic anterior hypothalamus by Martin and Bacino (28), is the occurrence of an elevation of core temperature. This raises the possibility of a β-endorphin influence upon thermoregulatory centres, and in the generation of body heat. Bläsig et al. (4) from our laboratory, have shown naloxone antagonism of the emotional hyperthermia accompanying handling stress, and, we have further observed that naloxone antagonizes the hyperthermia produced by foot-shock stress. Whether this hyperthermia is a directed physiological aim or an epiphenomenon of some other underlying processes remains in need of clarification.

Analgesia and hyperthermia have been considered above, and whilst peripheral opiate receptors, for example in the gut or in the vas deferens, are possibly susceptible to influence by circulating β-endorphin, a limited amount of evidence suggests that β-endorphin may penetrate to the brain from the blood by an, as yet, unknown mechanism. Thus, Pezalla et al. (30), after previous introduction of β-endorphin into the blood of rabbits, have detected it in the CSF of rabbits. In a preliminary study, using an antiserum which does not recognize rabbit β-endorphin (probably different from that of the rat), Merin has measured, in a similar design, β-endorphin in both the CSF and brain of rabbits. These studies have shown that β-endorphin slowly penetrates to and accumulates in brain structures (Merin, *unpublished*). A critical question which remains unresolved, however, is whether β-endorphin cannot only enter the brain (and CSF), but whether it can reach the appropriate receptor in an adequate concentration to exert a physiological effect.

Evidence presented above suggests that the intermediate lobe is not a contributor to the stress-initiated rise of blood β-endorphin levels. Irrespective of the fact that the cause of stress-induced analgesia and hyperthermia is still not fully elucidated, it is noteworthy that removal of the intermediate lobe (in our laboratory), in contrast to the ablation of its anterior counterpart, affects neither foot-shock evoked analgesia nor hyperthermia. The possibility that the intermediate lobe is a, or the, major determinator of basal β-endorphin levels in the blood has been raised, but the significance, if any, of modulation in these levels remains obscure, as does, in fact, the role of intermediate lobe β-endorphin.

REFERENCES

1. Akil, H., Madden, J., Patrick, R. L., and Barchas, J. D. (1976): Stress-induced increase in endogenous opiate peptides: Concurrent analgesia and its partial reversal by naloxone. In: *Opiates and Endogenous Opioid Peptides,* edited by H. W. Kosterlitz. Elsevier, Amsterdam.
2. Baumgarten, H. G., Björklund, A., Holstein, A. F., and Nobin, A. (1972): Organization and ultrastructural identification of the catecholamine nerve terminals in the neural lobe and pars intermedia of the rat pituitary. *Z. Zellforsch. Mikrosk. Anat.,* 126:483–517.
3. Björklund, A. (1968): Monoamine-containing fibres in the intermediate lobe of the pig and rat. *Z. Zellforsch.,* 89:573–589.
4. Bläsig, J., Höllt, V., Bäuerle, U., and Herz, A. (1978): Involvement of endorphins in emotional hyperthermia of rats. *Life Sci.,* 23:2525–2532.
5. Bloom, F., Battenberg, E., Rossier, J., Ling, N., and Guillemin, R. (1978): Neurons containing β-endorphin in rat brain exist separately from those containing enkephalin: Immunocytological studies. *Proc. Natl. Acad. Sci. USA,* 3:1591–1595.
6. Bloom, F., Battenberg, E. L. F., Rossier, J., Ling, N., Leppaluoto, J., Vargo, T. M., and Guillemin, R. (1977): Endorphins are located in the intermediate and anterior lobes of pituitary gland, not in the neurohypophysis. *Life Sci.,* 20:43–48.
7. Bodnar, R. J., Kelly, D. D., Spiaggia, A., Ehrenberg, C., and Glusman, M. (1978): Dose-dependent reductions by naloxone of analgesia induced by cold-water stress. *Pharmacol. Biochem. Behav.,* 8:667–672.
8. Bradbury, A. F., Feldberg, W. F., Smyth, D. G., and Snell, C. R. (1976): Lipotropin C-fragment: An endogenous peptide with potent analgesic activity. In: *Opiates and Endogenous Opioid Peptides,* edited by H. W. Kosterlitz. North-Holland, Amsterdam.
9. Cheng, R., Pomeranz, B., and Yü, G. (1979): Dexamethasone partially reduces and 2% saline-treatment abolishes electroacupuncture analgesia: These findings implicate pituitary endorphins. *Life Sci.,* 24:1481–1486.
10. Duka, Th., Höllt, V., Przewłocki, R., and Wesche, D. (1978): Distribution of methionine- and leucine-enkephalin within the rat pituitary gland measured by highly specific radioimmunoassays. *Biochem. Biophys. Res. Commun.,* 85:1119–1127.
11. Feldberg, W. J., and Smyth, D. G. (1977): Analgesia produced in cats by C-fragment of lipotropin and by a synthetic pentapeptide. *J. Physiol. (Lond.),* 265:25P–27P.
12. Gráf, L., Ronai, A. Z., Bajusz, S., Cseh, G., and Szekely, J. I. (1976): Opioid agonist activity of β-lipotropin fragments: A possible biological source of morphine-like substances in the pituitary. *FEBS Lett.,* 64:181–184.
13. Gramsch, Ch., Höllt, V., Mehraein, P., Pasi, A., and Herz, A. (1978): Regional distribution of endorphins in human brain and pituitary. In: *Developments in Neuroscience, Vol. 4: Character-*

istics and Function of Opioids, edited by J. M. van Ree and L. Terenius. Elsevier/North-Holland, Amsterdam.

14. Gramsch, Ch., Höllt, V., Mehraein, P., Pasi, A., and Herz, A. (1979): Regional distribution of methionine-enkephalin and beta-endorphin-like immunoreactivity in human brain and pituitary. *Brain Res.,* 171:261–270.

15. Greer, M. A., Allen, C. F., Panton, P., and Allen, J. P. (1975): Evidence that the pars intermedia and pars nervosa of the pituitary do not secrete functionally significant quantities of ACTH. *Endocrinology,* 96:718–724.

16. Guillemin, R., Vargo, T., Rossier, J., Minick, S., Ling, S., Rivier, C., Vale, M., and Bloom, F. (1977): β-endorphin and adrenocorticotropin are secreted concomitantly by pituitary gland. *Science,* 197:1367–1369.

17. Hayes, R. L., Bennett, G. J., Newlon, P. G., and Mayer, D. J. (1978): Behavioral and physiological studies of nonnarcotic analgesia in the rat elicited by certain environmental stimuli. *Brain Res.,* 155:69–90.

18. Herz, A., Höllt, V., Przewłocki, R., Duka, Th., Gramsch, Ch., and Emrich, H. (1978): Distribution in and release of endorphins from brain and pituitary under normal and pathological conditions and after chronic opiate treatment. In: *Endorphins '78,* edited by L. Gráf, H. Palkovits, and A. Z. Rónai. Akademiai Kiadó, Budapest.

19. Hosobuchi, Y., and Li, C. H. (1979): Demonstration of the analgesic activity of human β-endorphin in six patients. In: *Endorphins in Mental Health Research,* edited by E. Usdin, W. E. Bunney, and N. S. Kline. MacMillan, London.

20. Hosobuchi, Y., Rossier, J., Bloom, F. E., and Guillemin, R. (1979): Stimulation of human periaqueductal gray for pain relief increases immunoreactive β-endorphin in ventricular fluid. *Science,* 203:279–281.

21. Höllt, V., and Herz, A. (1978): In vivo receptor occupation by opiates and correlation to the pharmacological effect. *Fed. Proc.,* 37:158–161.

22. Höllt, V., Przewłocki, R., and Herz, A. (1978): Radioimmunoassay of β-endorphin. Basal and stimulated levels in extracted rat plasma. *Naunyn Schmiedebergs Arch. Pharmacol.,* 303:171–174.

23. Höllt, V., Przewłocki, R., and Herz, A. (1978): β-Endorphin-like immunoreactivity in plasma, pituitaries and hypothalamus of rats following treatment with opiates. *Life Sci.,* 23:1057–1066.

24. Li, C. H., and Chung, D., (1976): Isolation and structure of an untriakontapeptide with opiate activity from camel pituitary glands. *Proc. Natl. Acad. Sci. USA,* 73:1145–1148.

25. Liotta, A. S., Suda, T., and Krieger, D. T. (1978): β-Lipotropin is the major opioid-like peptide of human pituitary and rat pars distalis: Lack of significant β-endorphin. *Proc. Natl. Acad. Sci. USA,* 75:2950–2954.

26. Loh, H. H., Tseng, L. F., Wei, E., and Li, C. H. (1976): β-Endorphin is a potent analgetic agent. *Proc. Natl. Acad. Sci. USA,* 73:2895–2898.

27. Mains, R. E., Eipper, B. A., and Ling, N. (1977): Common precursor to corticotropins and endorphins. *Proc. Natl. Acad. Sci. USA,* 74:3014–3018.

28. Martin, G. E., and Bacino, C. B. (1978): Action of intrahypothalamically injected β-endorphin on the body temperature of the rat. In: *Abstracts Society for Neuroscience, Vol. 4: Neuropeptides.* Society of Neurosciences, Bethesda, Maryland.

29. Osborne, H., Przewłocki, R., Höllt, V., and Herz, A. (1979): Release of β-endorphin-like immunoreactivity from rat hypothalamus in vitro. *Eur. J. Pharmacol.,* 55:425–428.

30. Pezalla, P. D., Lis, M., Seidah, N. G., and Chrétien, M. (1978): Lipotropin, melanotropin and endorphin in vivo catabolism and entry into cerebrospinal fluid. *J. Can. Sci. Neurol.,* 3:183–188.

31. Przewłocki, R., Höllt, V., Duka, Th., Kleber, G., Gramsch, Ch., Haarmann, I., and Herz, A. (1979): Long-term morphine treatment decreases endorphin levels in rat brain and pituitary. *Brain Res.,* 174:357–361.

32. Przewłocki, R., Höllt, V., and Herz, A. (1978): Release of β-endorphin from rat pituitary in vitro. *Eur. J. Pharmacol.,* 51:179–181.

33. Przewłocki, R., Höllt, V., and Herz, A. (1978): Substances modulating the release of β-endorphin-like immunoreactivity (β-EI) from rat pituitary in vitro. In: *Characteristics and Function of Opioids,* edited by J. M. van Ree and L. Terenius. Elsevier/North-Holland, Amsterdam.

34. Przewłocki, R., Höllt, V., Voigt, K. H., and Herz, A. (1979): Modulation of in vitro release of β-endorphin from separate lobes of the rat pituitary. *Life Sci.,* 24:1601–1608.

35. Rossier, J., Battenberg, E., Pittman, Q., Bayon, A., Koda, L., Miller, R., Guillemin, R., and Bloom, F. E. (1979): Hypothalamic enkephalin neurones may regulate the neurohypophysis. *Nature,* 277:653–655.
36. Rossier, J., French, E. D., Rivier, C., Ling, N., Guillemin, R., and Bloom, F. E. (1977): Foot-shock induced stress increases β-endorphin levels in blood but not brain. *Nature,* 270:618–620.
37. Rossier, J., Vargo, T. M., Minick, S., Ling, N., Bloom, F. E., and Guillemin, R. (1977): Regional dissociation of β-endorphin and enkephalin contents in rat brain and pituitary. *Proc. Natl. Acad. Sci. USA,* 74:5162–5165.
38. Vale, W., Rivier, C., Yang, L., Minick, S., and Guillemin, R. (1978): Effects of purified hypothalamic corticotropin-releasing factor and other substances on the secretion of adrenocorticotropin and β-endorphin immunoreactivities in vitro. *Endocrinology,* 103:1911–1915.
39. Watson, S. J., Huda, A., Richard III, Ch. W., and Barchas, J. P. (1978): Evidence for two separate opiate peptide neuronal systems. *Nature,* 275:226–228.
40. Weber, E., Voigt, K. H., and Martin, R. (1978): Concomitant storage of ACTH- and endorphin-like immunoreactivity in the secretory granules of anterior pituitary corticotrophs. *Brain Res.,* 157:385–390.

Neuropeptides and Neural Transmission,
edited by C. Ajmone Marsan and W. Z. Traczyk.
Raven Press, New York © 1980.

Disinhibitory Role of Endorphins/Enkephalins in the Release of Oxytocin and Vasopressin Controlled by Dopamine: Effects on axon terminals

E. S. Vizi and V. Volbekas

Department of Pharmacology, Semmelweis University of Medicine, H-1445 Budapest, Hungary

Neurochemical and morphological data published in the last few years suggest that the construction of the nervous system is more complex than has previously been assumed. It has been proposed that, in addition to the classical view of neurochemical transmission, a modulator system may be in operation whereby modulators such as noradrenaline, dopamine, etc. are released from nonsynaptic axonal varicosities and, by diffusion, reach remote receptors located on neurons thereby modulating transmitter release (48). This long-range type of modulation also operates discriminantly, as the localization of receptors sensitive to modulators determine the site of action.

Studies on the interaction between hormone release and neurotransmitters have centered mainly on the entire hypothalamo-neurohypophysial system. It was found (9) that acetylcholine or dopamine are able to release hormones and that the site of their action is on the cell bodies. In addition, the effect of neurohypophysial hormones on brain neurotransmitter levels was also studied (43). No study has been made, however, analysing the possible interaction between monoamines and neurohypophysial hormone release in a preparation in which only the nerve terminals are present.

The fact that the release of neurohypophysial hormones (oxytocin and vasopressin) from the nerve endings of the hypothalamo-neurohypophysial tract can readily be studied (14) *in vitro* provided an opportunity to study the axon terminal modulation of hormone release. In this study evidence has been presented on isolated neural lobes of hypophysis which contain only the nerve terminals of the hypothalamo-hypophysial system (8,9,13) in favor of an intrinsic physiological neuromodulatory role of endorphins and dopamine in oxytocin (50,51) and vasopressin release.

MATERIALS AND METHODS

Male and female Wistar rats weighing 140 to 160 g were used. Rats were killed by decapitation and brains quickly removed. The neural and intermediate

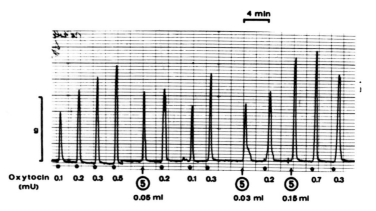

FIG. 1. Assay of oxytocin on isolated uterus horn. Organ bath, 3.5 ml; modified Tyrode solution (μg concentration doubled, Ca concentration halved). Isometrical recording. Note that sample 5 was assayed in three different volumes.

lobes of the pituitary gland were dissected from the anterior lobe under a stereo-microscope and immersed in a phosphate-buffered Locke solution (NaCl, 154 mM; $CaCl_2$, 2.2 mM; $MgCl_2$, 1.1 mM; KCl, 5.6 mM; NaH_2PO_4, 2.15 mM; and glucose, 10 mM). Four neurointermediate lobes were pooled and incubated in 1 ml of the solution at 37°C. The bath fluid was gassed with 5% CO_2 in O_2. After 30 min incubation the fluid was removed and replaced by fresh solution. The samples obtained were bioassayed (see Figs. 1 and 2) on isolated uterus preparation of the rat. Young Wistar rats weighing 100 to 130 g were used. Stilboestrol (0.1 mg/kg) was injected subcutaneously 24 hr before the experiment

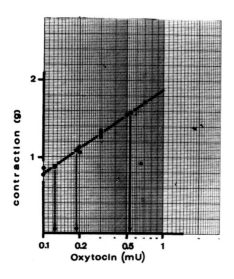

FIG. 2. Dose-response curve of oxytocin. Data taken from experiment shown in Fig. 1. The oxytocin content of sample 5 was calculated by interpolation: 0.03 ml contains 0.12 mU (4 mU/ml), 0.05 ml 0.19 mU (3.8 mU/ml), and 0.15 ml 0.54 mU (3.6 mU/ml); the release was 3.8 mU.

to bring the rats into oestrus. The horn of the uterus was set up in an organ bath of 5 ml. The solution was bubbled with 5% CO_2 in O_2.

The contractions of the uterus were recorded isometrically. The responses increase fairly sharply with increases in log dose. A modified Tyrode solution was used: Ca^{2+} concentration was halved and Mg^{2+} concentration doubled in order to reduce spontaneous activity of the uterus. The dose-response curve was made with standard oxytocin and the sample was tested in three different volumes (Fig. 1). The calculation of oxytocin content of the sample was made as shown in Fig. 2 by interpolation from a dose-response curve.

The media containing ouabain, dopamine, or opioid peptides were found to be without effect on the assay at the concentration used. The release of oxytocin and vasopressin was expressed in mU/4 lobes/10 min. Evidence for the identity of oxytocin activity assayed was obtained by gel filtration. A Sephadex G-50 column was used. Standard oxytocin and lyophilized samples were eluted through the column. The eluted fractions were then tested. The elution profiles of oxytocin-like substance and standard oxytocin were identical, indicating that the substance assayed was oxytocin. When vasopressin release was measured the lobes were halved. The rat blood pressure method was used for bioassay of vasopressin.

Results of assays are expressed as mean $\pm$ SEM and statistical analysis was performed using Student's *t*-test. The following drugs were used: oxytocin (Syntocinon®, Sandoz Ltd.); dopamine HCl (Sigma); β-endorphin [synthetic and isolated (1)]; naloxone (Endo Lab.); α-methyl-*p*-tyrosine methylester HCl (Axel Kistner AB); noradrenaline bitartrate (Koch-Light Lab.); D-Ala²-Pro⁵-NH-Et and D-Met²-Pro⁵-enkephalinamide [Institute for Drug Research, Budapest (1,2)]; Synthetic lysin-vasopressin (Sandoz).

RESULTS

Effect on Oxytocin Release

In 65 experiments the average release of oxytocin from the isolated neurointermediate lobe was 2.03 ± 0.23 mU/4 lobes/10 min. The release alternated for the first 30 min of incubation, remained constant for the next 50 to 60-min period, and tended to decline thereafter. Jakubowska-Naziemblo and Cyrkowicz (25) have also observed that the resting release alternates with time.

Effect of Ouabain

Ouabain, a selective inhibitor of Na^+-K^+-activated ATPase which has been shown to release transmitters (47) and neurohypophysial hormones (13), in a concentration of 2×10^{-5} M significantly enhanced the release of oxytocin from 2.5 ± 0.4 to 8.0 ± 1.1 mU/4 lobes/10 min ($p < 0.001$, $N = 6$). When ouabain was applied in a concentration of 2×10^{-4} M, the release was higher

TABLE 1. *Calcium dependence of oxytocin release from neurointermediate lobe of rat pituitary*

| Treatment | Oxytocin release[a] (mU/4 lobes/10 min) | | p |
	Ca^{2+} (2.2mM)	Ca-free[b]	
Resting	2.03 ± 0.23 (65)	1.58 ± 0.6 (4)	< 0.05
Ouabain (2 × 10^{-5} M)	7.96 ± 1.14 (6)	2.47 ± 1.0 (3)	< 0.02
Ouabain (2 × 10^{-4} M)	18.8 ± 0.90 (3)	10.6 ± 1.4 (5)	< 0.01
K-excess (49.7 mM)	23.8 ± 2.4 (4)	3.6 ± 0.5 (6)	< 0.001

[a] Number of experiments expressed in parentheses.
[b] Ca was removed and 1 mM EGTA was added.

(26.4 mU/4 lobes/10 min) and persisted even in the absence of Ca^{2+} and in the presence of 1 mM EGTA (Table 1). The removal of Ca^{2+} and the administration of 1 mM EGTA did not affect the resting release. A similar observation was made by Dicker (13).

Effect of Dopamine

Dopamine (2 × 10^{-4} M), which by itself failed to affect the resting release, prevented the effect of ouabain. α-Methyl-*p*-tyrosine, which, according to Godden et al. (20), reduces dopamine content in the pituitary, was injected 120 min before the experiments to study the effect of dopamine-deficiency on oxytocin release. The resting release of oxytocin (5.5 ± 0.31 mU/4 lobes/10 min, $N = 5$) was significantly higher in neural lobes obtained from rats that had been pretreated with α-methyl-*p*-tyrosine than in those from control rats (2.5 ± 0.4 mU/lobes/10 min, $p < 0.01$, $N = 10$).

The effect of ouabain was also much more marked (14.2 ± 0.6 mU/4 lobes/10 min) in preparations obtained from rats that had been pretreated with α-methyl-*p*-tyrosine. While dopamine in the concentration used (2 × 10^{-4} M) did not affect the resting release of oxytocin from lobes from untreated rats, it significantly reduced the amount of oxytocin from 4.95 ± 0.3 to 2.2 ± 0.6 mU/4 lobes/10 min ($p < 0.05$, $N = 5$) in dopamine-deficient lobes.

Effect of Opioid Peptides

β-Endorphin (10^{-6} M) significantly enhanced the release of oxytocin induced by ouabain (Fig. 3 and Table 2); however, it did not affect the resting secretion. A similar effect was observed with D-Ala^2-Pro^5-NH-Et and D-Met^2-Pro^5-enkephalinamide administered in a concentration of 10^{-6} M (51).

Naloxone (10^{-5} M) a pure opiate antagonist, reduced the resting release (Table 1) and prevented the enhancing effect of β-endorphin (Fig. 3) on oxytocin release in response to ouabain administration (51). The effect of ouabain was also prevented by naloxone.

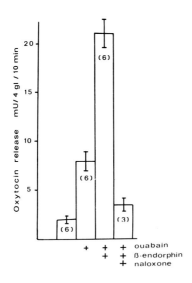

FIG. 3. Effect of β-endorphin on oxytocin release from isolated neurointermediate lobe of the rat. Note that naloxone (10^{-6} M) prevented the effect of β-endorphin (10^{-6} M) on ouabain (2×10^{-5} M)-induced release of oxytocin. Number of experiments expressed in parentheses. *Vertical bars* represent the SEM. Collection time: 20 min; organ bath: 1 ml, 37°C. Four lobes were pooled in 1 ml solution. For details see *Methods.*

Effect of Excess Potassium

Much evidence supports the idea that the "stimulus-secretion coupling" involves depolarization of the neurosecretory terminals followed by some calcium-dependent link (14). The presence of calcium in the external medium is required for hormone release. Table 1 shows that K-evoked oxytocin release also requires Ca_0, as was already shown by Douglas and Poisner (14).

While dopamine and opioid peptides were capable of affecting oxytocin release evoked by ouabain, the release induced by K-excess was not affected (Table 2).

TABLE 2. *Effect of different drugs on oxytocin release induced by ouabain and excess potassium[a]*

Treatment	Oxytocin release (SEM)[b] (mU/4 lobes/10 min)		
	Resting	Ouabain-induced (2×10^{-5} M)	K-excess (49.3 mM)
Control	2.03 ± 0.23 (65)	7.96 ± 1.14 (6)[d]	29.9 ± 1.8 (4)
Dopamine (2×10^{-4} M)	2.3 ± 0.18 (4)	3.1 ± 0.41 (4)[d]	26.9 ± 1.2 (4)
β-endorphin (10^{-6} M)	3.8 ± 1.6 (3)	23.6 ± 6.9 (6)	30.0 (2)
Leu-enkephalin (10^{-6} M)	4.1 ± 0.9 (4)	18.8 ± 2.1 (4)	—
Clonidine (10^{-6} M)[c]	1.85 ± 0.35 (4)	4.8 ± 0.3 (4)[d]	28.9 ± 6.4 (4)
Naloxone (10^{-5} M)	1.2 ± 0.2 (7)	3.1 ± 0.9 (7)[d]	27.3 ± 4.36 (4)

[a] Isolated neurointermediate lobe of rat pituitary.
[b] Number of experiments expressed in parentheses.
[c] Clonidine is an α-adrenoceptor stimulant.
[d] The difference is significant at the level of $p < 0.01$, in comparison with control.

In the presence of 1 mM EGTA and in the absence of calcium 49.3 mM, potassium failed to release oxytocin from nerve endings.

Effect on Vasopressin Release

The amount of vasopressin released during four successive periods of 30 min was measured. The resting release of vasopressin from halved neurointermediate lobe of the rat is 2.95 ± 0.10 mU/4 lobes/10 min ($N = 21$). This is consistent with previous observations. The release remained constant over a period of 90 min. A similar observation was made by Traczyk (46).

Effect of Ouabain

Ouabain enhanced the release of vasopressin and its action proved to be concentration-dependent (Fig. 4). In a concentration of 2×10^{-4} M, ouabain enhanced the release from 4.8 ± 0.82 to 36.5 ± 4.51 mU/4 lobes/10 min ($N = 5$). The increase is significant at the level of $p < 0.01$. A further increase in the concentration of ouabain did not result in higher release (Fig. 4).

Effect of Dopamine

In concentration of 10^{-4} M, dopamine failed to affect the resting release of vasopressin, but significantly inhibited the release evoked by ouabain (Fig. 5).

DISCUSSION

In the classical experiments of Harris (23) and Cross and Harris (11), evidence was presented that stimulation of supraoptic and paraventricular nuclei or the infundibular stem produced effects on urine flow, uterine contractility and milk

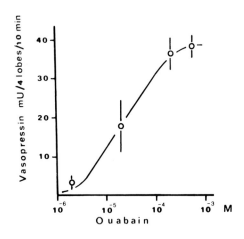

FIG. 4. Release of vasopressin from isolated neurointermediate lobe of the rat as a function of ouabain concentration. Collection time: 30 min. *Vertical bars* represent SEM, five experiments.

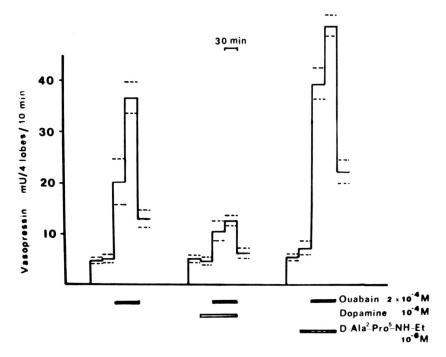

FIG. 5. Effect of dopamine (10^{-4} M) and an enkephalin analog (D-Ala^2-Pro^5-NH-Et, 10^{-6} M) on the release of vasopressin from isolated neurointermediate lobe of the rat. Collection time, 30 min. Five identical experiments. SE of the mean. For details see text.

ejection, which could be matched by neurohypophysial hormones, oxytocin, and vasopressin. The results obtained by determination of changes in blood concentrations of neurohypophysial hormones in response to different experimental conditions provided no adequate information concerning the site of action of drugs and the rate of hormone release.

The neurosecretory neurons of the supraoptic and paraventricular nuclei in the hypothalamus and their nerve terminals in the neural lobe of the pituitary were the subject of different investigations (Table 3). Using isolated neural lobe of pituitary, which contains only the nerve terminals of the hypothalamo-neurohypophysial system, it was possible to show the direct inhibitory effect of dopamine on axon terminals and to study the site of action of dopamine and opioid peptides on the release of oxytocin and vasopressin.

Effect of Neurotransmitters on the Perikaryon

Evidence has been presented (9) that stimulation of dopamine and acetylcholine receptors in isolated hypothalamus results in the increase of both vasopressin and oxytocin release. The maximally effective concentration (6.5×10^{-12} M)

TABLE 3. *Effect of different transmitters/modulators and experimental conditions on the release of neurohypophysial hormones from neural lobe of rat pituitary gland*

Different transmitters and drugs	Oxytocin release		Vasopressin release	
	Effect	Refs.	Effect	Refs.
Acetylcholine	None	13	None	(12–14,26)
Dopamine	Inhibits	49,50, this chapter	Inhibits	This chapter
K-excess	Enhances (112 mM)	13	Enhances (112 mM)	13
	Enhances (56 mM)	15	Enhances (56 mM)	12,14–16,29
			Enhances (60 mM)	26
Ouabain (inhibition of membrane ATPase)[a]	Enhances	13,50, this chapter	Enhances	13,50, this chapter
ATP[a]	Inhibits	13	Inhibits	13

[a] ATP, adenosine triphosphate.

of dopamine produced a fivefold increase over the basal level. Acetylcholine (10^{-11} M) caused a similar action. In isolated preparation where the neurohypophysis and the supraoptic and paraventricular nuclei of the hypothalamus were involved, acetylcholine enhanced the hormone release (12). Since the nerve endings of the supraoptico- and paraventriculo-hypophysial system are excluded in this preparation, it was suggested that the site of action is proximal to the nerve terminals and that cholinergic and dopaminergic receptors are involved in the stimulation of the hypothalamo-neurohypophysial system. Consistent with this is the fact that haloperidol, a dopamine antagonist, inhibits the release of oxytocin in *in vivo* experiments (34).

Effect of Dopamine on Nerve Endings of Hypothalamo-Hypophysial Neuron

Table 3 shows the effect of different modulators and experimental conditions on oxytocin and vasopressin release. In our experiments it has been shown (50,51) that dopamine presynaptically controls the release of oxytocin and vasopressin. The finding that the resting release of oxytocin is about two times higher from lobes dissected from α-methyl-*p*-tyrosine pretreated (dopamine-deficient) rats than from normal rats indicates that there is a continuous inhibition of oxytocin release by endogenous dopamine.

It has been observed that dopamine-containing nerve terminals are heavily concentrated in the neural lobe (Table 4) of the pituitary (40). Therefore, it is very probable that dopamine released from neurons originating from the rostral zone of the arcuate nucleus (5) exerts a direct modulatory control over the secretion of oxytocin and vasopressin. The dopaminergic terminals are frequently situated in close proximity to the neurosecretory axons and processes of pituicytes, but membrane thickenings **have not been demonstrated** (4). It is therefore suggested that dopamine released from these nerve terminals reaches its target cells by diffusion (Fig. 6). It has been shown that action potentials generated in cells cultured from intermediate lobes of the rat can be suppressed by dopamine. In addition, dopamine has been shown to inhibit the release of adrenocorticotropic hormone (18) and melanophore-stimulating hormone (7) from intermediate lobe cells *in vitro*. Holzbauer et al. (24) suggested that the dopaminergic innervation of the pituitary gland may modulate the release of oxytocin and vasopressin. In their experiments, which were performed during the release of increased amounts of pituitary hormones, a decrease in pituitary dopamine content and an increase in its turnover was observed, indirectly suggesting an enhanced release of hormones.

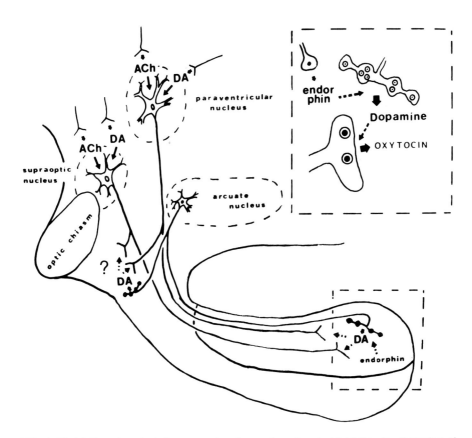

FIG. 6. Modulation of oxytocin/vasopressin release. Axon terminal inhibition by dopamine of oxytocin/vasopressin release. Dopamine released inhibits the release of hormones. Endorphin/enkephalin released inhibits the release of dopamine: disinhibitory phenomenon. Dopamine (DA) and acetylcholine (ACh) stimulate cell body of hypothalamo-neurohypophysial neuron which in fact leads to hormone release (9). It is suggested that dopamine is involved at two different sites in the hypothalamo-neurohypophysial system: it stimulates the transmission at the hypothalamic synapses and inhibits hormone release from nerve terminals via a direct action on axon terminals.

Effect of α-Adrenoceptor Stimulation on Oxytocin Release

A typical α-adrenoceptor stimulant, clonidine (Catapresan®),[1] significantly reduced the ouabain-induced release of oxytocin but failed to affect those evoked by K-excess (Table 2).

Effect of Opioid Peptides on Oxytocin and Vasopressin Release

In our earlier work (50,51) it has been shown that β-endorphin and enkephalins (D-Met²-Pro⁵-enkephalinamide, D-Ala²-Pro⁵-NH-Et) enhanced the release of oxytocin evoked by ouabain, their effect being antagonized by naloxone, a pure opiate antagonist. This fact indicates that the effect of opioid peptides is mediated via opiate receptors. Although evidence has accumulated for disinhibitory effect of opioid peptides on oxytocin release by removing dopaminergic control inhibiting dopamine release (51) (Fig. 6), there is another possibility that requires discussion: peptides have a direct action on nerve terminals contributing to the attenuation of the high rate of hormone release. This possibility is, however, not favoured by the fact that stimulation of opiate receptors fails to increase further the release from dopamine-deficient neural lobes (51) where the indirect effect of peptides can be excluded. The question arises now as to what is the physiological role of enkephalins and/or endorphins.

Endorphins have now been shown to produce all the effect of the opiates. It is well known that morphine causes a release of antidiuretic hormone and thereby a decrease in urinary output. There is evidence that all endorphins which have so far been identified are present and synthetized in the pituitary (10). β-Endorphin (18,21,31), α-Endorphin (22), and γ-endorphin (32) have been isolated from pituitary glands, and α- and β-endorphin have been identified in pituitary tissue by radioimmunoassays and by immunohistochemical techniques (6).

Detailed study on the precise localization (41,44) of the endorphins in the pituitary gland showed that the pars intermedia is very rich in α- and β-endorphin (6,29), but the pars nervosa does not contain any (6). However, receptors sensitive to opioid peptides have been shown to exist (41,42) in the neurohypophysis. It has been reported that endorphins are released in the pituitary (28,35, 42,45).

In addition, it has been shown that significant amounts of immunoreactive Met- and Leu-enkephalin were present in extracts of neural lobe of the pituitary (38). Therefore, it seems very likely that the inhibitory action of enkephalin and endorphin on dopamine release (51) is of physiological importance. Opioid peptides released either *in loco* or from the intermediate lobe may reduce the release of dopamine, thereby disinhibiting the dopaminergic "brake" system on oxytocin and vasopressin release.

---

[1] 2-(2,6-Dichloroanilino)-2-imidazoline

TABLE 4. *Biogenic amines and acetylcholine content of rat pituitary[a]*

Lobes	ACh[b]	NA[c]	Dopamine[c]	5-HT[c]	Histamine[c]
Anterior		0	0.20 ± 0.02	1.85 ± 0.3	3.03 ± 0.67
Intermediate	0^d	0.15 ± 0.10	1.78 ± 0.79	3.69 ± 0.44	17.15 ± 4.5
Posterior	0^d	0.80 ± 0.28	7.16 ± 0.91	4.05 ± 1.0	13.75 ± 2.06

[a] Content: ng/mg protein. ACh, acetylcholine; NA, noradrenaline; 5-HT, 5-hydroxytryptamine.
[b] Acetylcholine content of lobes was measured as described by Vizi et al. (49).
[c] Data from Vizi et al., ref. 49.
[d] Less than 0.01 ng/mg protein.

Lack of Modulatory Effect of Acetylcholine on Oxytocin and Vasopressin Release from Isolated Neural Lobe

On morphological grounds it has been suggested that acetylcholine occurs in the neural lobe of pituitary (19,36). Koelle (27) has made the interesting speculation that the action potential may first cause the terminal to release acetylcholine which then depolarizes its own axon terminals to produce release of peptide.

In addition, de Robertis (37) has also suggested that the neural lobe is a cholinergic organ where the nerve endings are able to release acetylcholine, which in fact leads to a release of hormones from the same terminals. If this were true, Dale's idea of one neuron-one transmitter would be challenged. It was found that acetylcholinesterase (33) and cholinacetyltransferase (17) are present in the neural lobe. Although Lederis and Livingston (30) have found that acetylcholine occurs in the neurohypophysis, we failed to measure any acetylcholine in the neural lobe of the rat (Table 4). In agreement with this finding, and in contrast to that of Feldberg and Vogt (17), Saavedra et al. (40) failed to show the presence of cholineacetyltransferase. Therefore, it is concluded that small (300–500 Å) clear synaptic vesicles identified by electron microscopy (3) could not contain acetylcholine, and acetylcholine cannot play any role in the modulation of hormone release in the neural lobe. In addition, it was found in *in vitro* experiments that acetylcholine did not affect hormone release (12–14,26).

SUMMARY

The results discussed in this chapter provide direct evidence that dopamine presynaptically controls the release of neurohypophysial hormones. Opioid peptides, however, inhibit the release of dopamine, thereby enhancing the release of oxytocin and vasopressin. It seems very likely that the main function of the opioid peptides both present and released, may be a disinhibitory modulation of the secretion of polypeptide hormones in neurohypophysis. A similar disinhibitory phenomenon has been observed in the striatum (49) where the release of acetylcholine is also controlled by an interaction of dopamine and opioid peptides. The stimulation of α-adrenoceptors also resulted in a decrease of oxytocin release. The release of oxytocin evoked by a high potassium concentration (49.3 mM) could not be affected by either dopamine or α-adrenoceptor or opiate receptor stimulation.

REFERENCES

1. Bajusz, S., Rónai, A. Z., Székely, J. I., Dunai-Kovács Z., Berzétei, I., and Gráf, L. (1976): Enkephalin analogs with enhanced opiate activity. *Acta Biochim. Biophys.*, 11:305–308.
2. Bajusz, S., Rónai, A. Z., Székely, J. I., Gráf, L., Dunai-Kovács, Z., and Berzétei, I. (1977): A superactive antinociceptive pentapeptide (D-Met^2,Pro^5)-enkephalinamide. *FEBS Lett.*, 76:91–92.
3. Barer, R., and Lederis, K. (1966): Ultrastructure of the rabbit neurohypophysis with special reference to the release of hormones. *Z. Zellforsch. Mikroskop. Anat.*, 75:201.
4. Baumgarten, H. G., Björklund A., Holstein A. F., and Nobin, A. (1972): Organization and ultrastructural identification of the catecholamine nerve terminals in the neural lobe and pars intermedia of the rat pituitary. *Z. Zellforsch. Mikrosk. Anat.*, 126:483–517.
5. Björklund, A., Moore, R. Y., Nobin, A., and Stenevi, U. (1973): The organization of the tubero-hypophysial and reticulo-infundibular catecholamine neuron system in the rat brain. *Brain. Res.*, 51:171–191.
6. Bloom, F., Battenberg, E., Rossier, J., Ling, N., Leppaluoto, J., Vargo, T. M., and Guillemin, R. (1977): Endorphins are located in the intermediate and anterior lobes of the pituitary gland not in the neurohypophysis. *Life Sci.*, 20:43–46.
7. Bower, A., Hadley, M. E., and Hruby, V. I. (1974): Biogenic amines and control of melanophore stimulating hormone release. *Science (NY)*, 184:70–72.
8. Bridges, T. E., Hillhouse, E. W., and Jones, M. T. (1975): The effect of dopamine on neurohypophysial hormone release *in vivo* and *in vitro*. *J. Physiol. (Lond.)*, 246:107–109.
9. Bridges, T. E., Hillhouse, E. W., and Jones M. T. (1976): The effect of dopamine on neurohypophysial hormone release in vivo and from the rat neural lobe and hypothalamus in vitro. *J. Physiol. (Lond.)*, 260:647–666.
10. Crine, P., Benjannet, S., Seidah, N. G., Lis, M., and Chrétien, M. (1977): In vitro biosynthesis of β-endorphin in pituitary glands. *Proc. Natl. Acad. Sci. USA*, 74:1403–1406.
11. Cross, B. A., and Harris, G. W. (1952): The role of the neurohypophysis in the milk ejection reflex. *J. Endocrinol.*, 8:148–161.
12. Daniel, A. R., and Lederis, K. (1967): Release of neurohypophysial hormones in vitro. *J. Physiol. (Lond.)*, 190:171–187.
13. Dicker, S. E. (1966): Release of vasopressin and oxytocin from isolated pituitary glands of adult and newborn rats. *J. Physiol. (Lond.)*, 185:429–444.
14. Douglas, W. W., and Poisner, A. M. (1964): Stimulus-secretion coupling in a neurosecretory organ: The role of calcium in the release of vasopressin from the neurohypophysis. *J. Physiol. (Lond.)*, 172:1–18.
15. Dreifuss, J. J., Grau, I. D., and Nordmann, A. (1973): Effects on the isolated neurohypophysis of agents which affect the membrane permeability to calcium. *J. Physiol. (Lond.)*, 96P–98P.
16. Dreifuss, J. J., Kalnin, I., Kelly, J. S., and Ruf, K. B. (1974): Action potentials and release of neurohypophysial hormones in vitro. *J. Physiol. (Lond.)*, 215:805–817.
17. Feldberg, W., and Vogt, M. (1948): Acetylcholine synthesis in different regions of the central nervous system. *J. Physiol. (Lond.)*, 107:372–381.
18. Fischer, I. L., and Moriarty, C. M. (1977): Control of bioactive corticotropin release from the neruo-intermediate lobe of the rat. *Endocrinology*, 100:1047–1054.
19. Gerschenfeld, H. M., Tramezzani, J. H., and De Robertis E. (1960): Ultrastructure and function of neurohypophysis of toad. *Endocrinology*, 66:741–762.
20. Godden, U., Holzbauer, M., and Sharman, D. F. (1977): Dopamine utilization in the posterior pituitary gland of the rat. *Br. J. Pharmacol.*, 59:478–479P.
21. Gráf, L., Rónai, A. Z., Bajusz, S., Cseh, G., and Székely, J. I. (1976): Opioid agonist activity

of β-lipotropin fragments: A possible biological source of morphine-like substances in the pituitary. *FEBS Lett.,* 64:181–184.

22. Guillemin, R., Ling, N., and Burgus, R. (1976): Endorphines, peptides, d'origine hypothalamique et neurohypophysaire à activité morphinomimetique. Isolament et structure moléculaire de l'β-endorphine. *C.R. Acad. Sci. (Paris),* 282:783–785.

23. Harris, G. W. (1947): The innervation and actions of the neurohypophysis; an investigation using the method of remote control stimulation. *Philos. Trans. R. Soc. Lond. (Biol. Sci.),* 323:385–441.

24. Holzbauer, M., Sharman, D. F., and Godden U. (1978): Observations on the function of the dopaminergic nerves innervating the pituitary gland. *Neuroscience,* 3:1251–1262.

25. Jakubowska-Naziemblo, B., and Cyrkowicz, A. (1978): Release of oxytocin from the rat posterior pituitary lobe incubated in situ and from the hypothalamic end of the cut pituitary stalk. *Acta Physiol. Pol.,* 29:2–105.

26. Kilbinger, H., Lohnes, I., and Muscholl, E. (1975): Absence of muscarinic modulation of vasopressin release from the isolated rat neurohypophysis. *Naunyn Schmiedebergs Arch. Pharmacol.,* 287:391–397.

27. Koelle, G. B. (1961): A proposed dual neurohumoral role of acetylcholine: Its functions at the pre- and postsynaptic sites. *Nature,* 190:208–209.

28. Kromer, W., Bläsig, J., Westenthanner, A., Haarmann, I., and Teschemacher, H. (1976): Characteristics of porcine pituitary peptides which act like opiate. Release from anterior lobes *in vitro*—relation between central effects and degradation by brain enzymes. In: *Opiates and Endogenous Opioid Peptides,* edited by H. W. Kosterlitz, pp. 1–8. Elsevier/North-Holland Biomedical Press, Amsterdam.

29. LaBella, F., Queen, G., Senyshyn, J., Lis, M., and Chrétien, M. (1977): Lipotropin: Localization by radioimmunoassay of endorphin precursor in pituitary and brain. *Biochem. Biophys. Res. Commun.,* 75:350–357.

30. Lederis, K., and Livingstone, A. (1966): Acetylcholine content in the rabbit neurohypophysis. *J. Physiol. (Lond.),* 185:37–38P.

31. Li, C. H., and Chung, D. (1976): Isolation and structure of an untriakontapeptide with opiate activity from camel pituitary glands. *Proc. Natl. Acad. Sci. USA,* 73:1145–1148.

32. Ling, N., Brugus, R., and Guillemin, R. (1976): Isolation primary structure and synthesis of β-endorphin and endorphin, two peptides of hypothalamohypophysial origin with morphinomimetic activity. *Proc. Natl. Acad. Sci. USA,* 73:3492–3946.

33. Livingstone, A. (1966): Acetylcholinesterase content of the rabbit neurohypophysis. *J. Physiol. (Lond.),* 187:37P.

34. Moos, F., and Richard, Ph. (1979): Effects of dopaminergic antagonist and agonist on oxytocin release induced by various stimuli. *Neuroendocrinology,* 28:138–144.

35. Przewłocki, R., Höllt, V., and Herz A. (1978): Release of β-endorphin from rat pituitary *in vitro. Eur. J. Pharmacol.,* 51:179–183.

36. de Robertis, E. (1962): Ultrastructure and function in some neurosecretory systems. In: *Neurosecretion,* edited by H. Heller and R. B. Clark, pp. 3–20. Academic, London, New York.

37. de Robertis, E. (1964): Histophysiology of synapses and neuro-secretion, Pergamon, Oxford.

38. Rossier, J., Battenberg, E., Pittman, Q., Bayon, A., Koda, L., Miller, R., Guillemin, R., and Bloom, F. (1979): Hypothalamic enkephalin neurones may regulate the neurohypophysis. *Nature,* 277:653–655.

39. Russel, J. T., and Thorn, N. A. (1974): Calcium and stimulus-secretion coupling in the neurohypophysis. *Acta Endocrinol.,* 76:471–487.

40. Saavedra, I. M., Palkovits, M., Kizer, I. S., Brownstein, M., and Zivin, J. A. (1975): Distribution of biogenic amines and related enzymes in the rat pituitary gland. *J. Neurochem.,* 25:257–260.

41. Simantov, R. (1978): Enkephalins, endorphins and opiate receptors: Studies in vitro and in vivo. In: *Endorphins '78,* edited by L. Gráf, M. Palkovits, and A. Z. Rónai, pp. 221–236. Akadémiai Kiadó, Budapest.

42. Simantov, R., and Snyder, S. H. (1977): Opiate receptor binding in the pituitary gland. *Brain Res.,* 124:178–184.

43. Telegdy, G., and Kovács, G. L. (1979): Role of monoamines in mediating the action of ACTH, vasopressin and oxytocin. In: *Central Nervous System Effects of Hypothalamic Hormones and Other Peptides,* edited by Collu et al. pp. 189–205. Raven Press, New York.

44. Teschemacher, H., Opheim, K. E., Cox, B. M., and Goldstein, A. (1975): A peptide-like substance from pituitary that acts like morphine. 1. Isolation. *Life Sci.,* 16:1771–1776.
45. Teschemacher, H., Westenthanner, A., Kromer, W., Csontos K., and Haarmann, I. (1977): Characteristics of opiate-like acting peptides (endorphins) released from porcine pituitaries in vitro. *Naunyn Schmiedebergs Arch. Pharmacol.,* 297(Suppl. II):R53.
46. Traczyk, W. Z. (1972): Vasopressin release from incubated in situ posterior pituitary lobe in rats. *Bull. Acad. Polon. Sci. Biol.,* 20:351–356.
47. Vizi, E. S. (1978): Na$^+$-K$^+$-activated adenosinetriphosphatase as a trigger in transmitter release. *Neuroscience,* 3:367–384.
48. Vizi, E. S. (1979): Presynaptic modulation of neurochemical transmission. *Prog. Neurobiol.,* 12:181–290.
49. Vizi, E. S., Hársing, L. G., Jr., and Knoll, J. (1977): Presynaptic inhibition leading to disinhibition of acetylcholine release from interneurons of the caudate nucleus: Effects of dopamine, β-endorphin and D-Ala^2-Pro^5-enkephalinamide. *Neuroscience,* 2:953–961.
50. Vizi, E. S., and Volbekas, V. (1978): Modulatory role of dopamine and β-endorphin in the release of oxytocin from neural lobe of pituitary. *Proceedings of the 7th International Congress of Pharmacology.* Paris, p. 562.
51. Vizi, E. S., and Volbekas, V. (1980): Inhibition by dopamine of oxytocin release from isolated posterior lobe of the hypophysis of the rat: Disinhibitory effect of β-endorphin/enkephalin. *Neuroendocrinology (in press).*

Neuropeptides and Neural Transmission,
edited by C. Ajmone Marsan and W. Z. Traczyk.
Raven Press, New York © 1980.

Effects of Leu-enkephalin on Certain Neurones in Snail, Helix pomatia L.

Lajos Erdélyi, *Ferenc Joó, and *József Soós

*Institute of Comparative Physiology, Attila József University, and *Institute of Biophysics, Biological Research Center, 6701 Szeged, Hungary*

Earlier results of Pert et al. (5) and Simantov et al. (8) in invertebrates, have failed to detect either enkephalin activity or opiate receptor binding. Although stereospecific opiate receptors are certainly not present in some invertebrates, the opiates themselves have been shown by Tremblay et al. (13) to be capable of eliciting a specific pharmacological response in invertebrates, which is quite similar to its effect in vertebrates.

The present study was undertaken to establish if Leu-enkephalin has any effect on the electrophysiological properties of snail neurones.

MATERIAL AND METHODS

Electron Microscopy

The suboesophageal ganglia were prepared from *Helix pomatia L.* Small cubes of tissue were cut by a razor blade and fixed in an aldehyde fixative (14) for 2 hr at 4°C. Samples were processed after post-fixation in buffered osmium tetroxide. After dehydration in graded series of alcohols, the samples were embedded in Durcupan® (Fluka). Sections of silver interference colours were stained with lead citrate (6). Sections were coated with carbon and viewed in a Jeol 100B transmission electron microscope.

Electrophysiology

Helix pomatia L. were collected locally and kept in the laboratory at room temperature. The circumoesophageal ganglions from the active snails were isolated and desheathed under visual control. The ganglions were pinned in an organ bath (volume 4 ml), which was mounted on the stage of a micromanipulator and illuminated using glass-fiber optics and observed with a Zeiss stereomicroscope. One or two potassium acetate-filled (1.5 M) microelectrodes were inserted into a selected neurone; one for recording the membrane potential and the second to pass current injections into the neurone. Sometimes, values for input resistance (R_{in}) were determined by passing a certain current through the recording microelectrode by means of a bridge circuit. Square or saw-tooth wave generators were used to supply the sufficient current injections for the measurement of reversal potential and the changes of input resistance evoked by the substance tested. Potentials were amplified and displayed on a Disa universal indicator 51 B 00 or Philips pen recorder PM 8202.

The ganglion preparation was maintained at room temperature and perfused with snail saline proposed by Kerkut and Thomas (4). After penetration of the neurones, the ganglion was allowed to rest and equilibrate with the snail saline for 20 min. Leu-enkephalin (E) from Serva and naloxone (N, Narcan®) from Winthrop were then added into the organ bath in 10^{-6} to 10^{-4} M final concentrations and the effects were recorded. Acetylcholine (ACh), atropine, d-tubocurare (D-TC) and tetraethylammonium (TEA) were also used in 5×10^{-5} to 10^{-4} M concentrations to characterize the cholinergic response.

RESULTS

Electron Microscopy

On the basis of fine structural appearance of the synaptic vesicles, three types of axonal endings could be readily distinguished in the neuropil of suboesophageal ganglia: (a) endings filled with clear synaptic vesicles of 50 nm diameter, (b) terminals containing dense-cored synaptic vesicles of 80 to 120 nm diameter, and (c) axons filled with large neurosecretory granules of 180 to 300 nm diameter (Fig. 1). The characteristics of neurosecretory granules were very similar to those observed in vertebrates, where these organelles are known to contain different types of neuropeptides.

Electrophysiology

The majority of neurones in this preparation responded to E and/or N with no changes of the membrane potential (E_m) or conductance (G_{in}) and they can be regarded as totally insensitive cells. Among the insensitive cells, silent, synaptically driven, and pacemaker cells were identified, which responded to ACh by either hyperpolarization (H-response) or depolarization (D-response).

A bursting pacemaker neurone, identified earlier (2) as a visceral Br cell and characterized as a D or DINHI neurone, responded to E with moderate depolarization, which accelerated the bursting pattern of neurone. The number of bursts increased from 8 to 13/min (163%) if 10^{-6} M E acted, and from 7 to 15/min (214%) if 10^{-5} M E was perfused; at the beginning of the washing period a 25% decrease of the burst activity was also observed. The interburst interval correspondingly decreased from 6.45 ± 1.13 sec (control) to 3.19 ± 0.65 sec (10^{-6} M E) and 2.48 ± 0.52 sec (10^{-5} M E), while it increased to 8.25 ± 3.77 sec ($N = 8$) during the washing period. But N (in 10^{-4} M concentra-

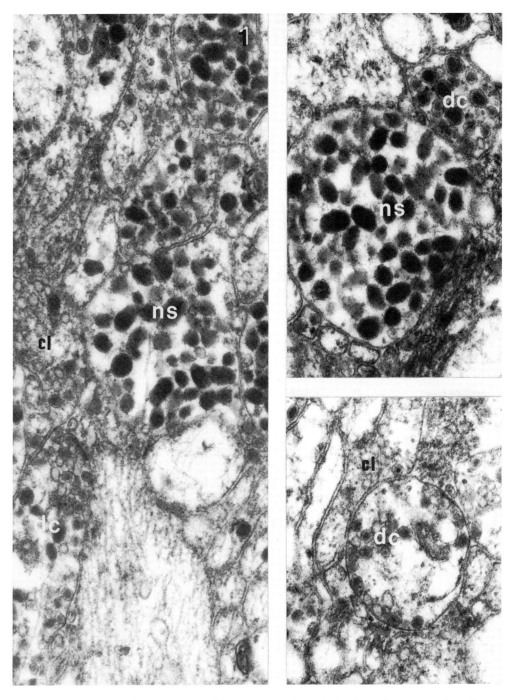

FIG. 1. Fine structural appearance of different nerve endings obtained from the suboesophageal ganglion of *Helix pomatia L.* cl, clear synaptic vesicles; dc, dense-cored vesicles; ns, neurosecretory granules. ×38,000.

tion) did not antagonize the E-evoked effects mentioned earlier. Instead, it also increased the burst pattern and decreased the interburst intervals significantly.

In a smaller number of the cases the response was hyperpolarizing if E acted and N antagonized the E-evoked effect on the membrane potential. The pen records of such experiments can be seen in Fig. 2 (a and b). Fig. 2a presents the activity pattern of a D-type synaptically influenced pacemaker neurone in which E (10^{-5} M) evoked moderate hyperpolarization and decreased the firing rate. N (10^{-5} M) antagonized the opiate pentapeptide-evoked hyperpolarization and accelerated the firing of the neurone. N alone also activated the neurone slightly (data not shown). In another D-type silent cell of the right parietal ganglion situated near the parietal burster, E (10^{-4} M) evoked 3 mV hyperpolarization of the E_m from -70 to -73 mV with a correspondent decrease of the R_{in} from 4.4 to 4.2 Mohm. The E_m was depolarized from -73 to -69 mV in the presence of N (10^{-5} M) and the R_{in} increased from 4.2 to 4.6 Mohm (Fig. 2b). The E_m stabilized at -69 mV and the R_{in} at 3.9 Mohm after washing in the control solution. When E + N were applied together the E_m did not change at the beginning of the experiment, but later it decreased from -69 to -65 mV and R_{in} increased from 3.9 to 4.6 Mohm. At the same time, the excitatory synaptic bombardment of the neurone increased. Reapplication of E + N or N produced gradual increase of the excitatory synaptic influence which, at last, reached the firing level and abortive excitatory post-synaptic potentials (EPSPs) and synaptically evoked spikes appeared. N alone or in the presence of E increased the membrane instability, as can be seen in Fig. 2b (small arrows). The E_m transiently decreased and the moderate postpulse depolarization decayed within two time constants when the hyperpolarizing pulse was released. The amplitude of this response increased and its time constant decreased under the action of E + N or N. The capacitive artefacts remained constant at the beginning and at the end of the pulses. R_{in} (4 Mohm) and E_m (-70 mV) were completely reversed on washing with E + N-free snail saline.

The actions of E and N were also studied in a series of experiments on ACh-evoked slow H-responses in order to determine whether the opiate pentapeptide could interact with the potassium-mechanism involved. Examples of the action of E and N are shown in Figs. 2c and 3. Fig. 2c shows the pen records of ACh (5×10^{-5} M) evoked H-response, which could be inhibited by 17% if E (10^{-4} M) was added. E + N (10^{-4} M) or N (10^{-4} M) alone did not influence significantly the amplitude of the ACh-evoked slow H-response. Duration and time course of the slow H-response were not significantly affected by E or E + N. The response to ACh of this cell was hyperpolarizing with high decrease of R_{in}, showing an apparent increase of the membrane conductance. The reversal potential (E_{ACh}) was -77 mV, which is very close to the equilibrium potential for K^+. Atropine (10^{-5} M) decreased the H-response by 70% while D-TC or TEA$^+$ (5×10^{-5} M) or Ba^{2+} (7 mM) did not attenuate it at all.

Another experiment also presented evidence for the modulation of the ACh-activated potassium mechanism (Fig. 3). ACh (10^{-5} M) also evoked hyperpolari-

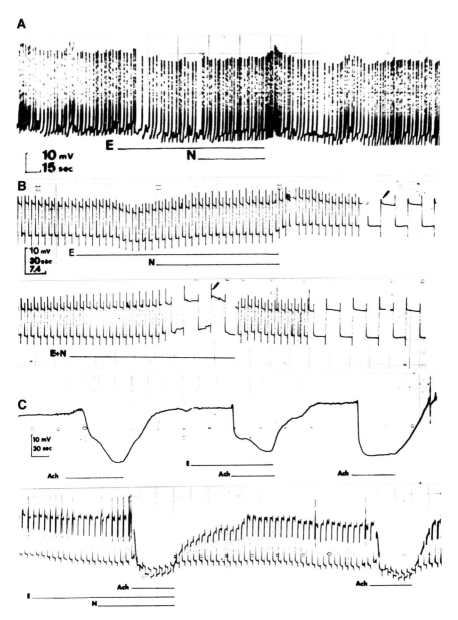

FIG. 2. a: Effects of E (10^{-4} M) and N (10^{-5} M) on the membrane potential and firing pattern of a synaptically driven neurone. The pen recorder attenuated the amplitude of the intracellular action potentials. **b:** Effects of E (10^{-4} M) and N (10^{-5} M) on the membrane potential and input resistance of a silent neurone located in the right parietal ganglion. *Arrows* show the transient postpulse depolarizations which indicate the changes of the membrane stability. Hyperpolarizing electrotonic potentials are superimposed on the membrane potential record evoked by constant (2.5 nA) square wave pulses. **c:** Effects of E (10^{-4} M) and N (10^{-4} M) on ACh (5×10^{-5} M) evoked slow H-responses in a silent cell of the right parietal ganglion. Intracellular action potentials are attenuated by the pen recorder. Hyperpolarizing electrotonic potentials are superimposed on the membrane potential record in the second row of the figure. Electrotonic potentials were induced by constant (2.5 nA) square wave pulses.

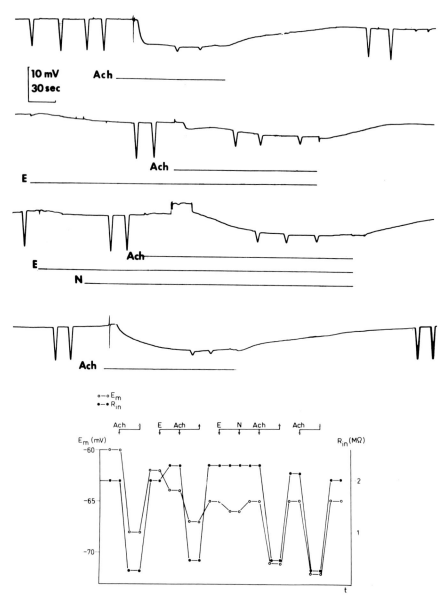

FIG. 3. Effects of E (10^{-4} M) and N (10^{-4} M) on ACh (10^{-5} M) evoked H-response in a silent cell of the visceral ganglion. Hyperpolarizing electrotonic potentials are superimposed on the membrane potential record induced by constant (4.4 nA) saw-tooth pulses before, during, and after the ACh actions.

zation (H-response) in this neurone with a correspondent increase of the conductance measured by constant (4.4 nA) hyperpolarizing saw-tooth pulses before, during, and after the ACh application. The reversal potential of the H-response (E_{ACh}) was −75 mV in this case. E_m and R_{in} slightly increased in the presence of E (10^{-4} M) and there was a significant decrease in the excitability of the neurone. Spike did not appear at the beginning of the ACh-evoked H-response in the presence of E. The H-response itself also decreased while R_{in} remained higher, relative to the control value: 0.43 and 0.22 Mohm, respectively. In the presence of E + N (10^{-4} M) the R_{in} was seemingly elevated and the time course of the H-response was slower in both cases, but the H-response was less attenuated when E + N acted. E_m and R_{in} or the ACh-evoked H-response were gradually reversed on washing with control solution.

We studied the effects of E and N on stimulus-evoked EPSPs and inhibitory post-synaptic potentials (IPSPs) in a series of experiments, but we could not demonstrate significant modulatory actions on the presynaptic mechanism present in vertebrates (see, for example, refs. 7, 15) or in *Aplysia* under the action of morphine (13). Even so, a presynaptic mechanism of the E action cannot be discarded, because we have found synaptically influenced neurones reacting to E by modification of the synaptically driven firing pattern. An example of the action of E on such a neurone is shown in Fig. 4. E (10^{-4} M) evoked two phasic actions in this neurone. One of them was acceleratory. The efficacy of the acceleratory phase decreased if E was applied repeatedly. The other phase was inhibitory, which slightly increased with the reapplication of the opiate

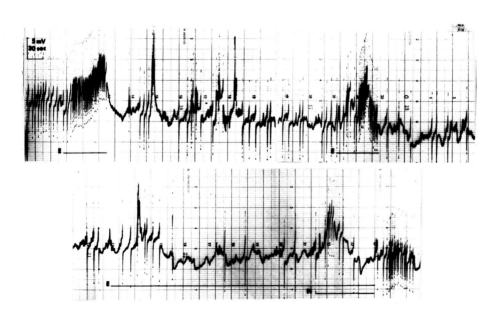

FIG. 4. Effects of E (10^{-4} M) and N (10^{-4} M) on a synaptically influenced neurone.

pentapeptide. N (10^{-4} M) antagonized only the inhibitory phase causing acceleration of the neuronal activity.

DISCUSSION

In these observations, the response to bath-applied E was seen to consist of various components in different neurones studied. In many of the cells, the response to E, or E + N, or N was very moderate showing rare density or lack of stereospecific opiate receptors as Pert et al. (5) have concluded for invertebrates. In other cases, the response to E could probably be peptidic in nature and peptide-sensitive receptors could have mediated the recorded responses without the involvement of opiate receptors. Although the reactivity of the visceral Br neurone was not tested by other peptides, there is evidence from various laboratories that Br activity can be modulated by peptide factors and hormones (1,12).

In a small number of cases, E evoked hyperpolarization of the membrane potential in synaptically influenced and silent cells. N antagonized some components of the E-evoked effects, while leaving other components unaffected or showing some agonistic action. Therefore, the agonistic activity of naloxone in *Helix* is consistent with some findings in vertebrates (9,10) or in *Aplysia* (13).

An interesting observation was that, in some experiments, the potassium-dependent ACh H-responses were modulated by E. N could antagonize some components of these E effects showing the presence of opiate receptors of certain *Helix* nerve cells. All neurones showing evidence for the presence of opiate receptors were ACh D- or H-cells (3,11). The actions are considered to have been mediated by opiate receptors, even though the effective concentrations of E or N were much higher than those used in vertebrate systems.

Presynaptic modulation of the transmitter release is not present in this system on stimulus-evoked EPSPs or IPSPs, but synaptically influenced neuronal activity also was biphasically modulated by E which can give the possibility of presynaptic modulation as well. The hyperpolarizing action of E was reversed only by changing the perfusion solution to one that contained both E and N, but N showed agonistic effect on the depolarizing action of the opiate pentapeptide.

From the present findings, it may be concluded that the potassium mechanism was modulated by E but the mode of the opiate receptor mediated actions is not yet clear.

CONCLUSIONS

Intracellular recordings were made from neurones of the snail brain. E effects exerted on the neuronal membrane were studied by adding the pentapeptide to the perfusing solution. The opioid pentapeptide elicits the following actions on various silent, synaptically influenced, and pacemaker neurones of the snail brain:

1. Most of the neurones studied were totally insensitive to E and/or the narcotic antagonist N.

2. Some neurones reacted with moderate hyperpolarizations (2–6 mV) to E, and N administration antagonized the E-evoked hyperpolarization.

3. ACh-evoked potassium-dependent hyperpolarizations were also modulated: decrease in amplitude and time course was seen as the effect of opioid pentapeptide. N antagonized these effects.

4. N did not antagonize all actions of E but might display some agonistic properties.

5. The active doses for both E and N were much higher than those reported in vertebrate systems.

In conclusion, the present results show that E exerts a dual effect in snail neurones: it induces hyperpolarizations of some neurones, and in addition, depresses the slow H-response in others. These effects can be interpreted as indicating low concentration or sensitivity of opioid receptors on the snail neuronal membranes.

Note added in proof: While this manuscript was in press, other publications have appeared indicating the presence of enkephalin-containing neurones in the earthworm (J. Aluments et al., *Nature,* 279:805, 1979) and in the leech (B. Zipser, *Nature,* 283:857–858, 1980). The existence of opiate-receptors on snail neurones was also evidenced by Dr. Katalin S.-Rózsa, Tihany, Hungary.

REFERENCES

1. Barker, J. L., Ifshin, M. S., and Gainer, H. (1975): Studies on bursting pacemaker potential activity in molluscan neurons. III. Effects of hormones. *Brain Res.,* 84:501–513.
2. Erdélyi, L. (1977): A new Br neurone in the visceral ganglion of Helix pomatia: Effects of Ach and Ba^{2+} on the firing pattern and I–V characteristics. *Comp. Biochem. Physiol.,* 56C:109–114.
3. Gerschenfeld, H. M. (1973): Chemical transmission in invertebrate central nervous systems and neuromuscular junctions. *Physiol. Rev.,* 53:1–119.
4. Kerkut, G., A., and Thomas, R. C. (1965): An electrogenic sodium pump in snail nerve cells. *Comp. Biochem. Physiol.,* 14:167–183.
5. Pert, C. B., Aposhian, D., and Snyder, S. H. (1974): Phylogenic distribution of opiate receptor binding. *Brain Res.,* 75:356–361.
6. Reynolds, E. S. (1963): The use of lead citrate as an electron dense stain in electron microscopy. *J. Cell Biol.,* 17:208–212.
7. Sakai, K. K., Hymson, D. L., and Shapiro, R. (1978): The mode of action of enkephalins in the guinea-pig myenteric plexus. *Neurosci. Lett.* 10:317–322.
8. Simantov, R., Goodman, R., Aposhian, D., and Snyder, S. H. (1976): Phylogenetic distribution of a morphine-like peptide 'enkephalin'. *Brain Res.,* 111:204–211.
9. Snyder, S. H., and Simantov, R. (1977): The opiate receptor and opioid peptides. *J. Neurochem.,* 28:13–20.
10. Soteropoulos, G. C., and Standaert, F. G. (1973): Neuromuscular effects of morphine and naloxone. *J. Pharmacol. Exp. Ther.,* 184:136–142.
11. Tauc, L. (1967): Transmission in vertebrate and invertebrate ganglions. *Physiol. Rev.,* 47:521–593.
12. Treistman, S. N., and Levitan, I. B. (1976): Alteration of electrical activity in molluscan neurones by cyclic nucleotides and peptide factors. *Nature,* 261:62–64.

13. Tremblay, J. P., Schlapfer, W. T., Woodson, P. B. J., and Barondes, S. H. (1974): Morphine and related compounds: Evidence that they decrease available neurotransmitter in *Aplysia californica. Brain Res.,* 81:107–118.
14. Winborn, W. B., and Seelig, L. L. (1970): Paraformaldehyde and s-collidine—a fixative for preserving large tissue blocks for electron microscopy. *Texas Rep. Biol. Med.,* 28:347–361.
15. Wouters, W., and Van den Bercken, J. (1979): Hyperpolarization and depression of slow synaptic inhibition by enkephalin in frog sympathetic ganglion. *Nature,* 277:53–54.

Neuropeptides and Neural Transmission,
edited by C. Ajmone Marsan and W. Z. Traczyk.
Raven Press, New York © 1980.

Electrophysiology of Vasopressinergic Neurons in the Hypothalamus

J. D. Vincent, D. Poulain, and E. Arnauld

Institut National de la Santé et de la Recherche Médicale, Unité de Recherches de Neurobiologie des Comportements, U 176, 33077 Bordeaux-Cedex France

A most interesting discovery to emerge recently from the electrophysiological studies of magnocellular neurosecretory cells is the observation of a bursting pattern of electrical activity displayed by vasopressinergic neurons. This so-called phasic or low frequency bursting activity is characteristic of neurons that are actively engaged in secreting vasopressin (VP). In spite of a common phylogenetic origin and many similarities between the two neurohormones VP and oxytocin, the neurons secreting the latter never exhibit a phasic pattern of discharge. This gives rise to the problem of the mechanism for this phasic activity and its functional significance. Since all of our electrophysiological knowledge about neurosecretory neurons in mammals is based on the observations of *extracellular* recording, any hypothesis about mechanism and function can only be made after extrapolation of the results obtained by *intracellular* recording in neurosecretory neurons of invertebrates.

ELECTROPHYSIOLOGICAL CHARACTERISTICS OF VASOPRESSINERGIC NEURONS

As a general feature, the stimulation of an axon or a nerve ending generates antidromically an action potential in the cell body. Kandel (32) used this property to identify neurosecretory cells in the preoptic nucleus of the goldfish by stimulating nerve endings in the posterior pituitary gland. Following the introduction of this technique in mammals by Yagi et al. (54), it has been possible to identify *in vivo* the magnocellular neurosecretory cells during spontaneous and stimulating conditions.

The first type of neurosecretory cells to be identified on electrophysiological parameters has been oxytonergic neurons, since a specific stimulus exists for the activation of these neurons: in the lactating rat *suckling* induces intermittent milk ejections every 5 to 15 min, caused by pulses of 0.5 to 1 mU of oxytocin. As has been shown by the work of Wakerley and Lincoln (52), before each milk ejection there is a high frequency discharge of action potentials usually followed by a few seconds of inhibition. This pattern of discharge is observed in about half the population of neurosecretory cells in the supraoptic and paraventricular nuclei (Fig. 1A).

The lack of a specific stimulus (under experimental conditions) for VP release has, for a long time, prevented the identification of vasopressin neurons *in vivo*. About half of the magnocellular neurons of the supraoptic and paraventricular nuclei do not react to suckling and this proportion correlates well with the percentage of magnocellular neurons which react with a specific antibody against VP (47,48). Further evidence that the cells unresponsive to suckling represent a population of vasopressin neurons has been obtained from experiments which have shown that, under conditions that stimulate the release of VP (and of oxytocin as well), oxytocin neurons and unresponsive cells display strikingly different patterns of electrical activity. Under normal conditions, the majority of the neurons showing no response to suckling have a slow irregular pattern of electrical activity ($<$ 3 spikes/sec) similar to the background activity of oxytocin neurons. During haemorrhage or intraperitoneal injection of hypertonic saline, the same neurone which did not react to suckling, showed a progressive increase in firing rate and the appearance of a bursting pattern of activity. This bursting pattern could not be induced in oxytocin neurones (7,46). The bursting pattern described in the rat (8,11,18,26,45,51,53), sheep (27), and monkey (1,2,29,30) consists of periodic bursts of action potentials followed by a period of quiescence (Fig. 1B). Several stimuli are capable of eliciting this bursting pattern in VP neurons: intracarotid injection (29–31,50), slow intravenous infusion (27), intraperitoneal injections (8) of hypertonic saline, and also, dehydration by water deprivation (1,2,45,53), haemorrhage (46), and carotid occlusion (11,26). However, the reaction of VP neurons is dependent upon the intensity of the stimulus: in the monkey, during progressive dehydration by water deprivation the number of bursting neurons increases progressively as plasma osmolality rises (1) (Fig. 2). In the lactating rat, after 12 hr of dehydration 80 to 100% of the VP neurons display this mode of firing (45,53). As the mean firing rate of VP neurons increases, one can also observe an increase in the frequency of action potentials inside the bursts and in the duration of these bursts. It should be noted that, in the same animal and under the same conditions, there is a great variability in the bursting pattern of electrical activity from one VP neuron to the next (1,53). This accounts for the absence of obvious synchronisation between bursts of neighbouring neurons, although a temporary synchronisation can be obtained under acute stimulation such as carotid occlusion.

MECHANISMS UNDERLYING THE PHASIC PATTERN

It has been suggested that the periodicity of phasically firing neurons may be produced by a negative feed-back action of a recurrent inhibition. After an antidromic shock the magnocellular neurons display an inhibition of electrical activity lasting from 50 to 150 msec (13,29,34,35,41,50). A possible hypothesis is that the neurosecretory product itself may mediate the recurrent inhibition.

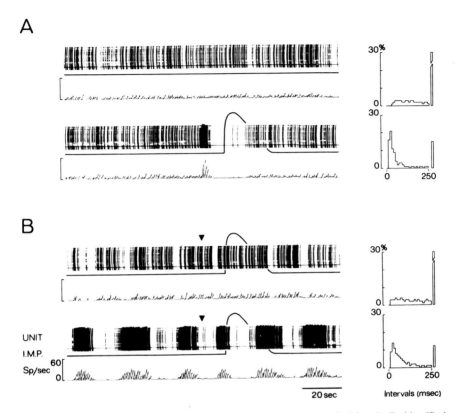

FIG. 1. Patterns of electrical activity of oxytocin and VP neurons. Antidromically identified neurosecretory cells were recorded in the supraoptic nucleus of anaesthetized lactating rats during suckling. On these polygraph records, action potentials represented by the polygraph pen deflections (UNIT) are drawn alongside the ratemeter output (spike/sec) and the intramammary pressure recording (I.M.P.) from a cannulated mammary gland. **A:** oxytocin neuron. **Top:** Background activity during suckling (note the flat intramammary pressure recording). **Bottom:** the same oxytocin neuron at the time of a milk ejection. The rise in intramammary pressure corresponds to 20 mmHg, equivalent to the response elicited by i.v. injection of 1 mU oxytocin. Note the brief high frequency discharge of action potentials occurring 14 sec before milk ejection (peak firing rate over a 0.5-sec period, 65 spikes/sec). Interspike interval histograms (Binwidth: 10 msec) have been drawn for the background activity **(top)** and for periods of 15 sec around the high frequency discharges **(bottom:** pooled data from 8 consecutive milk ejections). **B:** VP neurons: examples of one VP neuron displaying a slow irregular pattern of electrical activity **(top)** and of another VP neuron displaying a bursting mode of firing **(bottom).** In the few seconds preceding the milk ejection induced by suckling, no high frequency discharges occurred *(arrowheads).* Note the similarity between the slow irregular activity of the oxytocin neuron outside the period of milk ejection and of the first VP neuron; in both cases, interspike interval histograms are flat. Despite the striking difference between the high frequency discharge of the oxytocin neuron and the bursting pattern of the VP neuron, those enhanced activities result in a shift of their interspike interval towards short intervals.

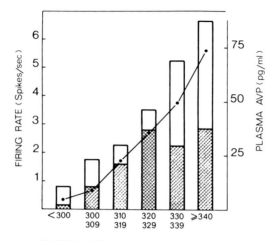

FIG. 2. Relation between plasma osmolality, VP release, and the electrical activity of supraoptic neurosecretory cells in the unanaesthetized monkey during water deprivation. Monkeys were deprived of drinking water for periods ranging from 1–5 days. Animals were classified into several groups according to the level of plasma osmotic pressure observed at the time of the experiments. The *black line* corresponds to the mean plasma arginine VP level (AVP) measured in each group by radioimmunoassay. For each group, the height of the blocks represents the mean firing rate of antidromically identified neurosecretory cells recorded in the supraoptic nucleus. The relative proportions of neurons displaying a bursting pattern of electrical activity are shown by the *shaded areas* (height of each block: 100% of the neurons in the group).

Therefore, according to Dale's principle of "one neuron-one transmitter" the neurosecretory product released in a neurohaemal organ must also be released from the recurrent terminals at the central synapses involved in recurrent inhibition. Nicoll and Barker tested this hypothesis by microiontophoretic application of VP in the vicinity of NSO magnocellular neurons (42). The majority of the cells (80%) were inhibited by the peptide. Vincent and Arnauld (49) observed that intracarotid injections of VP in monkeys depress the spontaneous firing of neurosecretory cells and their response to osmotic stimulation. Against this hypothesis is the observation that recurrent inhibition exists in both oxytocin and VP neurons and that iontophoretically applied oxytocin excites magnocellular neurons (40). Furthermore, serious doubt has been raised as to whether VP participates in the synaptic events that mediate recurrent inhibition since the demonstration of recurrent inhibition in the homozygous strain of Brattleboro rats which have an absolute deficiency in VP synthesis (14,16). However, this observation does not exclude the possibility that a VP-like peptide, which possesses synaptic activity but lacks any hormonal function, may exist in magnocellular neurons of the Brattleboro rat.

Recurrent inhibition could explain the long period of inhibition apparent in oxytocin neurons following high frequency discharge (37,52). It could also account for the similar inhibition displayed by neurosecretory cells after a volley of antidromic stimulation (9,49) or after activation by intracarotid injection of hypertonic saline (30,31,50). Its possible effects on bursting activity are unclear. That this particular property of the magnocellular neuron results from the activity of an intranuclear neuronal network is supported by anatomical studies showing that two-thirds of the synaptic boutons impinging on supraoptic neurons have an intranuclear origin (36). The fact that phasic NSO neurons can be recorded in rat hypothalamic slices (23), or in culture explants of the supraoptic nucleus area (20), also suggests that the mechanism capable of generating the phasic pattern lies very close to or within the nucleus itself.

An alternative hypothesis would be provided by the endogenous property of magnocellular neurons to generate the bursting pattern of spike activity. Such an intrinsic pacemaker is currently observed in invertebrate neurosecretory cells (21). The endogenously generated bursts of spikes are caused by slow membrane potential oscillations. The spikes are triggered when the depolarization phase of the oscillation reaches the threshold level for spike generation. During the hyperpolarizing phase of the oscillation the spikes are not generated. Using the voltage-clamp technique, it has been possible to study the membrane property of snail neurosecretory cells which exhibit bursting pacemaker potentials (4,5). When the snail is dormant, the cell is either silent, generates randomly occurring spikes, or exhibits a beating pattern and does not synthetize a neurosecretory product. On the other hand, when the snail is active, the cell typically generates bursting pacemaker activity. It is also possible to induce bursting pacemaker activity in "dormant" cells by injecting VP or related peptides close to the membrane (3,4).

When analyzed by the voltage clamp technique, spontaneously or VP-induced bursting neurons display a relatively linear current voltage relation (IV curve) at membrane potentials greater than -40 mV. However, when the membrane potential is decreased below this value the membrane develops a slowly inactivating inward current carried by Na^+. At lower membrane potentials (-10 mV), a slowly inactivating outward current carried by K^+ is generated. This membrane potential domain (between -40 and -10 mV) corresponds to a negative inflexion in the IV curve and represents an electrically unstable zone which forms the basis of the pacemaker potential oscillation. When the membrane potential is depolarized to the critical level (-40 mV), it develops a self-generating inward current which brings the membrane to the level of spike initiation. Following a series of spike currents, the polarity of the current is reversed and the slope conductance becomes positive again. The periodicity of the pacemaker oscillations appears to be determined mainly by the inactivating kinetics of the hyperpolarizing K^+ conductance. The slower the inactivation, the more prolonged is the slow depolarization and the longer is the period of depolarization. Ca^{2+} appears to play an important role in the sequence of events. The spike generation leads to a pulsatile increase of internal Ca^{2+} which, in turn, leads to the activation of K^+ conductance. As such, the successive Na^+-inward and K^+-outward slow, inactivating and voltage-dependent currents may account for the regenerative cycle of depolarization-repolarization supporting the bursting activity. It is sufficient to depolarize the cell to the critical level (−40 mV) in order to induce a self-sustaining pacemaker activity. Nevertheless, it is important to point out that such an activity cannot be induced by depolarizing the membrane of a cell which is not spontaneously generating bursting pacemaker potentials. As seen in Fig. 3, the cell in a resting state does not exhibit the N-shaped current/ voltage relationship. Addition of VP is able to change the shape of the curve and so induce bursting pacemaker activity.

Different arguments favour the existence of such an endogenous mechanism in vertebrate magnocellular neurons. When depolarized to a sufficient level by application of glutamate, neurosecretory neurons recorded in hypothalamic slices are able to generate sustained bursting activity (23). The fact that bursting activity is dependent on the internal properties of the cell and not exclusively on the synaptic input is supported by the observation that acetylcholine, which is able to excite NSO cell and to trigger a single burst in phasically firing cell (7), has never been shown to induce phasic activity in a silent or an irregularly firing cell even after a long application. In the case of a strong stimulation of neurosecretory cells such as that evoked by haemorrhage, the cells do not turn to phasic activity immediately but after a more or less prolonged period of fast continuous firing. As a tentative hypothesis it can be proposed that the intrinsic properties of the membrane have to change before the phasic activity may appear. An external factor such as a peptide, i.e., VP or a related substance released by a recurrent collateral pathway, may cause this change in membrane property.

This hypothesis does not explain why oxytocin cells never display phasic activity and respond to stimulation by fast continuous firing or by a single

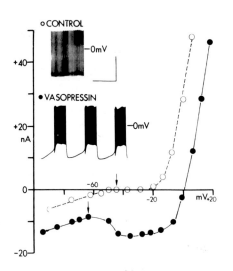

FIG. 3. Recording from a peptide-sensitive cell from the snail before (CONTROL) and after bath application of 1 μM VP (VASOPRESSIN). CONTROL shows a regular beating activity and VASOPRESSIN a bursting pacemaker activity. Current voltage (IV) curves during control and VP application. Calibration: 50 mV, 20 sec. (From Barker and Smith, ref. 5, with permission.)

high frequency burst. Different factors can alter the ion conductances and maintain the membrane polarization outside the critical domain of pacemaker initiation: variable coupling by electrical junctions may account for such alterations. A maximal degree of coupling of oxytocin cells in the lactating rat may also give a support for the synchronous discharge of these cells during the milk ejection reflex.

FUNCTIONAL SIGNIFICANCE OF THE PHASIC PATTERN

Relation Between the Action Potential and Hormone Release

Since the original work of Haterius and Fergusson (28), many studies have confirmed that the release of neurohypophysial hormones can be evoked by electrical stimulation of the hypophysial tract (24,25,39). Douglas observed that depolarization of the neurosecretory axons by an excess of K^+ in the bathing medium causes hormone liberation from isolated neurohypophysis (10). He further demonstrated that the presence of calcium was necessary in the medium and that hormone release increased when the external Ca^{2+} was raised. Douglas proposed that hormone release is initiated on arrival of impulses which, by depolarizing the axon endings, promote Ca^{2+} influx. The amount of hormone release and the $^{45}Ca^{2+}$ are both stimulated by increasing K^+ depolarization, although prolonged K^+ depolarization leads to a decline in hormonal output by inactivation of Ca^{2+} entry (43). Subsequent reactivation of Ca^{2+} entry by veratridine is able to retard hormone release (17). Further information showing the importance of calcium has been obtained from studies with the squid giant synapse preparation. Using the voltage clamp technique, it was found that an inward Ca^{2+} current in the presynaptic fiber preceded the excitatory post-synaptic potential (38). The calcium current evoked by depolarization is slow in onset, rapidly decaying with hyperpolarization, and does not appear to inactivate. There is a linear relationship between peak calcium current and the amplitude of the post-synaptic potential, i.e., the amount of transmitter released.

As for the presynaptic terminal (33), calcium activation and the resulting hormone release in the neurosecretory terminals are not exclusively dependent on the action potential per se. Tetrodotoxin, which abolishes action potentials, does not inhibit hormonal release induced by K^+ depolarization (12). When the neurosecretory endings are directly stimulated by current pulses (2 msec duration) in Na^+ free Locke solution, which precludes action potential generation, a clear-cut dependence of hormone release on frequency of stimulation can be observed (44); an identical number of pulses will release more hormone when delivered at a higher frequency. Thus, from these *in vitro* experiments, it can be concluded that hormone release depends both on the amplitude of the depolarization and on the frequency of the depolarizing pulses.

The action potential per se, however, plays a role in the mechanisms of hormone release. When the isolated neurohypophysis is stimulated in normal Locke solution (12), such that depolarization is generated in the endings by action potentials, the results are different from those obtained in Na⁺ free Locke solution. With a frequency of stimulation below 35 Hz, the hormone release was found to depend on the total number of stimuli applied as well as on the frequency of stimulation. Above 35 Hz, an identical number of stimuli were progressively less effective as the frequency of stimulation was increased. The inefficiency of a long train of high frequency stimulation is probably due to the inability of the fibers to conduct action potentials at a frequency higher than 35 Hz. Gainer (22) has pointed out that the frequency potentiation of hormone release for frequencies under 35 Hz is considerably greater than that already observed in the absence of action potential (Fig. 4). This observation suggests that the frequency potentiation of hormone release may be dependent upon frequency per se and in addition upon a frequency dependent property of the spike.

Significance of the Phasic Pattern

As discussed above, numerous *in vivo* studies have demonstrated a correlation between the extent of phasic activity in the magnocellular neurons and their secretory activity. The only direct evidence that the bursting pattern is highly efficient in inducing hormone release (15,19) has been obtained by stalk stimulation of isolated neurohypophysis. Clustering stimulus pulses with an overall frequency of 5.5 Hz released the same amount of hormone as a regular stimulation at 20 Hz (19). In a further experiment action potentials of phasically firing units recorded *in vivo* were used to trigger pulses delivered to neurohypophysis

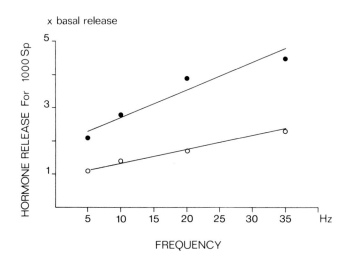

FIG. 4. Release of neurohypophysial hormone *in vitro* from isolated neurohypophysis stimulated at varying frequencies. *Open circles,* in Na⁺ free Locke solution; *closed circles,* in normal Locke solution. Graph based on ref. 22.

in vitro (15); more VP was released by pulses driven from phasic neurons than by regularly spaced pulses at the same overall frequency. Moreover, the amount of hormone release was correlated to the number of short interspike intervals ($<$ 100 msec) within the bursts. Under physiological conditions, the phasic pattern may represent the most economical way of obtaining short interspike intervals and thus producing frequency potentiation of hormone release.

The mechanism of potentiation is not clear. It has been shown by voltage clamp in invertebrate neurosecretory cells that the repolarization of action potentials is regulated by their frequency of discharge (6). The higher the frequency, the more rapid and thorough is the depression of the repolarization. This leads to a progressive augmentation of the duration of action potentials during the burst. Since Ca^{2+} entry is directly related to depolarization with a slow onset and without inactivation, the slower the repolarization and the longer the spike duration, the greater is the entry of calcium into the cell body. Finally, if we assume that action potentials recorded at the cell body are conducted unaltered down to the axon endings and that the membrane of the terminals has the same properties as that of the cell body, then the bursting pattern would facilitate Ca^{2+} entry, thereby facilitating neurohormone release.

ACKNOWLEDGMENTS

This work was supported by grants from INSERM (CR 176056.6) CNRS (ERA 493), and Phillipe Foundation.

REFERENCES

1. Arnauld, E., Dufy, B., and Vincent, J. D. (1975): Hypothalamic supraoptic neurones: Rates and patterns of action potential firing during water deprivation in the unanaesthetized monkey. *Brain Res.,* 100:315–325.
2. Arnauld, E., Vincent, J. D., and Dreifuss, J. J. (1974): Firing patterns of hypothalamic supraoptic neurons during water deprivation in monkeys. *Science,* 185:535–537.
3. Barker, J. L., and Gainer, H. (1974): Peptide regulation of bursting pacemaker activity in molluscan neurosecretory cell. *Science,* 184:1371–1373.
4. Barker, J. L., Ifshin, M., and Gainer, H. (1975): Studies on bursting pacemaker potential activity in molluscan neurons. III. Effects of hormones. *Brain Res.,* 84:501–513.
5. Barker, J. L., and Smith, T. G. (1976): Peptide regulation of neuronal membrane properties. *Brain Res.,* 103:167–170.
6. Barker, J. L., and Smith, T. G. (1977): Peptides as neurohormones. In: *Society for Neurosciences Symposia, Vol. 2: Approaches to the Cell Biology of Neurons,* edited by W. M. Cowan and J. A. Ferrendelli, pp. 340–373, Society for Neurosciences, Bethesda, Maryland.
7. Bioulac, B., Gaffori, O., Harris, M., and Vincent, J. D. (1978): Effects of acetyl-choline, sodium glutamate and GABA on the discharge of supraoptic neurons in the rat. *Brain Res.,* 154:159–162.
8. Brimble, M. J., and Dyball, R. E. J. (1977): Characterisation of the responses of oxytocin and vasopressin-secreting neurones in the supraoptic nucleus to osmotic stimulation. *J. Physiol. (Lond.),* 271:253–271.
9. Cross, B. A., Dyball, R. E. J., Dyer, R. G., Jones, C. W., Lincoln, D. W., Morris, J. F., and Pickering, B. T. (1975): Endocrine neurons. In: *Recent Progress in Hormone Research, Vol. 31,* pp. 243–293. Academic, New York.

10. Douglas, W. W. (1963): A possible mechanism of neurosecretion: Release of vasopressin by depolarization and its dependance on calcium. *Nature,* 197:81–84.
11. Dreifuss, J. J., Harris, M. C., and Tribollet, E. (1976): Excitation of phasically firing hypothalamic supraoptic neurones by carotid occlusion in rats. *J. Physiol. (Lond.),* 257:337–354.
12. Dreifuss, J. J., Kalnins, I., Kelly, J. S., and Ruf, K. B. (1971): Action potentials and release of neurohypophyseal hormones *in vitro. J. Physiol. (Lond.),* 215:805–817.
13. Dreifuss, J. J., and Kelly, J. S. (1972): Recurrent inhibition of antidromically identified rat supraoptic neurons. *J. Physiol. (Lond.),* 220:87–103.
14. Dreifuss, J. J., Nordmann, J. J., and Vincent, J. D. (1974): Recurrent inhibition of supraoptic neurosecretory cells in homozygous Brattleboro rats. *J. Physiol. (Lond.),* 237:25–27P.
15. Dutton, A., Dyball, R. E. J., Poulain, D. A., and Wakerley, J. B. (1978): The importance of short interspike intervals in determining vasopressin release from isolated neurohypophysis. *J. Physiol. (Lond.),* 280:23P.
16. Dyball, R. E. J. (1974): Single unit activity in the hypothalamo-neurohypophyseal system of Brattleboro rats. *J. Endocrinol.,* 60:135–143.
17. Dyball, R. E. J., and Nordmann, J. J. (1977): Reactivation by veratridine of hormone release from the K^+-depolarized rat neurohypophysis. *J. Physiol. (Lond.),* 269:65P.
18. Dyball, R. E. J., and Poutney, P. S. (1973): Discharge patterns of supraoptic and paraventricular neurones in rats given a 2 percent NaCl solution instead of drinking water. *J. Endocrinol.,* 56:91–98.
19. Dyball, R. E. J., and Thomson, R. J. (1977): Augmentation of vasopressin release from the electrically stimulated rat neurohypophysis by clustering of stimulus pulses. *J. Physiol. (Lond.),* 271:13P.
20. Gahwiller, B. H., Sandoz, P., and Dreifuss, J. J. (1978): Neurones with synchronous bursting discharges in organ cultures of the hypothalamic supraoptic nucleus area. *Brain Res.,* 151, 245–253.
21. Gainer, H. (1972): Electrophysiological behavior of an endogenously active neurosecretory cell. *Brain Res.,* 39:403–418.
22. Gainer, H. (1978): Input-output relations of neurosecretory cells. In: *Comparative Endocrinology,* edited by P. J. Gaillard and H. H. Boer, pp. 293–304. Elsevier/North Holland, Amsterdam.
23. Haller, E. W., Brimble, M. J., and Wakerley, J. D. (1978): Phasic discharge in supraoptic neurones recorded from hypothalamic slices. *Exp. Brain Res.,* 33:131–134.
24. Haller, E. W., Sachs, H., Sperelakis, N., and Share, L. (1965): Release of vasopressin from isolated guinea pig posterior pituitaries. *Am. J. Physiol.,* 209:79–83.
25. Harris, G. W. (1947): The innervation and the actions of the neurohypophysis; an investigation using the method of remote control stimulation. *Phil. Trans. R. Soc. Lond. (Biol. Sci.),* 232:385–441.
26. Harris, M. C., Dreifuss, J. J., and Legros, J. J. (1975): Excitation of phasically firing supraoptic neurones during vasopressin release. *Nature,* 258:80–82.
27. Haskins, J. T., Jennings, D. P., and Rogers, J. M. (1975): Response of neuroendocrine cell firing pattern types to measured changes in plasma osmolality. *Physiologist (Lond.),* 18:240.
28. Haterius, O., and Fergusson, J. K. B. (1938): Evidence for the hormonal nature of the oxytocic principle of the hypophysis. *Am. J. Physiol.,* 124:314–329.
29. Hayward, J. N., and Jennings, D. P. (1973): Activity of magnocellular neuroendocrine cells in the hypothalamus of unanesthetized monkeys. I. Functional cell types and their anatomical distribution in the supraoptic nucleus and the internuclear zone. *J. Physiol. (Lond.),* 232:515–543.
30. Hayward, J. N., and Jennings, D. P. (1973): Activity of magnocellular neuroendocrine cells in the hypothalamus of unanesthetized monkeys. II. Osmosensitivity of functional cell types in the supraoptic nucleus and the internuclear zone. *J. Physiol. (Lond.),* 232:545–572.
31. Hayward, J. N., and Vincent, J. D. (1970): Osmosensitive single neurones in the hypothalamus of unanesthetized monkeys. *J. Physiol. (Lond.),* 210:947–972.
32. Kandel, E. R. (1964): Electrical properties of hypothalamic neuroendocrine cells. *J. Gen. Physiol.,* 47:691–717.
33. Katz, B., and Miledi, R. (1967): A study of synaptic transmission in the absence of nerve impulses. *J. Physiol. (Lond.),* 192:407–436.
34. Kelly, J. S., and Dreifuss, J. J. (1970): Antidromic inhibition of identified rat supraoptic neurons. *Brain Res.,* 22:406–409.
35. Koizumi, K., and Yamashita, H. (1972): Studies of antidromically identified neurosecretory

VASOPRESSINERGIC NEURONS 291

cells of the hypothalamus by intracellular and extracellular recordings. *J. Physiol. (Lond.),* 221:683–705.

36. Leranth, C., Zaborski, L., Marton, J., and Palkovits, M. (1975): Quantitative studies on the supraoptic nucleus in the rat. I. Synaptic organisation. *Exp. Brain Res.,* 22:509–523.

37. Lincoln, D. W., and Wakerley, J. B. (1974): Electrophysiological evidence for the activation of supraoptic neurones during the release of oxytocin. *J. Physiol. (Lond.),* 242:533–554.

38. Llinas, R. R. (1977): Calcium and transmitter release in squid synapse. In: *Approaches to Cell Biology of Neurons,* edited by W. M. Cowan and J. A. Ferrendelli, pp. 139–155. Society for Neuroscience, Bethesda, Maryland.

39. Mikiten, T. M., and Douglas, W. W. (1965): Effect of calcium and other ions on vasopressin release from rat neurohypophysis stimulated electrically *in vitro. Nature,* 207:302–303.

40. Moss, R. L., Dyball, R. E. J., and Cross, B. A. (1972): Excitation of antidromically identified neurosecretory cells of the paraventricular nucleus by oxytocin applied iontophoretically. *Exp. Neurol.,* 34:95–102.

41. Negoro, H., and Holland, R. C. (1972): Inhibition of unit activity in the hypothalamic paraventricular nucleus following antidromic activation. *Brain Res.,* 42:385–402.

42. Nicoll, R. A., and Barker, J. L. (1971): The pharmacology of recurrent inhibition in the supraoptic neurosecretory system. *Brain Res.,* 35:501–511.

43. Nordmann, J. J. (1976): Evidence for calcium inactivation during hormone release in the rat neurohypophyses. *J. Exp. Biol.,* 65:669–695.

44. Nordmann, J. J., and Dreifuss, J. J. 1972): Hormone release evoked by electrical stimulation of rat neurohypophysis in the absence of action potentials. *Brain Res.,* 45:604–607.

45. Poulain, D. A., and Wakerley, J. B. (1977): Effects of dehydration on oxytocin and vasopressin neurons in the suckled rat. *J. Endocrinol.,* 72:6–7P.

46. Poulain, D. A., Wakerley, J. B., and Dyball, R. E. J. (1977): Electrophysiological differentiation of oxytocin and vasopressin cells during suckling and haemorrhage. *Proc. R. Soc. Lond. (Biol. Soc.),* 196:367–384.

47. Swaab, D. F., Nihveledt, F., and Pool, C. W. (1975): Distribution of oxytocin and vasopressin in the rat supraoptic and paraventricular nucleus. *J. Endocrinol.,* 67:461–462.

48. Vandesade, F., and Dierickx, K. (1975): Identification of the vasopressin producing and of the oxytocin producing neurons in the hypothalamic magnocellular neurosecretory system of the rat. *Cell Tissue Res.,* 164:153–162.

49. Vincent, J. D., and Arnauld, E. (1975): Vasopressin as a neurotransmitter in the central nervous system: Some evidence from the supraoptic neurosecretory system. In: *Progress in Brain Research, Vol. 42: Hormones Homeostasis and the Brain,* edited by W. H. Giepsen, Tj. B. Van Wimersma-Greidanus, R. Bohus, and D. De Wied, pp. 56–66. Elsevier, Amsterdam.

50. Vincent, J. D., Arnauld, E., and Nicolescu-Catargi, A. (1972): Osmoreceptors and neurosecretory cells in the supraoptic complex of the unanesthetized monkey. *Brain Res.,* 45:278–281.

51. Wakerley, J. B., and Lincoln, D. W. (1971): Phasic discharge of antidromically identified units in the paraventricular nucleus of the hypothalamus. *Brain Res.,* 25:192–194.

52. Wakerley, J. B., and Lincoln, D. W. (1973): The milk ejection reflex of the rat: A 20 to 40 fold acceleration in the firing of paraventricular neurones during oxytocin release. *J. Endocrinol.,* 57:477–493.

53. Wakerley, J. B., Poulain, D. A., and Brown, D. (1978): Comparison of firing patterns in oxytocin and vasopressin releasing neurons during progressive dehydration. *Brain Res.,* 148:425–440.

54. Yagi, K., Azuma, T., and Matsuda, K. (1966): Neurosecretory cell: Capable of conducting impulse in rats. *Science,* 154:778–779.

Neuropeptides and Neural Transmission,
edited by C. Ajmone Marsan and W. Z. Traczyk.
Raven Press, New York © 1980.

Neurohypophyseal Peptides and Avoidance Behavior: The Involvement of Vasopressin and Oxytocin in Memory Processes

Tj. B. van Wimersma Greidanus, J. M. van Ree, and D. H. G. Versteeg

Rudolf Magnus Institute for Pharmacology, 3521 GD Utrecht, The Netherlands

Peptides originating from the hypothalamus or from the posterior lobe of the pituitary have been shown to affect several types of behavior. Vasopressin is best known in this respect and systemic administration of this peptide delays extinction of active avoidance behavior and of behavior that is positively reinforced. Moreover, vasopressin improves passive avoidance behavior (1,28,31,40). The fact that a single injection of vasopressin exerts a long-lasting behavioral effect, which may extend far beyond the actual presence of the injected material in the organism, suggests that vasopressin affects the maintenance of a learned response probably by facilitation of consolidation processes (29,32). Time gradient studies performed using various paradigms reveal a promoting influence of vasopressin on retrieval processes as well (2).

Extensive structure–activity relationship studies with analogs and fragments of vasopressin in the pole-jump active avoidance procedure (28) indicate that arginine[8]-vasopressin (AVP) is among the most potent behaviorally active neurohypophyseal peptides. Upon intracerebroventricular injection of vasopressin, rather small amounts (25 pg) are sufficient to delay extinction of the pole-jump avoidance response (30). Using this route of administration, it appears that oxytocin has an effect opposite to that of vasopressin; i.e., oxytocin facilitates extinction of the avoidance response (2,3). This is in accordance with the earlier observations by Schulz et al. (19), who reported a competition-like effect between vasopressin and oxytocin or an opposite action of the two hormones on the central nervous system upon systemic administration. Also in the passive avoidance procedure these opposite effects are found after intracerebroventricular administration of neurohypophyseal hormones (2,3). Vasopressin improves passive avoidance behavior, which is reflected by prolonged avoidance latencies during retention of the response, whereas oxytocin impairs passive avoidance behavior, as indicated by decreased latency scores (23). From these and other data vasopressin has been suggested to improve memory function, while oxytocin has been designated as an amnestic peptide. An influence of vasopressin on memory has recently been demonstrated in humans as well (12,15).

Development of tolerance to and physical dependence on morphine may be regarded as a form of learning or memory (see ref. 17). Interestingly, vasopressin and analogs of this neurohypophyseal peptide appear to facilitate the development of tolerance to morphine and the physical dependence on this drug (11,18). Further experimentation has revealed that particularly the C-terminal tripeptide of oxytocin, prolyl-leucyl-glycinamide (PLG), is the most potent peptide in this respect (18). Thus, neurohypophyseal hormones and their fragments may be modulators of development of tolerance to morphine. Similar data have been recently reported for ethanol tolerance (6).

VASOPRESSIN LEVELS IN RELATION TO AVOIDANCE BEHAVIOR

In order to obtain evidence for a possible physiological role of endogenous vasopressin in acquisition and maintenance of avoidance behavior, levels of this hormone were measured in plasma of rats submitted to acquisition and retention of active and passive avoidance behavior. Although a correlation was found between passive avoidance behavior and the level of bioactive vasopressin in eye plexus blood (23), no correlation was observed between peripheral levels of vasopressin as measured by radioimmunoassay and the behavioral performance of the animals, either in active or passive avoidance behavior (36). An elevation in plasma vasopressin levels was only found in rats with the longest latencies during retention of a passive avoidance response (36). Also in the cerebrospinal fluid vasopressin levels seem to be unaltered during retention of passive avoidance behavior (36). Thus, it may be that vasopressin-containing neurons, which connect the site(s) of synthesis of vasopressin and its sites of behavioral action in limbic midbrain structures (4,5,10), are of primary importance for the behavioral effect of the peptide.

INHIBITION OF CENTRALLY AVAILABLE NEUROHYPOPHYSEAL HORMONES

A different approach to examine the possible involvement of endogenous peptides in behavior is to study the effect of reduction of their bioavailability in the brain by specific antisera. Intracerebroventricular injection of antisera to vasopressin or to oxytocin during acquisition and/or retention of active and passive avoidance behavior results in marked behavioral disturbances, depending on the dose and on the time of administration. Oxytocin antiserum delays extinction of an active avoidance response and increases passive avoidance latency scores (3), whereas vasopressin antiserum induces facilitation of extinction of active avoidance behavior (3,33) and attenuation of passive avoidance latencies (38). In a learned helplessness procedure, treatment with antiserum to vasopressin interferes with long-term memory as well (13). Mice treated intracerebroventricularly with antiserum do not show the escape deficits which are displayed after an initial period of inescapable footshocks by control animals. These data suggest that temporary neutralization or inactivation of neurohypophyseal peptides in the brain interferes with memory function and that vasopressin and oxytocin may be physiologically involved in memory processes; vasopressin facilitating consolidation and/or retrieval processes, oxytocin being an amnestic hormone.

Similar data as in avoidance behavior were obtained when investigating the influence of administration of vasopressin antiserum on the development of tolerance of the analgesic action of morphine. This development was studied in rats using an electric footshock (EFS) test procedure. Animals were tested for their responsiveness to EFS by scoring the percentage of jerks, flinches, or no responses displayed by the animal during exposure to EFS of different shock levels. Two different treatment schedules were used.

At first, rats received an initial intraperitoneal injection of either saline or morphine (40 mg/kg), followed by a second injection of morphine (10 mg/kg) 17 hr later. Thirty minutes after the latter injection animals were tested for their responsiveness to EFS. Antiserum to vasopressin, or normal rabbit serum as control, was injected intracerebroventricularly (2 μl) either 1 hr after the first morphine injection (storage processes) or 30 min prior to the second one (retrieval). Control animals showed about 30% no responses, 10% flinches,

TABLE 1. Effect of repeated administration of morphine on responsiveness to EFS

N	Respon-siveness	Day 1	Day 2	Day 3	Treatment (i.p./i.c.v.)
10	J	65.0 ± 2.6	62.5 ± 3.0	63.3 ± 2.9	Saline/NRS
	Fl	25.0 ± 2.1	27.1 ± 1.7	30.0 ± 2.6	
	0	10.0 ± 2.5	10.4 ± 2.2	6.7 ± 1.9	
10	J	27.9 ± 6.2[c]	36.2 ± 5.2[c]	47.1 ± 4.4[a,d]	M/NRS
	Fl	36.2 ± 3.3[d]	37.1 ± 3.3[d]	33.3 ± 2.6	
	0	35.9 ± 5.9[c]	26.6 ± 3.7[c]	19.6 ± 4.4[a,d]	
14	J	33.3 ± 4.1	25.9 ± 3.5	28.0 ± 2.2[b]	M/Anti-AVP
	Fl	35.1 ± 2.1	38.4 ± 2.6	38.4 ± 1.9	
	0	31.6 ± 1.8	35.7 ± 3.3	33.6 ± 3.0[b]	
12	J	62.2 ± 1.8	62.9 ± 2.7	60.8 ± 2.7	Saline/Anti-AVP
	Fl	25.3 ± 1.8	24.0 ± 1.9	28.1 ± 1.6	
	0	12.5 ± 1.8	13.1 ± 2.5	11.1 ± 2.6	

[a] $p < .05$ vs same group on day 1.
[b] $p < .02$ vs group M/NRS.
[c] $p < .001$ vs group Saline/NRS.
[d] $p < .02$ vs group Saline/NRS.
Rats were treated i.c.v. on days 1 and 2 with antivasopressin serum (anti-AVP) or with normal rabbit serum (NRS) immediately after morphine (M) administration (30 mg/kg i.p.). The responsiveness to EFS is expressed as percentages ± SEM of jerks (J), flinches (Fl), or no responses (0).

and 60% jerks. An acute injection of morphine (10 mg/kg) changed this pattern significantly to about 30% no responses, 30% flinches, and 40% jerks. After two morphine injections tolerance had been developed: the percentages of no responses, flinches, and jerks were similar to those after control treatment. Administration of antivasopressin serum either after the first morphine injection or prior to the second one inhibited the development of tolerance to morphine; the rats displayed a similar responsiveness to EFS as after acute morphine treatment.

Secondly, morphine (30 mg/kg i.p.) or saline was injected once daily for 3 consecutive days, 20 min prior to testing for the responsiveness to EFS. Antivasopressin serum or control serum was injected intracerebroventricularly immediately after the EFS test on days 1 and 2. In control rats development of tolerance to morphine was observed on days 2 and 3, in that an increasing percentage of jerks and a decreasing percentage of no responses were observed on these days as compared with day 1 (see Table 1). However, animals treated with antivasopressin serum showed on days 2 and 3 a similar responsiveness to EFS as on day 1, indicating that tolerance did not develop in these animals (see Table 1). Thus, like in memory processes, vasopressin may be of importance for storage and/or retrieval of information with respect to development of morphine tolerance.

BRAIN SITES OF ACTION

The behavioral effects of local application of vasopressin or vasopressin analogs in different limbic system structures during extinction of an active avoidance response suggest that the parafascicular thalamic region plays an important role in the effectiveness of vasopressin. The results of lesion studies and of microinjection experiments indicate that, in addition to the parafascicular nuclei, the rostral septal area, the dorsal hippocampal complex, the dorsal raphe nucleus, and the amygdala are essential in this respect (8,34,35,39). Knife cuts through the fornix, transecting pre- and postcommissural fibers and the stria terminalis do not block the behavioral effect of vasopressin. A single injection of the vasopressin analog des-glycinamide^9-lysine^8 vasopressin (DG-LVP) induces a dose-dependent long-lasting inhibition of a pole-jumping avoidance response (Fig. 1), in animals with a fornix transection as well as in sham-operated rats. This suggests that vasopressin can improve memory function in rats with a disrupted limbic system and that the limbic structures involved may act as more or less independent anatomical substrates for the behavioral effects of vasopressin (37).

MODE OF ACTION

Recently evidence has been accumulating which strongly suggests that vasopressin acts in the brain as a neuromodulator, i.e., that it amplifies or dampens

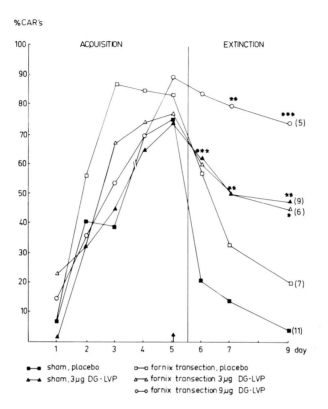

FIG. 1. Effect of s.c. injection of graded doses of DG-LVP on extinction of a pole-jump avoidance response in rats with fornix transections and in sham-operated animals. *Arrow* signifies injection. *Parentheses* enclose number of animals per group. DG-LVP vs placebo: *.02 $< p <$ .05; **.01 $< p <$ .02; ***$p <$ .01.

the activity of particular transmitter systems in the brain. It has been found that, following intracerebroventricular administration of nanogram quantities of vasopressin, regional catecholaminergic nerve impulse flow is changed (16, 20,21). For instance, norepinephrine turnover, as estimated from the rate of disappearance of this amine following inhibition of its synthesis with α-methyl-p-tyrosine, is enhanced after vasopressin administration in a number of brain regions rich in projections of the coeruleotelencephalic norepinephrine system. Dopamine turnover is increased after vasopressin treatment in terminal areas of the nigrostriatal and tuberoinfundibular dopamine systems (9,20,21). Subsequently, it has been observed that in situations in which the amount of bioavailable vasopressin in the brain is low, catecholamine turnover is decreased in brain regions in which it has been found to be enhanced after vasopressin administration (25,26). This is noted in rats of the Brattleboro strain which are deficient in vasopressin synthesis (26) as well as in normal Wistar rats following intracerebroventricular administration of antivasopressin serum (25).

These results suggest a relation between the effects of manipulation of the amount of bioavailable vasopressin in the brain on memory processes and on regional catecholaminergic activity in the brain. This has led to the hypothesis that vasopressin might exert its regulatory influence on memory processes by modulating catecholaminergic neurotransmission in distinct systems or particular terminal areas of the brain (17,25–27). Further experiments yielded results that support this hypothesis. It has been shown that vasopressin influences memory consolidation via various terminal areas of the coeruleotelencephalic norepinephrine system. In rats in which the dorsal noradrenergic bundle, which contains the norepinephrine-containing fibers originating in the locus coeruleus and projecting to a variety of telencephalic structures (14,24), had been lesioned with 6-hydroxydopamine, administration of vasopressin did not facilitate passive avoidance behavior (7). Furthermore, it appeared that microinjections of minute amounts of vasopressin in the dorsal hippocampus, the dorsal septal nucleus, or the dorsal raphe nucleus, regions which all contain projections of the coeruleotelencephalic system, result in a facilitation of passive avoidance behavior, whereas microinjections of vasopressin in the locus coeruleus, which contains the cell bodies of this system, failed to do so (8).

Although evidence in favor of a neuromodulator role of vasopressin in the brain seems quite convincing, to date only few data are available concerning oxytocin in this respect. Recently, Telegdy and Kovacs (22) reported that oxytocin altered regional catecholaminergic neurotransmission in some brain regions in a direction opposite to that induced by vasopressin. Results obtained in our institute, however, do not justify the conclusion to be drawn as yet that the opposite effects of vasopressin and oxytocin on memory processes are the result of the opposite action on brain catecholaminergic systems (Versteeg et al., *unpublished results*). Nevertheless, it seems reasonable to assume that both vasopressin and oxytocin act as neuromodulators. Moreover it seems likely that, in addition to norepinephrine and dopamine, other neurotransmitters in the brain may be modulated by the neurohypophyseal peptides as well. In fact, data related to this possibility have been presented for serotonin (16) and epinephrine (27).

CONCLUDING REMARKS

In conclusion it seems reasonable to suggest that an optimal function of the brain with respect to memory depends on an equilibrium between the amounts of centrally available vasopressin and oxytocin. The neurohypophyseal peptides may exert their influence on memory function by modulating catecholaminergic neurotransmission in the limbic system. Future research should elucidate whether other processes, in addition to memory function, are dependent on modulation of brain neurotransmission by vasopressin and oxytocin as well.

REFERENCES

1. Ader, R., and Wied, D. de (1972): Effect of lysine vasopressin on passive avoidance learning: *Psychon. Sci.,* 29:46–48.
2. Bohus, B., Kovács, G. L., and Wied, D. de (1978): Oxytocin, vasopressin and memory: Opposite effects on consolidation and retrieval processes. *Brain Res.,* 157:414–417.
3. Bohus, B., Urban, I., Wimersma Greidanus, Tj. B. van, and Wied, D. de (1978): Opposite effects of oxytocin and vasopressin on avoidance behaviour and hippocampal theta rhythm in the rat. *Neuropharmacology,* 17:239–247.
4. Buys, R. M. (1978): Intra- and extrahypothalamic vasopressin and oxytocin pathways in the rat. *Cell Tissue Res.,* 192:423–435.
5. Buys, R. M., Swaab, D. F., Dogterom, J., and Leeuwen, F. W. van (1978): Intra- and extrahypothalamic vasopressin and oxytocin pathways in the rat. *Cell. Tissue Res.,* 186:423–433.
6. Hoffman, P. L., Ritzmann, R. F., Walter, R., and Tabakoff, B. (1978): Arginine vasopressin maintains ethanol tolerance. *Nature,* 276:614–616.
7. Kovács, G. L., Bohus, B., and Versteeg, D. H. G. (1979): Facilitation of memory consolidation by vasopressin: Mediation by terminals of the dorsal noradrenergic bundle? *Brain Res.,* 172:73–85.
8. Kovács, G. L., Bohus, B., Versteeg, D. H. G., Kloet, E. R. de, and Wied, D. de (1979): Effect of oxytocin and vasopressin on memory consolidation: Sites of action and catecholaminergic correlation after local microinjection into limbic-midbrain structures. *Brain Res.,* 175:303–314.
9. Kovács, G. L., Vécsei, L., Szabó, G., and Telegdy, G. (1977): The involvement of catecholaminergic mechanisms in the behavioral effects of vasopressin. *Neurosci. Lett.,* 5:337–344.
10. Kozlowski, G. P., Brownfield, M. S., and Hostetter, G. (1978): Neurosecretory supply to extrahypothalamic structures: Choroid plexus, circumventricular organs and limbic system. In: *Neurosecretion and Neuroendocrine Activity,* edited by W. Bargmann, A. Oksche, A. Polenov, and B. Scharrer, pp. 217–227. Springer Verlag, Berlin.
11. Krivoy, W. A., Zimmermann, E., and Lande, S. (1974): Facilitation of development of resistance to morphine analgesia by desglycinamide-lysine-vasopressin. *Proc. Natl. Acad. Sci. USA,* 71:1852–1856.
12. Legros, J. J., Gilot, P., Jeron, X., Claessens, J., Adam, A., Moeglen, J. M., Audibert, A., and Berchier, P. (1978): Influence of vasopressin on learning and memory. *Lancet,* I:41–42.
13. Leshner, A. I., Hofstein, R., Samuel, D., and Wimersma Greidanus, Tj. B. van. (1978): Intraventricular injections of anti-vasopressin serum blocks learned helplessness in rats. *Pharmacol. Biochem. Behav.,* 9:889–892.
14. Lindvall, O., and Björklund, A. (1974): The organization of the ascending catecholamine neuron system in the rat brain. *Acta Physiol. Scand. (Suppl.)* 412:1–48.
15. Oliveros, J. C., Yandali, M. K., Timsitt-Berthier, M., Remy, R., Bengezal, A., Audibert, A., and Moeglen, J. M. (1978): Vasopressin in amnesia. *Lancet,* I:42.
16. Ramaekers, F., Rigter, H., and Leonard, B. F. (1977): Parallel changes in behaviour and hippocampal serotonin metabolism in rats following treatment with desglycinamide lysine vasopressin. *Brain Res.,* 120:485–492.
17. Ree, J. M. van, Bohus, B., Versteeg, D. H. G., and Wied, D. de (1978): Neurohypophyseal principles and memory processes. *Biochem. Pharmacol.,* 27:1793–1800.
18. Ree, J. M. van, and Wied, D. de (1976): Prolyl-leucyl-glycinamide (PLG) facilitates morphine dependence. *Life Sci.,* 19:1331–1340.
19. Schulz, H., Kovács, G. L., and Telegdy, G. (1974): Effect of physiological doses of vasopressin and oxytocin on avoidance and exploratory behaviour in rats. *Acta Physiol. Acad. Sci. Hung.,* 45:211–215.
20. Tanaka, M., Kloet, E. R. de, Wied, D. de, and Versteeg, D. H. G. (1977): Arginine-vasopressin affects catecholamine metabolism in specific brain nuclei. *Life Sci.,* 20:1799–1808.
21. Tanaka, M., Versteeg, D. H. G., and Wied, D. de (1977): Regional effects of vasopressin on rat brain catecholamine metabolism. *Neurosci. Lett.,* 4:321–325.
22. Telegdy, G., and Kovács, G. L. (1979): Role of monoamine in mediating the action of hormones on learning and memory. In: *IBRO Monograph Series, Vol. 4: Brain Mechanisms in Memory and Learning: From Single Neuron to Man,* edited by M. A. B. Brazier, pp. 249–268. Raven Press, New York.

23. Thompson, E. A., and Wied, D. de (1973): The relationship between the antidiuretic activity of rat eye plexus blood and passive avoidance behavior. *Physiol. Behav.,* 11:377–380.
24. Ungerstedt, U. (1971): Stereotaxic mapping of the monoamine pathways in the rat brain. *Acta Physiol. Scand.,* 367:1–49.
25. Versteeg, D. H. G., Kloet, E. R. de, Wimersma Greidanus, Tj. B. van, and Wied, D. de (1979): Vasopressin modulates the activity of catecholamine containing neurons in specific brain regions. *Neurosci. Lett.,* 11:69–73.
26. Versteeg, D. H. G., Tanaka, M., and Kloet, E. R de (1978): Catecholamine concentration and turnover in discrete regions of the brain of the homozygous Brattleboro rat deficient in vasopressin. *Endocrinology,* 103:1654–1661.
27. Versteeg, D. H. G., Tanaka, M., Kloet, E. R. de, Ree, J. M. van, and Wied, D. de (1978): Prolyl-leucyl-glycinamide (PLG): Regional effects on α-MPT induced catecholamine disappearance in rat brain. *Brain Res.,* 143:561–566.
28. Walter, R., Ree J. M. van, and Wied, D. de (1978): Modification of conditioned behavior of rats by neurohypophyseal hormones and analogues. *Proc. Natl. Acad. Sci. USA,* 75:2493–2496.
29. Wied, D. de (1971): Long term effect of vasopressin on the maintenance of a conditioned avoidance response in rats. *Nature,* 232:58–60.
30. Wied, D. de (1976): Behavioral effects of intraventricular administered vasopressin and vasopressin fragments. *Life Sci.,* 19:685–690.
31. Wied, D. de, Bohus, B., Urban, I., Wimersma Greidanus, Tj. B. van, and Gispen, W. H. (1975): Pituitary peptides and memory. In: *Peptides: Chemistry, Structure and Biology. Proceedings of the IVth American Peptide Symposium,* edited by R. Walter and J. Meienhofer, pp. 635–643. Ann Arbor Science Publishers, Ann Arbor, Michigan.
32. Wied, D. de, Wimersma Greidanus, Tj. B. van, Bohus, B., Urban, I., and Gispen, W. H. (1976): Vasopressin and memory consolidation. In: *Progress in Brain Res., Vol. 45: Perspectives in Brain Research,* edited by M. A. Corner and D. F. Swaab, pp. 181–194. Elsevier, Amsterdam.
33. Wimersma Greidanus, Tj. B. van, Bohus, B., and Wied, D. de (1975): The role of vasopressin in memory processes. In: *Progress in Brain Research, Vol. 42: Hormones, Homeostasis and the Brain,* edited by W. H. Gispen, Tj. B. van Wimersma Greidanus, B. Bohus, and D. de Wied, pp. 135–141. Elsevier, Amsterdam.
34. Wimersma Greidanus, Tj. B. van, Bohus, B., and Wied, D. de (1975): CNS sites of action of ACTH, MSH and vasopressin in relation to avoidance behavior. In: *Anatomical Neuroendocrinology,* edited by W. F. Stumpf and L. D. Grant, pp. 284–289. Karger, Basel.
35. Wimersma Greidanus, Tj. B. van, Croiset, G., Bakker, E. A. D., and Bouman, H. (1979): Amygdaloid lesions block the effect of neuropeptides (vasopressin, ACTH 4–10) on avoidance behavior. *Physiol. Behav.,* 22:291–295.
36. Wimersma Greidanus, Tj. B. van, Croiset, G., Goedemans, H., and Dogterom J. (1979): Vasopressin levels in peripheral blood and cerebrospinal fluid during passive and active avoidance behavior in rats. *Horm. Behav.,* 12:102–111.
37. Wimersma Greidanus, Tj. B. van, Croiset, G., and Schuiling, G. A. (1979): Fornix transection: Discrimination between neuropeptide effects on attention and memory. *Brain Res. Bull.,* 4:625–629.
38. Wimersma Greidanus, Tj. B. van, and Wied, D. de (1976): Modulation of passive avoidance behavior of rats by intracerebroventricular administration of antivasopressin serum. *Behav. Biol.,* 18:325–333.
39. Wimersma Greidanus, Tj. B. van, and Wied, D. de (1976): Dorsal hippocampus: A site of action of neuropeptides on avoidance behavior? *Pharmacol. Biochem. Behav.,* 5 (Suppl. 1):29–33.
40. Wimersma Greidanus, Tj. B. van, and Wied, D. de (1977): The physiology of the neurohypophysial system and its relation to memory processes. In: *Biochemical Correlates of Brain Structure and Function,* edited by A. N. Davison, pp. 215–248. Academic, London.

Neuropeptides and Neural Transmission,
edited by C. Ajmone Marsan and W. Z. Traczyk.
Raven Press, New York © 1980.

Effects of Neurohypophyseal Hormone Analogs and Fragments on Learning and Memory Processes in Behavioral Tests

I. Krejčí, B. Kupková, E. Kasafírek, *T. Barth, and *K. Jošt

*Research Institute for Pharmacy and Biochemistry, 194 04 Prague 9, and
*Institute of Organic Chemistry and Biochemistry, Czechoslovak Academy of Sciences,
166 10 Prague 6, Czechoslovakia*

Several groups of vasopressin and oxytocin analogs, designed as metabolically more stable compounds, reveal protracted effects in specific biologic systems. The aim of this study was to determine whether the increased half-life of some of these analogs would be reflected in the effects on learning and memory processes. The main group of vasopressin analogs consisted of "deamino-carba-vasopressins," considered to be resistant to aminopeptidases as well as to the reductive opening of the ring. Two other analogs, N^α-glycyl-glycyl-glycyl(8-lysine) vasopressin and its des-glycinamide derivative behave as "hormonogens" in the organism, which means that they release the free hormone (or its des-glycinamide), while the additional amino acids are split off by enzyme action (11). Furthermore, we studied the effects of the C-terminal linear part of the oxytocin molecule and its analogs.

MATERIALS

Lysine-vasopressin (LVP) (commercial preparation), [8-L-lysine] des-9-glycinamide-vasopressin (DG-LVP) (2), [8-L-arginine] deamino-6-carba-vasopressin (dC⁶AVP), [8-D-arginine] deamino-6-carba-vasopressin (dC⁶DAVP), [8-L-ornithine] deamino-6-carba-vasopressin (dC⁶OVP) (6), [8-L-arginine] deamino-1-carba-vasopressin (dC¹AVP) (9), [8-L-arginine] deamino-6-carba-des-9-glycinamide-vasopressin (DG-dC⁶AVP) (Barth, *unpublished results*), N^α-glycyl-glycyl-glycyl [8-lysine] vasopressin (Trigly-LVP), N^α-glycyl-glycyl-glycyl [8-lysine] des-9-glycinamide-vasopressin (DG-Trigly-LVP) (10), deamino-6-carba-oxytocin (dC⁶OT) (7), Pro-Leu-Gly-NH₂, Pro-Leu-β-Ala-NH₂, Z-Gly-Pro-Leu-Gly-NH₂, EUC-Leu-Gly-NH₂, EUC-Leu-β-Ala-NH₂, EUC-Leu-NH₂ (EUC,2-oxoimidazolidine-1-carboxylic acid) (8).

EFFECTS ON PASSIVE AVOIDANCE BEHAVIOR

Passive avoidance behavior was studied in a "step through" type of apparatus described by Ader et al. (1). This consisted of a dark box equipped with a grid floor, to which an elevated illuminated runway was attached. Male rats (weighing 180–210 g) were placed on the runway and their latency to enter the dark box was recorded. Two such trials were performed on day 1 and day 2. Upon the last entering of the second day animals received an electric footshock. They were tested for retention 1 to 13 days after the acquisition trial. Peptides or saline were administered subcutaneously either after the footshock or 20 min before the test trial. In another series of experiments animals underwent an amnesic treatment immediately after the footshock. Amnesia was induced by halothane anesthesia. The drugs were injected 20 min before the footshock and their ability to attenuate amnesia was estimated in a retrieval trial after 24 hr.

Because the passive avoidance test did not allow us to estimate dose-response curves for individual peptides, we could make only an assessment of relative potencies on the basis of approximate threshold doses. All vasopressin analogs significantly increased avoidance latencies, both when injected after the shock and before the test trial, and they were effective in attenuating amnesia induced by halothane. Four representatives of carba vasopressins, namely dC⁶AVP, dC¹AVP, dC⁶DAVP, and dC⁶OVP were effective in 0.1 μg doses administered after the shock, whereas 3 to 10 times higher doses of LVP or DG-LVP (depending on the interval between learning and test) were required to obtain a significant increase of avoidance latencies. No marked differences between the potency of hormonogens and LVP could be detected. The results are summarized in Table 1.

TABLE 1. *Effects of vasopressin analogs on retention of passive avoidance behavior tested 24 hr till 13 days after the acquisition trial*

Treatment (μg)	Threshold doses (μg)[a]		
	After shock trial	Prior to test trial	Prior to amnesia induction (halothane)
LVP	0.3–1.0	0.3	1.0
DG-LVP	0.3–1.0	0.3	1.0
dC⁶OVP	0.1	0.1	1.0
dC⁶AVP	0.1	0.1	1.0
dC⁶DAVP	0.1	—	—
DG-dC⁶AVP	1.0	1.0	—
DC¹AVP	0.1	—	1.0
Trigly-LVP	1.0	—	—
DG-Trigly-LVP	1.0	1.0	1.0

[a] Approximated threshold doses necessary for enhancing avoidance latencies. $p < 0.05$.

There is, however, another interesting feature of the effect of carba vasopressins: their sedative action on rats. 1 μg of dC⁶AVP, dC¹AVP, or dC⁶OVP reduced ambulation, rearing, and grooming and increased the time spent in immobility in the open field test. Higher doses induced sleep-like immobility; nevertheless, sound and touch stimuli awoke the sleeping rats immediately. The sedation culminated 20 to 30 min after the subcutaneous injection. It has commonly been accepted that excitation, rather than sedation, affects positively learning and memory processes (see, for example, refs. 3, 12). Nevertheless, even 20 μg dC⁶AVP given after shock facilitated retention of the passive avoidance response. It was only when preacquisition treatment was used (20–30 min before the shock) that the carba analogs did not increase the avoidance latencies (Fig. 1).

Bohus et al. (4) have recently shown that intracerebroventricularly administered oxytocin impaired retention of passive avoidance response. Ten micrograms of dC⁶OT also induced impairment of retention when injected subcutaneously 20 min before the test trial.

Pro-Leu-Gly-NH₂ and its analogs increased avoidance latencies both when injected after the acquisition or before the test trial and they also attenuated the amnesic effect of halothane anesthesia. However, they had to be administered in 100 to 1000-fold higher doses than those used in the case of vasopressins; the studied modifications of Pro-Leu-Gly-NH₂ did not bring about an enhancement of potency (Table 2).

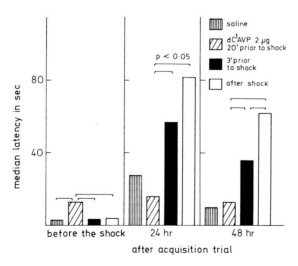

FIG. 1. Effects of dC¹AVP (2 μg) on retention of the passive avoidance response (footshock = 0.3 mA for 3 sec). Columns in the left part represent latencies of the last entering of rats into the dark box where they received the footshock. Each group consisted of 10 animals.

TABLE 2. *Effects of hormone fragments on retention of passive avoidance behavior tested 24 hr after the acquisition trial*

| | Threshold doses (mg)[a] | | |
| | After acquisition trial | Prior to test trial | Prior to amnesia induction (halothane) |
Treatment (mg)			
Pro-Leu-Gly-NH$_2$	0.2	0.2	0.2
Pro-Leu-β-Ala-NH$_2$	0.2	0.2	0.2
EUC-Leu-Gly-NH$_2$	0.2	0.2	0.2
EUC-Leu-β-Ala-NH$_2$	0.2	0.2	0.2
EUC-Leu-NH$_2$	—	—	1.0
Z-Gly-Pro-Leu-Gly-NH$_2$	0.2	0.6	0.2

[a] Approximated threshold doses necessary for enhancing avoidance latencies. $p < 0.05$.

INFLUENCE OF PEPTIDES ON LEARNING FOR WATER REWARDS

Operant behavior was studied using rats maintained on a 23-hr water deprivation schedule. During the first part of the experiment, rats were trained to

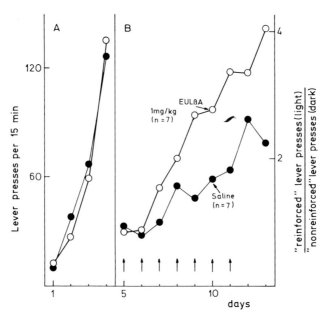

FIG. 2. Acquisition of lever-pressing by rats for water reinforcement. **A:** Continuous reinforcement schedule. **B:** Lever-presses rewarded only during the "light" cycles. *Arrows* denote days when peptide or saline were administered. The area below the curve representing the performance of rats treated with EUC-Leu-β-Ala-NH$_2$, differs significantly from the area below the curve representing the performance of the control group. Note that the difference in performance persisted even after the treatment had been interrupted.

press a lever in a Skinner box on a continuous reinforcement schedule (CRF) for water reinforcement (each lever-press was followed by the presentation of a small amount of water). The session lasted 15 min. After 4 days of training, the schedule was changed. Short periods (24 sec) of the original schedule, during which a white light was present in the box, were alternated regularly with periods of the same duration, during which neither reinforcement nor light signal was presented. The performance of rats was expressed as the following ratio:

$$\frac{\text{Mean number of responses during ``reinforced'' lever-pressing}}{\text{Mean number of responses during ``nonreinforced'' lever-pressing}}$$

Treatment started on the first day of the second part of the experiment, half of the rats being injected with either saline or peptide 20 min before the session. In rats treated with 1 mg/kg EUC-Leu-β-Ala-NH$_2$, the estimated ratio increased at a higher rate than in control animals (Fig. 2). By contrast, treatment with DG-LVP and DG-Trigly-LVP (5 μg/kg) failed to influence the rate of acquisition of the task.

DISCUSSION

The results obtained with several deamino-carba vasopressins supported our assumption that metabolically more stable vasopressin analogs could have high activity in tests concerning memory processes. Furthermore, we found that some of them exerted a sedative effect which interfered with their facilitatory influence on retention if the animals experienced the shock in the drugged state. We may speculate that sedation had to be sufficiently pronounced at the time when the process of memory consolidation became sensitive to the facilitatory effects of the peptide, or that the integrity of the perceptional ability of animals was impaired by the time of the painful experience. State dependency should also be considered.

Regarding the activities of hormonogens, we must take into account the activation–inactivation kinetics of these analogs. We must assume that the plasma levels of free hormone are lower after the application of a hormonogen compared with an identical dose of LVP itself. The determination of threshold doses is apparently not a suitable criterion for evaluating the activity of this type of analog.

Although dC^{6}OT impaired retention, the linear part of its molecule (Pro-Leu-Gly-NH$_2$) and analogs of this tripeptide had facilitatory effects on memory retention of the passive avoidance response and attenuated amnesia; however, much higher doses had to be used as compared with vasopressins. Furthermore, EUC-Leu-Gly-NH$_2$ enhanced the rate of learning of lever pressing for water reward, whereas DG-LVP and DG-Trigly-LVP did not. This is another example of drug specificity required by receptors responsible for mediating the effects of different analogs of neurohypophyseal hormones in different behavioral testing paradigms. Thus, for example, both oxytocin and Pro-Leu-Gly-NH$_2$ attenuated puromycin-induced amnesia in the active avoidance test performed with mice (5), both peptides increased the resistance to extinction of a pole-jumping avoidance response in rats (14) and facilitated morphine dependence in rats (13). On the contrary, intracerebroventricularly administered oxytocin attenuated the retention of passive avoidance in rats (4).

REFERENCES

1. Ader, R., Weijnen, J. A. W. M., and Moleman, P. (1972): Retention of a passive avoidance response as a function of the intensity and duration of electric shock. *Psychon. Sci.,* 26:125–128.
2. Barth, T., and Kluh, I. (1974): Des-glycinamide⁹-vasopressin and des-lysine,glycinamide⁹-vasopressin: Some pharmacological properties. *Coll. Czech. Chem. Commun.,* 39:506–508.
3. Bloch, V. (1970): Facts and hypothesis concerning memory consolidation processes. *Brain Res.,* 24:561–575.
4. Bohus, B., Kovács, G. L., and Wied, D. de (1978): Oxytocin, vasopressin and memory: Opposite effects on consolidation and retrieval processes. *Brain Res.,* 157:414–417.
5. Flexner, J. B., Flexner, K. B., Hoffman, P. L., and Walter, R. (1977): Dose-response relationships in attenuation of puromycin-induced amnesia by neurohypophyseal peptides. *Brain Res.,* 134:139–144.
6. Jošt, K., Procházka, Z., Cort, J. H., Barth, T., Škopková, J., Prusík, Z., and Šorm, F. (1974): Synthesis and some biological activities of deaminovasopressin with disulphide bridge altered to thioether bridge. *Coll. Czech. Chem. Commun.,* 39:2835–2848.
7. Jošt, K., and Šorm, F. (1971): The effect of the presence of sulphur atoms on the biological activity of oxytocin; synthesis of deamino-carba⁶-oxytocin and deamino-dicarba-oxytocin. *Coll. Czech. Chem. Commun.,* 36:234–242.
8. Kasafírek, E., Krejčí, I., and Felt, V. (1979): Analogues of melanostatine. *Coll. Czech. Chem. Commun.,* 45:294–297.
9. Procházka, Z., Barth, T., Cort, J. H., Jošt, K., and Šorm, F. (1978): Synthesis and some pharmacological properties of 8-L-arginine-deamino-1-carba vasopressin. *Coll. Czech. Chem. Commun.,* 43:655–663.
10. Procházka, Z., Krejčí, I., Kupková, B., Slaninová, J., Bojanovská, V., Prusík, Z., Vosekalná, I. A., Maloň, P., Barth, T., Frič, I., Bláha, K., and Jošt, K. (1978): Synthesis and properties of the Nα-glycyl-glycyl-glycyl-vasopressin and its desglycinamide derivative. *Coll. Czech. Chem. Commun.,* 43:1285–1299.
11. Rudinger, J., Pliška, V., and Krejčí, I. (1972): Oxytocin analogs in the analysis of some phases of hormone action. *Rec. Prog. Horm. Res.,* 28:131–172.
12. Urban, I., and Wied, D. de (1978): Neuropeptides: Effects on paradoxical sleep and theta rhythm in rats. *Pharmacol. Biochem. Behav.,* 8:51–59.
13. Van Ree, J. M., and Wied, D. de (1976): Prolyl-leucyl-glycinamide facilitates morphine dependence. *Life Sci.,* 19:1331–1340.
14. Walter, R., van Ree, J. M., and Wied, D. de (1978): Modification of conditioned behavior of rats by neurohypophyseal hormones and analogues. *Proc. Natl. Acad. Sci. USA,* 75:2493–2496.

Neuropeptides and Neural Transmission,
edited by C. Ajmone Marsan and W. Z. Traczyk.
Raven Press, New York © 1980.

Vasopressin and Oxytocin Distribution in Rat Brain: Radioimmunoassay and Immunocytochemical Studies

J. Dogterom and R. M. Buijs

Netherlands Institute for Brain Research 1095 KJ Amsterdam, The Netherlands

Peptide hormones of hypothalamic and hypophyseal origin exert behavioral effects if administered to man or laboratory animals (1,6,9). The presence of peptide hormones as neurohypophyseal hormones, releasing factors, and cleavage products of the adrenocorticotropic hormone (ACTH), lipotropin hormone (LPH) family in a variety of brain regions (2,4) raises a number of questions concerning their possible physiological involvement in brain functions.

The neurohypophyseal hormones vasopressin and oxytocin play a role in behavioral processes (15). These peptide hormones reach their target sites in the brain, e.g., the limbic system, via a network of vasopressin- or oxytocin-containing fibers (3), which probably provided the anatomical basis for their central action. This possibility is supported by the finding that local microinjections of minute amounts of vasopressin altered the turnover of aminergic neurotransmitters in nuclei of the limbic system and other brain regions which have been implicated in the behavioral action of vasopressin (8,14). As a result of these and other findings (16) it has been proposed that vasopressin and oxytocin function as neurotransmitters, thus regulating behavioral processes. Such a suggestion implies that vasopressin and oxytocin are released upon a behavioral stimulus from peptidergic synapses in the brain and subsequently metabolized, possibly resulting in a change in peptide concentration in well-defined brain regions. In order to test this possibility, basal vasopressin and oxytocin concentrations were determined in samples of rat brain and compared with the concentrations of these hormones in brain samples from rats that had been trained for passive avoidance behavior. In addition, immunoelectronmicroscopic studies have been performed to reveal the existence of peptidergic synapses in brain regions which are of importance for the behavioral effects of vasopressin (14).

MATERIALS AND METHODS

Radioimmunoassay

Male rats of an inbred Wistar strain (CPB/TNO, Zeist, The Netherlands) weighing 160 to 180 g were used. The animals were housed 5 per cage on sawdust and had food and water *ad libitum* (light on from 7.00 A.M. to 7.00 P.M.). Two groups of rats, which had been handled for 5 days, were used:

1. Control group: These animals were decapitated between 10.30 and 11.30 A.M., directly after being taken from their home cage.

2. Experimental group: These animals were decapitated also between 10.30 and 11.30 A.M. after being trained for passive avoidance behavior. The training procedure consisted of five adaptation trials on 2 consecutive days and one learning trial, including electric footshock (1 mA, 2 sec). The latency to enter of each animal during the learning trial was recorded and shock was applied immediately after the animal had entered the dark compartment. Five minutes after the beginning of the learning trial the animals were decapitated.

Immediately after decapitation the brains were removed and frozen in Freon-12 ($-80°C$). In a previous study (4) animals were anesthetized and perfused with saline in order to remove the blood. Since in a pilot study the values in perfused and non-perfused brain were similar, perfusion was omitted in the present study.

Transverse 300-μm sections of whole brain were cut at $-10°C$ in a cryostat on the same day. The sections were then lyophilized overnight. The following day, punched dry samples were obtained according to the method of Lowry and Passoneau (10) and of Palkovits (11) and placed in 0.1 N HCl after weighing on a Mettler UM 7 balance. The samples were sonified for 1 min at 20 kHz and 4°C and stored at $-70°C$ until the next day when vasopressin and oxytocin were extracted from the tissues and their levels determined by radioimmunoassay (RIA) (4). Minor modifications have been introduced in both assays; bovine serum albumin has been substituted with human serum albumin (Sigma, No. 9511); 325 mesh Vycor glass was used for extraction, and 80% aqueous acetone was used for the elution of the peptides from the glass. Recovery of standard vasopressin and oxytocin, added to the extraction medium, was about 80 and 70%, respectively. Little, if any, nonspecific activity was measured in blank tubes containing only medium. The detection limit of the vasopressin-RIA was 1 pg/sample and of the oxytocin-RIA 2 pg/sample. The RIA data were corrected for recovery and expressed in picograms hormone per milligram dry weight.

Immunoelectronmicroscopy

Male Wistar rats (TNO, Zeist), weighing 180 to 200 g, were anesthetized with Nembutal® (0.1 ml/100 g body weight i.p.), perfused intracardially with saline followed by 2.5% glutaraldehyde, 1% paraformaldehyde in 0.1 M cacodylate buffer pH 7.25 (all chemicals from Merck). The desired brain regions were isolated free-hand in slices of approximately 2 mm and subsequently immersed in the same fixative for 2 to 3 hr at 4°C.

The tissue blocks were sectioned using a vibratome (Oxford Instruments) 20 to 80 μm into 0.05 M Tris/HCl buffer pH 7.6 in 0.9 NaCl. Sections were handled with a paint brush and placed into glass vials. The immunocytochemical procedures were essentially the same as described previously (3), and consisted of subsequent incubations at 4°C in (a) 10% swine serum plus 0.1% Triton X-100 for 30 min; (b) rabbit vasopressin no. 125 or oxytocin no. 02C antiserum purified (1:400) or nonpurified (1:1,000) plus 0.1% Triton X-100 for 16 hr. (c) washed in Tris/saline for 1 hr; (d) swine antirabbit IgG (Fc fragment) serum (1:40) (Nordic) for 2 hr; (e) washed in Tris/saline for 1 hr; (f) peroxidase antiperoxidase (PAP) (1:200) for 2 hr; (g) washed in Tris/saline for 4 hr; (h) 0.5 mg/ml 3,3-diaminobenzidine (DAB) (Sigma) 0.01% H_2O_2 (Merck) in Tris/saline for 3 to 8 min, (i) washed in Tris/saline for 30 min; (j) 2% OsO_4 in Tris/saline for 30 min; (k) washed in Tris/saline for 60 min; (l) dehydrated in graded ethanol series; and (m) flat embedded in Epon 812.

Ultrathin sections were cut with a diamond knife, examined in Philips EM 200 electron microscope both with and without staining in uranyl acetate and lead citrate. Specificity controls used were (a) replacement of the first antiserum by normal rabbit serum; (b) vasopressin antiserum and oxytocin antiserum were adsorbed to, respectively, vasopressin- and oxytocin-containing agarose beads; (c) Ho-DI rat brain sections of the lateral septum as a control for the specificity of the vasopressin antiserum; and (d) SCN sections for the specificity of the oxytocin antiserum.

RESULTS AND DISCUSSION

In the lateral septum, lateral habenular nucleus, and medial nucleus of the amygdala, vasopressin synapses could frequently be demonstrated. In addition, oxytocin-containing synapses were also observed in the medial nucleus of the amygdala. The majority of the terminations were seen on dendrites (Fig. 1), although some synapses were found on cell bodies. In the lateral septum and lateral habenular nucleus, structures were sometimes seen resembling synapses "en passage" (Fig. 2). The demonstration of these peptidergic profiles in the limbic system makes it plausible that the described exohypothalamic vasopressin and oxytocin pathways (3) are the morphological basis for the reported effects of these neuropeptides on avoidance behavior (1). For an understanding of this peptide–neuron interaction it is important to know what transmitter is present in the structures these synapses are terminating upon. That vasopressin does influence neurotransmitter metabolism is demonstrated in studies in which local injected vasopressin influenced turnover of monoamines. These neurotransmitters, however, are not present in the neurons of the limbic system.

Table 1 summarizes the basal vasopressin and oxytocin concentration in samples from 25 distinct regions of the rat brain. The neurohypophyseal hormone-synthesizing nuclei of the hypothalamus were found to contain the highest concentration of hormone. Relatively high concentrations were also observed in the septum, lateral habenula, and nucleus tractus solitarius. Low concentrations were found in the cortex, cerebellum, and hippocampus. Generally, vasopressin

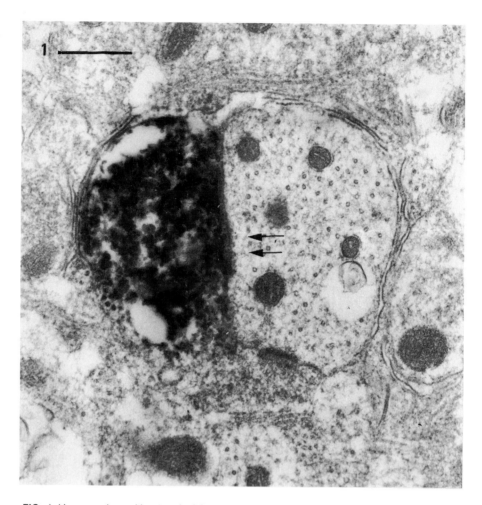

FIG. 1. Vasopressin positive terminal forms a synapse *(double arrow)* with a dendrite in the lateral habenular nucleus. Contrasted with uranyl acetate and lead citrate. Bar = 1 μm.

concentrations were higher than the oxytocin concentrations with exception of nuclei from the medulla oblongata, where the oxytocin concentrations exceeded those of vasopressin. Both hormones were also measured in samples from 11 brain regions of rats that had been submitted to training for passive avoidance behavior (Table 1). In no case were the vasopressin and oxytocin levels significantly different from those found in the corresponding regions of control brains (Student's t-test: $p > 0.05$). The median latency to enter of the trained group was 14 sec.

A previous study (4) had already shown that vasopressin and oxytocin may be determined in relatively large brain samples. However, in the present experi-

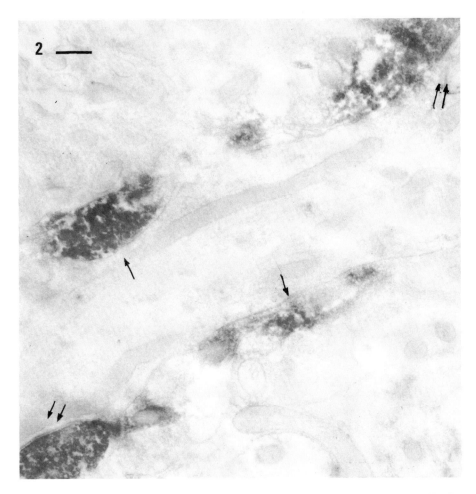

FIG. 2. Vasopressin positive fiber *(arrow)* forms synapses *(double arrow)* with a dendrite in the lateral septum. Bar = 2 μm.

ment the use of individually punched-out brain nuclei enabled a more specific quantitative localization of the hormones to be achieved. Using this technique, it was possible to select for study, regions which our extensive immunocytochemical observations have shown to be rich in peptidergic fibers (3). The observation that the concentrations of vasopressin and oxytocin in the present study were generally higher than those previously reported may be accounted for by this much more precise localization of the punched samples. In addition, the improvement in the RIA technique enabled us to demonstrate the presence of oxytocin in the choroid plexus, amygdala, hippocampus, and cortex and of both hormones in the cerebellum.

TABLE 1. *Vasopressin and oxytocin content of brain regions of control and trained rats*

	N	Control values			Values 5 min after the learning trial		
		Sample wt (μg)	Vasopressin (pg/mg dry wt)	Oxytocin	Sample wt (μg)	Vasopressin (pg/mg dry wt)	Oxytocin
Plexus choroideus	6	163 ± 34	228 ± 76	181 ± 40	nd	nd	nd
Bulbus olfactorius	6	538 ± 39	43 ± 9	nd	nd	nd	nd
Nucleus caudatus	5	3,028 ± 678	und	und	nd	nd	nd
Septum lateralis/dorsalis	5	318 ± 32	396 ± 92	49 ± 10	353 ± 35	465 ± 73	74 ± 20
Septum medialis/fimbrialis/triangularis	5	107 ± 11	554 ± 131	161 ± 61	115 ± 12	1,100 ± 340	313 ± 134
Organus vasculosum laminae terminalis	6	23 ± 3	2,770 ± 1,100	2,100 ± 600	nd	nd	nd
Organum subfornicale	5	18 ± 6	1,600 ± 460	nd	nd	nd	nd
Nucleus suprachimaticus	5	59 ± 13	157,000 ± 66,000	und	nd	nd	nd
Nucleus supraopticus	6	271 ± 45	520,000 ± 208,000	6,800 ± 2,100	nd	nd	nd
Cortex singularis	5	537 ± 62	102 ± 12	130 ± 64	364 ± 70	238 ± 159	62 ± 17
Cortex frontalis	5	480 ± 63	326 ± 135	25 ± 3	456 ± 49	157 ± 57	138 ± 79
Nucleus paraventricularis	5	487 ± 101	198,000 ± 60,000	4,100 ± 950	nd	nd	nd
Area amygdaloidea	6	312 ± 72	187 ± 65	nd	nd	nd	nd
Nucleus amygdaloideus	5	448 ± 40	164 ± 18	79 ± 46	367 ± 67	326 ± 91	155 ± 72
Hippocampus dorsalis	5	564 ± 207	121 ± 37	62 ± 25	286 ± 27	388 ± 98	58 ± 22
Hippocampus lateralis/ventralis	5	743 ± 92	67 ± 19	44 ± 35	685 ± 147	195 ± 64	56 ± 19
Habenula lateralis	5	115 ± 7	892 ± 146	97 ± 43	130 ± 11	1,350 ± 180	278 ± 107
Nucleus parafascicularis	6	143 ± 23	110 ± 31	159 ± 72	nd	nd	nd
Substantia grisea centralis	6	336 ± 137	337 ± 86	158 ± 24	nd	nd	nd
Substantia nigra	5	179 ± 12	206 ± 113	179 ± 51	191 ± 32	327 ± 184	268 ± 115
Organum subcommissurale	5	8 ± 1	und	nd	nd	nd	nd
Nucleus tractus solitarius	5	191 ± 20	388 ± 104	984 ± 185	157 ± 44	444 ± 151	884 ± 118
Nucleus ambiguus	6	358 ± 47	37 ± 12	197 ± 46	nd	nd	nd
Area postrema	5	33 ± 7	490 ± 225	nd	nd	nd	nd
Cerebellum	6	401 ± 76	217 ± 101	23 ± 16	521 ± 163	323 ± 130	24 ± 9

Values are given as mean ± SEM. *N*, number of samples; nd, not determined; und, undetectable.

The experiment also confirmed the previous finding that vasopressin concentrations were generally higher than oxytocin concentrations in brain tissue, while in the medulla oblongata the reverse was found. If it is assumed that the protein content of the dried brain samples is approximately 50% of the total dry weight, it can be calculated that the hormone concentrations in the supraoptic and paraventricular nuclei appeared approximately 4 times lower than the values reported by George and Forest (5) in Long Evans rat. The vasopressin concentration in the suprachiasmatic nucleus is similar in both studies. Differences in the exact part of the nuclei that were dissected, RIA procedures, and species might explain the discrepancies. The vasopressin level in the subfornical organ in our study is approximately 10 times higher than the level reported by Summy-Long et al. (12), which can be explained by differences in the dissected areas. The latter study used samples that contained the subfornical organ and some adjacent tissue, which will result in lower concentrations on weight basis.

Although no differences in hormone concentrations were found when the animals were killed 5 min after the onset of the behavioral stimulus, it remains possible that a rapid release of hormone might occur in the brain upon such a stimulus. It could be that the behavioral stimulus is too mild to cause demonstrable central release of vasopressin. In cerebrospinal fluid and in plasma no vasopressin release was detected at 5 min after a similar behavioral stimulus (13), while a more severe stimulus, such as vagal stimulation, caused a simultaneous release of vasopressin into the cerebrospinal fluid and blood stream (7). It is also possible that the time lag between stimulus application and sacrifice of the animals is too short.

Finally it may be possible that the amount of hormone released is too small to produce a demonstrable change in the basal levels. Similar problems were encountered in studies on the release and breakdown of aminergic neurotransmitters in the brain during behavioral experiments. These problems were only solved by the use of inhibitors of synthesis (8). Unfortunately, compounds that act selectively on peptide synthesis in the brain are not available at present.

The demonstration of a wide-spread peptidergic fiber system including synaptic contacts, the quantification of these peptides in a variety of brain regions, together with the electrophysiological and behavioral effects of these hormones nevertheless support the concept that they play a physiological role as neurotransmitter in central nervous system processes.

ACKNOWLEDGMENTS

The Foundation for Medical Research FUNGO is acknowledged for financial support. Dick Swaab is acknowledged for his stimulating comments during the preparation of the manuscript. The authors are indebted to Hans van Oyen, Peter de Groot, Frank Snijdewint, and Sonja van der Zwan for skillful technical assistance.

REFERENCES

1. Bohus, B., Urban, I., Van Wimersma Greidanus, Tj. B., and de Wied, D., (1978): Opposite effects of oxytocin and vasopressin on avoidance behavior and hippocampal theta rhythm in the rat. *Neuropharmacology,* 17:239–247.
2. Brownstein, M. J. (1977): Biologically active peptides in mammalian central nervous system. In: *Peptides in Neurobiology,* edited by H. Gainer, pp. 145–170. Plenum, New York.
3. Buijs, R. M. (1978): Intra- and extrahypothalamic vasopressin and oxytocin pathways in the rat: Pathways to the limbic system, medulla oblongata and spinal cord. *Cell Tiss. Res.,* 192:423–435.
4. Dogterom, J., Snijdewint, F. G. M., and Buijs, R. M. (1978): The distribution of vasopressin and oxytocin in the rat brain. *Neurosci. Lett.,* 9:341–346.
5. George, J. M., and Forest, J. (1976): Vasopressin and oxytocin content of microdissected hypothalamic areas in rats with hereditary diabetes insipidus. *Neuroendocrinology,* 21:275–279.
6. Guillemin, R., (1978): Peptides in the brain: The new endocrinology of the neuron. *Science,* 202:390–402.
7. Heller, H., Hasan, S. A., and Saifi, A. Q. (1968): Antidiuretic activity in the cerebrospinal fluid. *J. Endocrinol.,* 41:273–280.
8. Kovács, G. L., Bohus, B., Versteeg, D. H. G., de Kloet, E. R., and de Wied, D. (1979): Effects of oxytocin and vasopressin on memory consolidation: Sites of action and catecholaminergic correlates after local microinjection into limbic-midbrain structures. *Brain Res.,* 175:303–314.
9. Legros, J. J., Gilot, P., Seron, X., Claessens, J., Adam, A., Moeglen, J. M., Audibert, A., and Berchier, B., (1978): Influence of vasopressin on learning and memory. *Lancet,* 1:41–42.
10. Lowry, O. H., and Passoneau, J. V. (1953): Some recent refinements of quantitative histochemical analysis. In: *Recent Advances in Quantitative Histo- and Cytochemistry,* edited by U. C. Dubach and U. Schmidt, pp. 63–84. Hans Huber, Berlin.
11. Palkovits, M., (1973): Isolated removal of hypothalamic or other brain nuclei of the rat. *Brain Res.,* 59:449–450.
12. Summy-Long, J. Y., Keil, L. C., and Severs, W. B. (1978): Identification of vasopressin in the subfornical organ region: Effects of dehydration. *Brain Res.,* 140:241–250.
13. Van Wimersma Greidanus, Tj. B., Croiset, G., Goedemans, H., and Dogterom, J. (1979): Vasopressin levels in peripheral blood and in cerebrospinal fluid during passive and active avoidance behavior in rats. *Horm. Behav.,* 12:103–111.
14. Van Wimersma Greidanus, Tj. B., and de Wied, D. (1975): CNS sites of action of ACTH, MSH and vasopressin in relation to avoidance behavior. In: *Anatomical Neuroendocrinology,* edited by W. E. Stumpf and L. D. Grant, pp. 284–289. Karger, Basel.
15. Van Wimersma Greidanus, Tj. B., and de Wied, D., (1977): The physiology of the neurohypophysial system and its relation to memory processes. In: *Biochemical Correlates of Brain Function,* edited by A. N. Davison, pp. 198–247. Academic, New York.
16. Vincent, J. D., and Arnauld, E. (1975): Vasopressin as a neurotransmitter in the central nervous system, some evidence from the supraoptic neurosecretory system. In: *Progress in Brain Research, Vol. 42: Hormones, Homeostasis and the Brain,* edited by W. H. Gispen, Tj. B. van Wimersma Greidanus, B. Bohus, and D. de Wied, pp. 57–66. Elsevier, Amsterdam.

Neuropeptides and Neural Transmission,
edited by C. Ajmone Marsan and W. Z. Traczyk.
Raven Press, New York © 1980.

Distribution of Immunoreactive Neurohypophyseal Peptides in the Rat Brain. Differential Response of Hypothalamic Nuclei Synthesizing Vasopressin Under Various Experimental Conditions

A. Burlet, M. Chateau, and F. Dreyfuss

Laboratoires d'Histologie et de Physiologie, Faculté de Médecine, BP184, 54500 Vandoeuvre, France

The hypothalamo-neurohypophyseal system (HNHS) of mammals has certainly been the system studied with the greatest variety of methods giving results that can be integrated into coherent interpretations. This system is composed of magnocellular neurosecretory neurons of which the most numerous axons reach the neurohypophysis. Two hormones at least are synthesized into perikaryons, transported within axons, and released from neurohaemal junctions of the neurohypophysis: vasopressin (VP) and oxytocin (OXY). Each hormone is associated *in vivo* with a carrier protein, a neurophysin (39). From the morphological point of view, numerous investigations have described the distribution of magnocellular neurosecretory neurons using classic techniques, staining hormones, and neurophysins under a similar aspect (3,17,21). Magnocellular neurons occur in different hypothalamic nuclei, the best-known being paraventricular and supraoptic nuclei. But in the rat, they also constitute the small intermediate groups named diffuse, fornical, commissural, and circular by Peterson (41).

In 1973, the application of the immunofluorescence method enabled us to affirm the presence of VP at the level of most of these hypothalamic nuclei and groups (12). In addition to the classic neurohypophyseal fibres, two regions showed pericapillary endings: the primary portal circulation of the external zone of the median eminence and the organum vasculosum of the lamina terminalis. Numerous immunological observations have confirmed these first results and extensive reports have described this "new cartography" of the hypothalamic neurohypophyseal centers (10,18,46,48,51,54).

From the physiological point of view, the multiplicity of the diencephalic locations of VP have suggested several hypotheses:

The main physiological function of VP in the adult mammal is a water-conserving function. All these groups or nuclei synthesizing VP are involved simultaneously or successively and progressively to assume the effectiveness of regulative mechanism of the hydro-osmotic function.

In addition to its antidiuretic activity, VP exercises other functions: it delays the extinction of active avoidance behavior and improves passive avoidance behavior (7,52); it is involved in the corticotropic function of adenohypophysis (14,24,53), although it is not the corticotropin-releasing hormone (32). Each group or nucleus can play a role in each particular function of VP.

These hypotheses integrate groups and nuclei synthesizing VP into hypo-thalamic circuits of regulation which are likely to be different. But Knaggs et al. (31) suggested that "accessory neurosecretory cell nuclei probably represent intermediate stages in the phylogenetic derivation of the paraventricular and supraoptic nuclei from the preoptic nucleus, and as such may well be functionally connected with the two main nuclei." Therefore, we verified the stereotaxic stability of these different stores of VP; then the variations of hormonal content at the level of magnocellular nuclei were measured during experimental conditions stimulating one or other of the VP functions. For this purpose, we used two methods: radioimmunoassay (RIA) of hormones in micro-dissected nuclei (33,40) and immunocytological localizations of hormones and neurophysins I and II (8,10).

STEREOTAXIC LOCALIZATIONS OF NEUROSECRETORY NEURONS

Stereotaxic marks were placed in the brains of anaesthetized rats (Wistar, 200–250 g) to determine several planes of reference (1). The cerebral tissues were fixed in the skull and cut in a cryostat following the stereotaxic axis. An immunoenzymatic technique was performed on serial frontal and sagittal sections.

Magnocellular Neurons

Two neuronal populations were present throughout the rat hypothalamus: the first synthesizing VP and stained by antibovine-neurophysin II (NII) antibodies; the second manufacturing OXY and stained by antibovine-neurophysin I (NI) antibodies (8). Diagrams regrouping data obtained on several serial sections summarize our observations (Figs. 1 and 2).

In the most anterior part of the hypothalamus, isolated OXY/NI neurons were numerous whereas isolated VP/NII neurons were relatively rare. These isolated neurons were scattered in the preoptica medialis and lateralis areas. A small dorsal group, the commissural nucleus of Peterson (41) was constituted by OXY/NI neurons only (Figs. 1A and 2C). At the level of the supraoptic crest, the most frequent neurons synthesized OXY and NI (Fig. 2C).

In the medial and posterior part of the supraoptic nuclei, VP/NII neurons had a ventral position and OXY/NI neurons a dorsal position. The retrochias-matic part of supraoptic nuclei was made up of numerous VP/NII neurons

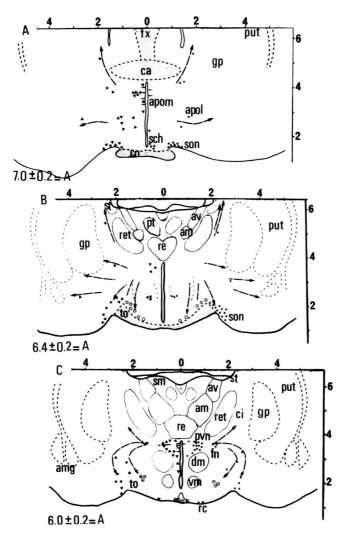

FIG. 1. Stereotaxic distribution of VP/N II *(stars)* and OXY/N I *(triangles)* neurons in frontal sections of rat brain: diagrams group observations obtained from serial sections situated on both sides of the drawn section. ahl, area hypothalamica lateralis; ahp, area hypothalamica posterior; am, nucleus anterior medialis thalami; amg, amygdala; an, nucleus arcuatus; apoa, area preoptica anterior; apol, area preoptica lateralis; apom, area preoptica medialis; av, nucleus anterior ventralis thalami; ca, commissura hippocampi; ci, capsula interna; cm, corpus mamilare; co, chiasma opticum; dbb, gyrus diagonalis; dm, nucleus dorsomedialis hypothalami; fld, fasciculus longitudinalis dorsalis; fn, fornicalis nucleus; fx, fornix; gp, globus pallidus; me, median eminence; pt, nucleus parateanialis; put, putamen; pvn, paraventricularis nucleus; rc, retrochiasmaticus supraopticus nucleus; re, nucleus reuniens; ret, nucleus reticularis thalami; sch, suprachiasmaticus nucleus; sm, stria medullaris; son, supraopticus nucleus; st, stria terminalis; thp, tractus habenulo interpedoncularis; tmt, tractus mamillo-thalamicus; to, tractus opticus; v, ventricle; vm, nucleus ventromedialis hypothalami; zi, zona incerta. *Dotted lines,* fibres carrying OXY or VP; *circles,* transversal sections of fibres; *arrows,* endings; *double arrows,* neurohaemal endings.

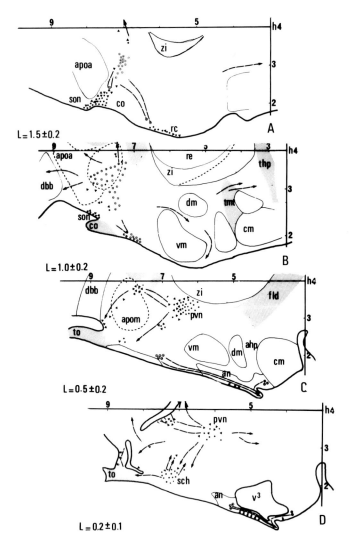

FIG. 2. Stereotaxic distribution of VP/N II *(stars)* and OXY/N I *(triangles)* neurons in sagittal sections of rat brain: diagrams group observations obtained from serial sections situated on both sides of the drawn section. See symbols and abbreviations from Fig. 1 legend.

and only few OXY/NI neurons (Figs. 1C and 2A). Circular nuclei including both neuronal populations had constant stereotaxic references; their anteroposterior extent was 200 μm. Neurons stained along the third ventricle synthesized OXY and NI.

In paraventricular nuclei, (Fig. 1C) VP/NII neurons were surrounded by OXY/NI neurons. Fornical nuclei included both types of neurons. Isolated magnocellular neurons were always numerous between the most anterior planes of supraoptic nuclei and the most posterior planes of the paraventricular nuclei.

Parvocellular Neurons

The most recent localizations of the neurohypophyseal hormones in the rat hypothalamus have shown the existence of a VP-like peptide in some of the suprachiasmatic neurons. Immunocytochemical results (11,50) were in agreement with radioimmunoassays (10,23). These parvocellular neurons also synthesized NII but not OXY or NI. Brattleboro rats genetically devoid of VP and NII at the level of the magnocellular system were also devoid of VP-like/NII suprachiasmatic synthesis. Several anti-VP antibodies, which did not bind OXY, were employed to detect the suprachiasmatic peptide. The first showed a cross-reactivity with lysine-VP but did not react with either arginine-VP or with arginine-vasotocin (serum N; ref. 14). This serum did not give immunostaining in the rat hypothalamus. The second (Fig. 3) showed the same affinity for arginine- and lysine-VP and for arginine-vasotocin. With this antiserum, magnocellular neurons and pathways were stained. In suprachiasmatic nuclei two types of immunostainings were observed: the perikaryons of neurons of internal and dorsal part of nuclei gave a positive reaction and positive varicosities appeared around the perikaryons of negative neurons (Fig. 4). The third antibody specifically bound arginine-VP but did not react with either lysine-VP or arginine-vasotocin. This serum stained the magnocellular neurons of the neurohypophyseal system and the varicosities surrounding the perikaryons of negative suprachiasmatic neurons. Suprachiasmatic neurons stained with anti-NII antibodies were not revealed by this antiarginine-VP antibody. In a preliminary study, it was verified that the acid extract prepared from suprachiasmatic nuclei of Wistar

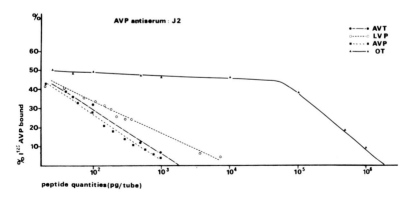

FIG. 3. Comparison of the cross-reaction of lysine-VP (LVP), vasotocin (AVT) and oxytocin (OXY), on the binding of ^{125}I-arginine-VP (AVP) to rabbit anti-AVP anti-serum. Increasing amounts of different peptides are added to the incubation medium (0.5 ml) containing constant amount of antibody (final dilution: 1: 100,000) and ^{125}I-AVP (8,000 to 10,000 cpm).

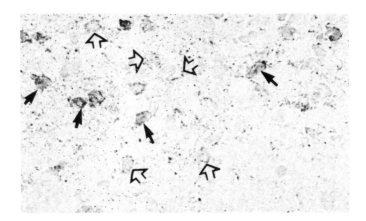

FIG. 4. Suprachiasmatic stainings obtained with the previous (Fig. 3) anti-AVP antiserum: peri-karyons of neurons *(filled arrows)* are stained as well as varicosities *(open arrows)* surrounding the negative neurons. ×270.

rats had antidiuretic activity (method of Jeffers et al., ref. 26, modified by Gharib, ref. 22), whereas no biological activity was found in the suprachiasmatic neurons of Brattleboro rats.

These biological and immunological properties of suprachiasmatic peptide have led us to consider the possibility that we had brought out the presence of arginine-VP in magnocellular neurons and arginine-vasotocin in parvocellular suprachiasmatic neurons.

Neurosecretory Pathways

Throughout the hypothalamus of rat, fibres carrying VP and NII and fibres carrying OXY and NI were always mixed: "pure" VP/NII or OXY/NI tracts did not exist. However, the relative number of each type of fibre could change in some regions. For example, the fibres arising from paraventricular and com-missural nuclei leading to the preoptic anterior area (Figs. 2C and D) were most frequently OXY/NI fibres. There were also numerous OXY/NI fibres below the ependymal cells and intruding into the third ventricle in the dorsal and anterior region of the hypothalamus (Fig. 5).

In order to verify some efferences of studied nuclei, partial deafferentations of the anterior hypothalamus were realized with Halazs' knife (extended anterior cut, from ref. 25). This frontal cut isolated the suprachiasmatic nuclei from their connections with medial and posterior hypothalamus. In these conditions, fibres carrying VP/NII and OXY/NI were numerous on the ventral part of the tractus opticus; they originated from paraventricular and supraoptic nuclei. It is possible that some of suprachiasmatic efferences also followed optic fibres, but the most numerous were found in the periventricular regions of the anterior hypothalamus. Extended anterior cut heavily loaded the organum vasculosum

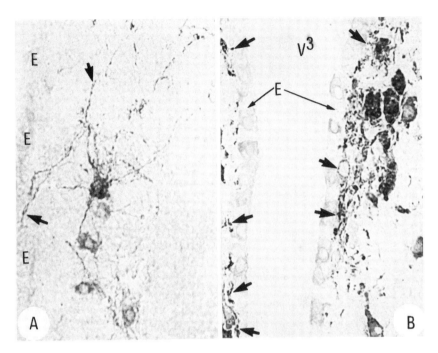

FIG. 5. Periventricular magnocellular neurons stained with anti-N I antiserum. Tangential **(A)** and frontal **(B)** sections of the third ventricle (V³) showing numerous fibres below and between ependymal cells (E). A, ×300; B, ×520.

of the lamina terminalis of VP and NII fibres and of a certain number of OXY/NI fibres. Both types of fibres terminated either around capillaries or between ependymal cells of the posterior wall of the organum vasculosum of the lamina terminalis (Fig. 2D).

In the intact rat, the main part of the supraoptic and paraventricular tracts reached the median eminence by an anteinfundibular pathway, whereas the retroinfundibular fibres were relatively rare (Fig. 2B). In the median eminence, the fibres were separated into two groups: an internal group—the hypothalamo-neurohypophyseal tract—carrying VP/NII and OXY/NI, and an external group terminating around the capillaries of the primary portal circulation—the VP/NII hypothalamo-infundibular tract (8). Only a few external fibres were stained with anti-NI or anti-OXY antibodies.

Extrahypothalamic pathways originated in the anterior and median areas of the hypothalamus (Fig. 1A and B). They carried VP and NII or OXY and NI; they were always associated with magnocellular neurons. As for intrahypothalamic tracts, there were no "pure" VP or OXY extrahypothalamic tracts. Most frequently, they did not compose true "tracts" but were scattered to the amygdalian and posterior areas. Only two symmetrical extrahypothalamic tracts could be described: the anterior and dorsal fibres appearing between the globus pallidus and the nucleus reticularis thalami (Fig. 1C). It was very difficult to specify which neurons gave rise to these extrahypothalamic fibres. Morphological criteria were not adequate: using such morphological criteria, the VP/NII infundibular tract was described as arising from suprachiasmatic nuclei (47) and the same authors proved the inaccuracy of their observations some months later (49).

HYPOTHALAMIC VP AND OSMOTIC STIMULATION

Among the hypotheses presented at the beginning of this text, the differential responses of paraventricular and supraoptic nuclei were studied during a stimulation of hydroosmotic function of VP induced by water deprivation. Morphological analysis suggested the involvement of both magnocellular nuclei (28–30,45); however, since the neurohypophysis releases VP and OXY simultaneously during such an experiment (27), the most classic explanation attributed variations in paraventricular nuclei to OXY release and variations in supraoptic nuclei to VP release. It was obvious that dehydration stimulated synthesis and release of hormones and neurophysins (38).

Table 1 showed that plasma VP increased during the first 5 days of dehydration whereas neurohypophyseal hormone decreased. After 1 week of experimentation, the neurohypophyseal vasopressin represented 5% of the initial content. At the supraoptic level, the variations were slight: VP content decreased at first, then statistically increased from the fifth day of stimulation. The changes revealed in paraventricular nuclei were the opposite: VP content continuously decreased. Immunocytochemical results corroborated the RIA only for certain aspects. At the level of paraventricular nuclei, the decrease in immunostaining was obvious but the increase at the supraoptic level was not evident. Ventral fibres were heavily loaded but the immunological charge of perikaryon was often low (13). Immunocytochemical staining of isolated neurons and intermediate groups was very stable.

To appreciate the hypothalamo-neurohypophyseal response to the restoration of a normal hydric balance, drinking water was given to another group of dehydrated rats. Twenty-four hours of rehydration counterbalanced the variations in hypothalamic hormones at the level of supraoptic and paraventricular nuclei. The changes in the neurohypophyseal content of VP and OXY are given in Table 2. Four days of dehydration depleted VP and OXY in the neurohypophysis but it was the VP decrease that was the highest. One day of rehydration did not stop OXY release but the restoration of the VP store was very rapid. In these experimental conditions, immunoultrastructural detections demonstrated that VP was stained in dilated fibres within several types of cellular elements: small scattered granules and tubular formations, anastomosing canalicules interconnected with small cisternae (Fig. 6). These formations had the size and the spatial organization of the cisternae of the smooth endoplasmic reticulum

TABLE 1. *Arginine-VP content in the hypothalamo-hypophyseal system during long-term water deprivation*

Hormonal localizations	Control rats N = 8	Dehydrated rats (1 day) N = 6	Dehydrated rats (3 days) N = 6	Dehydrated rats (5 days) N = 8	Dehydrated rats (7 days) N = 6	Dehydrated rats (10 days) N = 8
			Experimental conditions			
SON (pmoles)	62.8 ± 3.5[a1]	55.8 ± 5.3[a2]	71.7 ± 8.8	78.9 ± 4.3[a1.2]	71.6 ± 9.3	80.7 ± 6.4[a1.2]
PVN (pmoles)	35.6 ± 2.2[a,b]	31.7 ± 5.9	26.6 ± 2.2	25.6 ± 2.7[b]	32.4 ± 6.0	14.6 ± 1.9[a]
ME (pmoles)	37.3 ± 3.1	41.4 ± 4.1	25.8 ± 4.5	23.8 ± 4.1	19.6 ± 2.4	24.5 ± 2.2
Neurohypophysis (pmoles)	3990 ± 201	3679 ± 478[a]	1166 ± 283[a]	369 ± 64[a]	188 ± 37[a]	172 ± 27[a]
PAH (μU/ml)	≤7	11 ± 0.8[a]	20 ± 2.3[a]	≤7	≤7	≤7

[a] $p < 0.001$.
[b] $p < 0.05$.
Mean ± SEM; comparison with multiple *t*-test; SON, supraoptic nuclei; PVN, paraventricular nuclei; ME, median eminence; PAH, plasmatic antidiuretic hormone.

TABLE 2. *VP and OXY concentration in rat neurohypophysis during rehydration following water deprivation*

Neurohormones	Experimental conditions[a,b]		
	Control rats $N=7$	Dehydrated rats (4 days) $N=7$	Rehydrated rats 24 hr $N=7$
VP	7218 ± 879[c]	1630 ± 263[c,d]	3239 ± 279[c,d]
(% control content)	100%	22.6%	44.8%
OXY	2648 ± 238[c]	1762 ± 165[c]	1452 ± 165[c]
(% control content)	100%	62.6%	54.7%

[a] Concentration given in pmoles/mg dry weight.
[b] Mean $\pm$ SEM; comparison of means with multiple t-test.
[c] Statistical difference between control rats and dehydrated or rehydrated rats; $p \leq 0.01$.
[d] Statistical difference between dehydrated and rehydrated rats; $p \leq 0.02$.
VP, vasopressin; OXY, oxytocin.

(20). During the same period, OXY was confined to small scattered granules of dilated fibres (Fig. 6C and D).

These observations suggested that during the first hours of rehydration, VP was rapidly transported from the perikaryon to the axon terminal of the neurosecretory cell within cisternae of the smooth endoplasmic reticulum.

The origin of these fibres (paraventricular or supraoptic nuclei) remains to be investigated. It appeared that during chronic stimulation of the hydroosmotic function, the paraventricular nuclei pool of VP was more rapidly releasable than the supraoptic nuclei pool of VP. Nevertheless, it could be emphasized that water deprivation was both an osmotic stimulation and a stress. Paraventricular VP was perhaps involved in the second aspect of the experiment, that is, the stress.

HYPOTHALAMIC VP AND CORTICOTROPIC FUNCTION

In normal corticotropic function, VP would be released from infundibular endings into primary portal circulation of adenohypophysis (14,55). Some data suggested that infundibular endings originated in paraventricular neurons (2,49).

Adrenalectomy stimulated the synthesis and release of adenohypophyseal adre-

FIG. 6. Neurohypophysis of the rat after 24 hr of rehydration. **a–c:** Incubations with anti-AVP antibodies. **a:** some fibres have a normal content in neurosecretory granules (NSG). Others are dilated *(stars)* and contain small scattered NSG. Negative fibres *(triangles)*, pituicyte (P). ×7,200. **b and c:** Abundant network of tubular elements in the axoplasm of some depleted nervous fibres; note immunoreactive formations *(arrows)*. Connections frequently exist between some granules and tubules. **b,** ×30,000; c, ×60,000. **c and d:** Incubations with the anti-OXY antibodies. **d:** Depleted fibres *(stars)*, negative fibres *(triangles)*. ×7,200. **e:** The axoplasm of dilated fibres presents a low density; immunoreaction is confined to the small scattered granules. ×60,000.

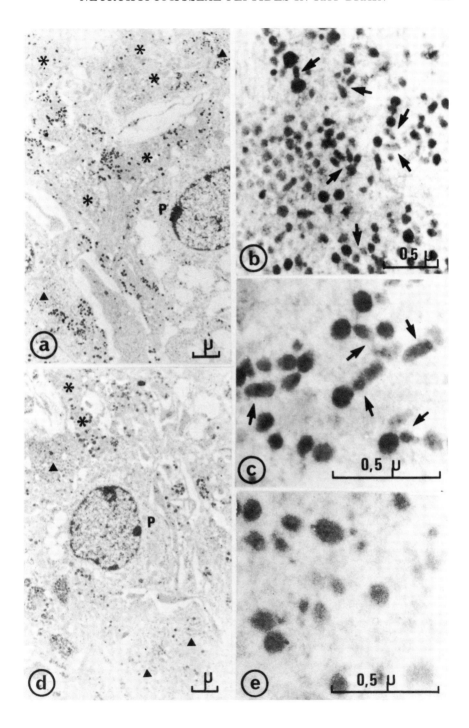

TABLE 3. *Arginine-VP content (pmoles) in the hypothalamo-hypophyseal system after adrenalectomy: Effect of hormonal therapy with dexamethasone*

	Region[a]			
Experimental conditions	SON	PVN	ME	Neurohypophysis (pmoles/mg dry wt)
Sham-operated rats	83.3 ± 11.3	47.8 ± 7.2[b]	13.8 ± 1.9[c]	6146 ± 423[d]
Rats: 15 days from adrenalectomy	73.8 ± 11.4	26.7 ± 3.8[b]	23.6 ± 2[c]	8373 ± 748[d]
Rats: 15 days from adrenalectomy, injected for 8 days with dexamethasone	85.6 ± 11.1	47.5 ± 9.3	20.7 ± 1.6[c]	6804 ± 512

[a] SON, supraoptic nuclei; PVN, paraventricular nuclei; ME, median eminence; NH, neurohypophysis. Values are means ± SEM; comparison with multiple t-test.
[b] Statistical difference between sham-operated rats and adrenalectomized rats; $p < 0.01$.
[c] Statistical difference between sham-operated rats and adrenalectomized rats with or without hormone therapy; $p < 0.01$.
[d] Statistical difference between sham-operated rats and adrenalectomized rats; $p < 0.02$.

nocorticotropic hormone (ACTH). Some arguments have suggested that synthesis of VP was also increased (34). Table 3 shows that 2 weeks after operation VP changes at the supraoptic level were not significant, whereas the VP content of paraventricular nuclei significantly decreased. Glucocorticoid therapy, consisting of twice daily injections of dexamethasone, restored the normal store of VP in paraventricular nuclei. Adrenalectomy also heavily loaded the median eminence of VP. Immunocytochemical stainings showed that VP had accumulated within pericapillary endings. At the same time, the passage of VP to the adenohypophysis, likely through the portal vessels, had increased (14). These two phenomena—eminential and adenohypophyseal—were abolished in operated rats treated by dexamethasone (8,14).

During the postnatal development of the rat, ACTH synthesis was stimulated (4,6,15). At the level of the median eminence, the immunohistological distribution of VP was similar to that described in the adrenalectomized rat: numerous endings terminating around portal capillaries were heavily loaded with VP and NII (9).

These observations suggested the involvement of VP in the corticotropic activity under certain experimental conditions and also during chronic physiological stimulations. They also brought evidence in favor of exclusive participation of paraventricular store of VP. In fact, as for dehydration, there were two possible explanations:

1. Under all situations requiring the release of VP, the paraventricular stock was more readily available than the supraoptic stock;

2. These important changes of paraventricular VP proved the rapid transport of the hormone from the perikaryon to the infundibular endings of the median eminence.

These two possibilities were examined under a third experimental situation, the total hypophysectomy.

HYPOTHALAMIC VP AND TOTAL HYPOPHYSECTOMY

Hypophysectomy induced a retrograde degeneration of many of nerve cells in magnocellular hypothalamic nuclei, but the number of surviving neurons was different for each nucleus. The chromatolytic changes affected 75 to 80% of supraoptic neurons and only 50% of paraventricular neurons (5,36,37,43,44). The number of intact cells appeared to remain constant over a long postoperative period. Daniel and Pritchard (16) proved that the differential extent of the cell loss in both paraventricular and supraoptic nuclei was related to the level of the transection in the stalk: the higher the level, the greater the loss. Therefore, it would appear that two types of neurosecretory magnocellular neurons exist in the hypothalamus: neurons with "long" axons terminating in the neurohypophysis, and neurons with "short" axons terminating in the stalk or in the median eminence.

On the other hand, the same operation increased the synthesis of hypothalamic corticotropic-releasing hormone (32) and the adrenal function of posterior-hypophysectomized rats has a normal regulation (35). Under these conditions it would be supposed that VP synthesized in surviving neurons whose axons terminated in the median eminence assumed the adrenocorticotropic function of operated rats. The hypophysectomy appeared to be a suitable situation for testing the hypotheses expressed at the end of the previous section.

In order to test the release of VP from the cut stalk of operated rats, all animals used for RIA were anaesthetized by chloroform vapors for 3 min. Antidiuretic activity of heparinized plasma was measured (22,26): it was always lower than 7 μUI/ml in operated rats for 1 to 21 days.

The evolution of hypothalamic VP is given in Table 4. During the first week after ablation the VP content of supraoptic and paraventricular nuclei continuously increased. Immunocytological staining in the perikaryon of neurons was very marked. Even in the absence of axon-terminal specializations of the neurohypophysis, there was a continued synthesis of the hormone. In the median eminence, the heavy loading which appeared during the same period was induced by simultaneous phenomena:

Intact neurons continued to synthesize hormones and neurophysins which were carried to the axon-terminals of the hypothalamo-neurohypophyseal system. There was a distal accumulation which preceded the massive capillary hypertrophy and the organization of a newly formed neurohypophysis (19,42). By immunocytology, VP, OXY, NI, and NII were revealed in this young neurohypophysis.

On the other hand, in the cephalic part of the median eminence, hypophysectomy induced the overloading of the pericapillary endings of VP and NII. This particular distribution was never seen with anti-OXY or anti-NI antibodies (Fig. 7).

TABLE 4. *Variations in the arginine-VP content in the hypothalamus after hypophysectomy*[a]

Hypothalamic nuclei (pmoles)	Control rats $N=8$	Experimental conditions[a]				
		Rats 1 day from operation $N=6$	Rats 3 days from operation $N=6$	Rats 7 days from operation $N=14$	Rats 14 days from operation $N=10$	Rats 21 days from operation $N=6$
SON	62.8 ± 3.9	98.4 ± 6.9[b]	116.1 ± 14.4[b]	87.9 ± 11.7[b]	21.9 ± 4.2[b]	33.5 ± 8.5[b]
PVN	35.6 ± 2.3	89.4 ± 16.6[b]	71.7 ± 11.2[b]	51.1 ± 6.6	15.4 ± 1.0	13.2 ± 2.9[b]
ME	37.3 ± 3.1	147.7 ± 13.6[b]	243.0 ± 31.5[b]	127.8 ± 26[b]	43.7 ± 5.9	35.9 ± 9.7

[a] Mean $\pm$ SEM; comparison of means with multiple t-test. Statistical difference between control rats and operated rats at various stages from hypophysectomy.
[b] $p < 0.001$.

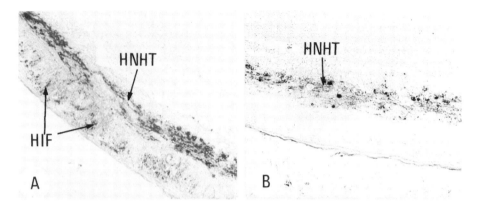

FIG. 7. Localization of VP **(A)** and OXY **(B)** in the rostral median eminence of an hypophysecto-mized rat killed 10 days after operation; VP only overloads the pericapillary endings. HNHT, hypothalamo-neurohypophyseal tract; HIF, hypothalamo-infundibular fibres. ×110.

Two weeks from operation, the distal accumulation of hormones and neuro-physins was assumed by the retroinfundibular fibres of the hypothalamo-neuro-hypophyseal system. In the rostral and medial parts of the median eminence, fibres of the hypothalamo-neurohypophyseal system had almost totally disap-peared but the infundibular loading of VP still remained obvious. At this moment, there was a reduction of hypothalamic stores of VP. The changes between the initial and the final content were just as great in supraoptic (58%) and paraven-tricular nuclei (63%). There were intact neurons in both nuclei and this experi-mental situation did not give any arguments to prove that VP infundibular endings originated in the paraventricular nuclei.

Ultrastructural studies (19,42) described the vascular reorganization of the stalk during the 2 weeks following ablation of the hypophysis. The loading of pericapillary endings of VP could have a functional significance and assume a normal control of the adrenocorticotropic function in posterior-lobectomized rats.

In conclusion, the use of immunological techniques proved that neurohy-pophyseal hormones had a large distribution in the hypothalamus and also in the extrahypothalamic areas. In the rat, two magnocellular populations were identified: the first synthesizing VP and a peptide related to bovine-neurophysin II, and a second synthesizing OXY and a peptide related to bovine-neurophysin I. Parvocellular neurons of the suprachiasmatic nuclei would appear to synthesize vasotocin and a peptide related to bovine-neurophysin II.

The osmotic stimulations of VP synthesis involved both magnocellular para-ventricular and supraoptic nuclei, whereas it was paraventricular nuclei that were involved in the corticotropic stimulations. The functional significance of the VP neuron in paraventricular nuclei and in supraoptic nuclei was different.

ACKNOWLEDGMENTS

The authors thank Dr. Czernichow for generous gifts of antioxytocin and antineurophysins antisera, and Dr. Kordon and Mrs. Pattou for the hypothalamic deafferentation of rats.

REFERENCES

1. Albe-Fessard, D., Stutinsky, F., and Libouban, S. (1966): *Atlas stéréotaxique du diencéphale du rat blanc.* Editions du C.N.R.S., Paris.
2. Alonzo, G., Balmefrezol, M., and Assenmacher, I. (1978): Etude de l'innervation monoaminergique et peptidergique de l'éminence médiane du rat par une combinaison, sur le même hypothalamus, des techniques d'histofluorescence, d'immunocytochimie et de radioautographie. *C. R. Soc. Biol. (Paris)*, 172:138–168.
3. Arizono, H., and Okamoto, S. (1957): Comparative neurologic study on the hypothalamo-neurohypophysial neurosecretory system. *Med. J. Osaka Univ.*, 8:195–228.
4. Bartova, A. (1967): Activity of the hypothalamo-pituitary-adrenal axis during the early postnatal period in rats. *Endocrinol. Exp. (Prague)*, 1:79–89.
5. Beck, E., Daniel, P. M., and Pritchard, M. M. L. (1969): Regeneration of hypothalamic nerve fibres in the goat. *Neuroendocrinology*, 5:161–182.
6. Beraud, G. (1977): Evolution suivant l'âge et le sexe de l'ACTH des pars distalis et neurointermedia de l'hypophyse de rat. *C. R. Acad. Sci. (Paris)*, 284:377–380.
7. Bohus, B., Kovacs, G. L., and de Wied, D. (1978): Oxytocin, vasopressin and memory: Opposite effects on consolidation and retrieval process. *Brain Res.*, 157:414–417.
8. Burlet, A., Chateau, M., and Czernichow, P. (1979): Infundibular localization of vasopressin, oxytocin and neurophysins in the rat; Its relationships with corticotrope function. *Brain Res.*, 168:275–286.
9. Burlet, A., Chateau, M., and Czernichow, P. (1979): Immunocytochemical study of neurohypophysial peptides during corticotropic maturation in infant rats. *Cell Tiss. Res.* 201:315–325.
10. Burlet, A., Chateau, M., and Marchetti, J. (1975): Contribution of immunoenzymatic technique to the study of diencephalic localization of vasopressin. In: *Immunoenzymatic Techniques,* edited by G. Feldman, P. Druet, J. Bignon, and S. Avrameas, pp. 333–343. North-Holland, New York.
11. Burlet, A., and Marchetti, J. (1975): La vasopressine immunoréactive du noyau suprachiasmatique. Observations préliminaires chez le rat. *C. R. Soc. Biol. (Paris)*, 169:148–150.
12. Burlet, A., Marchetti, J., and Duheille, J. (1973): Etude par immunofluorescence de la répartition de la vasopressine au niveau du système hypothalamo-neurohypophysaire du rat. *C. R. Soc. Biol. (Paris)*, 167:924–927.
13. Burlet, A., Marchetti, J., and Duheille, J. (1974): Immunohistochemistry of vasopressin study of the hypothalamo-neurohypophysial system of normal, dehydrated and hypophysectomized rat. In: *Neurosecretion: The Final Neuroendocrine Pathway,* edited by F. Knowles and L. Vollrath, pp. 24–30. Springer Verlag, Berlin.
14. Chateau, M., Marchetti, J., Burlet, A., and Boulangé, M. (1979): Evidence of vasopressin in adenohypophysis: Research into its role in corticotrope activity. *Neuroendocrinology*, 28:25–35.
15. Chiappa, S. A., and Fink, G. (1977): Releasing factor and hormonal changes in the hypothalamic-pituitary-gonadotrophin and adrenocorticotrophin systems before and after birth and puberty in male, female and androgenized female rats. *J. Endocrinol.*, 72:211–224.
16. Daniel, P. M., and Pritchard, M. M. L. (1975): Studies of the hypothalamus and the pituitary gland with special reference to the effects of transection of the pituitary stalk. *Acta Endocrinol. (Kbh)*, 80 (Suppl. 201):1–216.
17. Dawson, A. B. (1966): Early secretory activity in the hypothalamic nuclei and neurohypophysis in the rat determined by selective staining. *J. Morphol.*, 118:549–564.
18. Defendini, R., and Zimmerman, E. A. (1978): The magnocellular neurosecretory system of the mammalian hypothalamus. In: *The Hypothalamus, Vol. 56,* edited by S. Reichlin, R. J. Baldessarini, and J. B. Martin, pp. 137–152. Raven Press, New York.

19. Delmann, H. D. (1973): Degeneration and regeneration of neurosecretory systems. *Int. Rev. Cytol.,* 36:215–315.
20. Dreyfuss, F., Burlet, A., Chateau, M., and Czernichow, P. (1979): Localisation ultrastructurale par immunocytochimie de la vasopressine non granulaire dans la neurohypophyse du rat: Rôle possible du réticulum endoplasmique lisse dans le transport de l'hormone. *Biol. Cell.,* 35:141–146.
21. Gabe, M. (1966): *Neurosecretion, Vol. 28,* edited by G. A. Kerputt, pp. 10–28. Pergamon, London.
22. Gharib, G. (1967): Le dosage de l'hormone antidiurétique. *Rev. Etud. Clin. Biol.,* 12:298–402.
23. George, J. M., and Jacobowitz, E. (1975): Localization of vasopressin in discrete areas of the hypothalamus. *Brain Res.,* 93:363–366.
24. Gonzalez-Luque, A., L'Age, M., Dhariwal, A. P. S., and Yates, F. E. (1970): Stimulation of corticotropin release by corticotropin releasing factor (CRF) or by vasopressin following intrapituitary infusions in unanesthetized dogs; inhibition of the response by dexamethasone. *Endocrinology,* 86:1134–1142.
25. Halasz, B., and Gorski, R. A. (1967): Gonadotrophic hormone secretion in female rats after partial or total interruption of neural afferents of the medial basal hypothalamus. *Endocrinology,* 80:608–622.
26. Jeffers, W. A., Livezey, M. M., and Austin, J. H. (1942): A method for demonstrating antidiuretic action of minute amounts of pitressin. Statistical analysis results. *Proc. Soc. Exp. Biol. Med.,* 50:184–188.
27. Jones, C. W., and Pikering, B. T. (1969): Comparison of water deprivation and sodium chloride inhibition on the hormone content of the neurohypophysis of the rat. *J. Physiol. (Lond.),* 203:449–458.
28. Kalimo, H. (1975): Ultrastructural studies on the hypothalamic neurosecretory neurons of the rat. III: Paraventricular and supraoptic neurons during lactation and dehydration. *Cell. Tiss. Res.,* 163:151–168.
29. Kekki, M., Attila, U., and Talanti, S. (1975): The kinetics of 35S-labelled cysteine in the hypothalamic-neurohypophysial neurosecretory system of the dehydrated rat. *Cell Tiss. Res.,* 158:439–450.
30. Klein, M. J., Porte, A., and Stutinsky, F. (1968): Comparaison ultrastructurale des noyaux neurosécrétoires hypothalamiques chez le rat normal ou en état de surcharge osmotique. *Bull. Assos. Anat.,* 142:1066–1072.
31. Knaggs, G. S., Tindal, J. S., and Turvey, A. (1971): Paraventricular-hypophysial neurosecretory pathways in the guinea-pig. *J. Endocrinol.,* 50:153–162.
32. Krieger, D. T., Liotta, A., and Brownstein, M. J. (1977): Corticotropin releasing factor distribution in normal and Brattleboro rat brain, and effect of deafferentation, hypophysectomy and steroid treatment in normal animals. *Endocrinology,* 100:227–237.
33. Marchetti, J. (1973): Immunoassay for lysine-vasopressin (LVP): Comparison of biological and immunological activity of lysine-vasopressin and some of its synthetic analogues. *Experientia,* 29:351–353.
34. Marchetti, J., Burlet, A., and Boulangé, M. (1978): Study of ADH secretion in adrenalectomized rats and effects of dexamethasone. *Acta Endocrinol. (Kbh),* 87:292–302.
35. Miller, R. E., Yueh-Chien, H., Wiley, M. K., and Hewitt, R. (1974): Anterior hypophysial function in the posterior hypophysectomized rat: Normal regulation of the adrenal system. *Neuroendocrinology,* 14:233–250.
36. Moll, J. (1957): Regeneration of the supraoptico-hypophysial and paraventriculohypophysial tracts in the hypophysectomized rat. *Z. Zellforsch.,* 46:686–707.
37. Moll, J., and de Wied, D. (1962): Observations on the hypothalamo-posthypophysial system of the posterior lobectomized rat. *Gen. Comp. Endocrinol.,* 2:215–218.
38. Norstrom, A., and Sjostrand, J. (1972): Effect of salt-loading, thirst and water-loading on transport and turnover of neurohypophysial proteins of the rat. *J. Endocrinol.,* 52:87–105.
39. North, W. G., Larochelle, F. T., Morris, J. F., Sokol, H. W., and Valtin, H. (1978): Biosynthesis specificity of neurons producing neurohypophysial principles. In: *Hypothalamic Function. Vol. 1: Hormones,* edited by K. Lederis and W. L. Vale, pp. 62–76. Karger, Basel.
40. Palkovits, M. (1973): Isolated removal of hypothalamic or other brain nuclei of the rat. *Brain Res.,* 59:449–450.
41. Peterson, R. P. (1966): Magnocellular neurosecretory centers in the rat hypothalamus. *J. Comp. Neurol.,* 128:181–190.

42. Raisman, G. (1973): Electron microscopic studies of the development of new neurohaemal contacts in the median eminence of the rat after hypophysectomy. *Brain Res.,* 55:245–261.
43. Raisman, G., (1973): An ultrastructural study of the effects of hypophysectomy on the supraoptic nucleus of the rat. *J. Comp. Neurol.,* 147:181–208.
44. Rasmussen, A. T., and Gardner, W. J. (1940): Effect of hypophysial stalk resection on the hypophysis and hypothalamus of man. *Endocrinology,* 27:219–226.
45. Scott, D. E., Dudley, G. K., Weindl, A., and Joynt, R. J. (1973): An autoradiographic analysis of hypothalamic magnocellular neurons. *Z. Zellforsch.,* 138:421–437.
46. Swaab, D. F., Pool, C. W., and Nijjvelt, F. (1975): Immunofluorescence of vasopressin and oxytocin in the rat hypothalamo-neurohypophysial system. *J. Neural Transmission,* 36:195–215.
47. Vandesande, F., de Mey, J., and Dierickx, K. (1974): Identification of neurophysin producing cells. I: The origin of the neurophysin-like substance-containing nerve fibres of the external region of the median eminence of the rat. *Cell Tiss. Res.,* 151:187–200.
48. Vandesande, F., and Dierickx, F. (1975): Identification of the vasopressin producing and of the oxytocin producing neurons in the hypothalamic magnocellular neurosecretory system of the rat. *Cell Tiss. Res.,* 164:153–162.
49. Vandesande, F., Dierickx, K., and de Mey, J. (1977): The origin of the vasopressinergic and oxytocinergic fibres of the external region of the median eminence of the rat hypophysis. *Cell Tiss. Res.,* 180:443–452.
50. van Leewen, F. W., Swaab, D. F., and Romijn, H. J. (1976): Light and electron microscopic localization of oxytocin and vasopressin in rats. In: *Immunoenzymatic Techniques,* edited by G. Feldman, P. Druet, J. Bignon, and S. Avrameas, pp. 345–353. North Holland, New York.
51. Watkins, W. B. (1975): Immunohistochemical demonstration of neurophysin in the hypo-thalamo-neurohypophysial system. *Int. Rev. Cytol.,* 41:241–284.
52. Wimersma Greidanus, T. B., and de Wied, D. (1977): The physiology of the neurohypophysial system and its relation to memory processes. In: *Biochemical Correlates of Brain Structure and Function,* edited by A. N. Davison, pp. 215–248. Academic, London.
53. Yates, F. E., Russel, S. M., Dallman, M. R., Hedge, G. A., McCann, S. M., and Dhariwal, A. P. S. (1971): Potentiation by vasopressin of corticotropin release induced by CRF. *Endocrinology,* 88:3–15.
54. Zimmerman, E. A., and Autunes, J. L. (1976): Organization of the hypothalamic-pituitary system: Current concepts from immunohistochemical studies. *J. Histochem. Cytochem.,* 24:207–215.
55. Zimmerman, E. A., Carmel, P. W., Husain, M. K., Ferin, M., Tannenbaum, M., Frantz, A. G., and Robinson, A. G. (1973): Vasopressin and neurophysin: High concentrations in monkey hypophyseal portal blood. *Science (NY),* 182:925–927.

Neuropeptides and Neural Transmission,
edited by C. Ajmone Marsan and W. Z. Traczyk.
Raven Press, New York © 1980.

Vasopressin and ACTH 4–10: Studies on Individual Giant Dopamine Neurons of the Snail *Planorbis Corneus*

W. Lichtensteiger and D. Felix

*Institute of Pharmacology and Brain Research Institute, University of Zürich,
CH-8006 Zürich, Switzerland*

Peptides may affect the functional state of neurons in various ways. Effects on ion conductance of the cell membrane, and hence on electrical activity of the neuron, are well documented (1), but additional actions on the metabolism of the neuron also seem conceivable, notably in the case of long-term effects. The giant dopamine (DA) neuron (GDN) of the European water snail *Planorbis corneus* (2) provides a model system where electrophysiological and histochemical or biochemical changes can be studied on the same identified neuron. We are presently using this model in investigations on the action of vasopressin, adrenocorticotropic hormone (ACTH) 4–10, and related peptides which influence the functional state of mammalian DA neuron groups (7). The DA metabolism of the snail neuron appears to correspond to that of mammalian systems (8); moreover, the GDN exhibits the same type of correlation between the intensity of catecholamine histofluorescence and firing rate as found in mammalian (nigral) DA neurons (4–6).

EFFECTS OF LYSINE VASOPRESSIN AND DESGLYCINAMIDE-LYSINE VASOPRESSIN ON THE ELECTRICAL ACTIVITY OF THE GDN

We studied the GDN of *Planorbis* in an *in vitro* preparation of the ring of circumoesophageal ganglia (5). The GDN could be reliably identified at the ventral surface of the left pedal ganglion (2). The cell was impaled with single micropipettes filled with 2 M KCl (tip diameter 0.1–1.0 μm, resistances 5–20 MΩ). Intracellular recordings were continuously monitored on an UV-oscillo-graph and the number of spikes per 10 sec was further counted by means of a programmable counter-timer (5,6). The preparation was frozen to $-195°$C by liquid propane cooled in liquid nitrogen during electrical recording, and subsequently processed for histochemical microfluorimetry (6).

When lysine vasopressin (LVP, Calbiochem) was administered to the bath

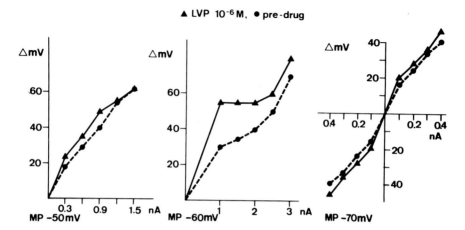

FIG. 1. LVP causes a slight but consistent increase in the change in membrane potential (ΔmV) elicited by injection of depolarizing or hyperpolarizing current (nA) into the GDN, which indicates increased membrane resistance. Data from three GDN studied before and 2–3 min after LVP administration. Current injected during 5 sec with 10-sec intervals. MP, resting membrane potential of the cell.

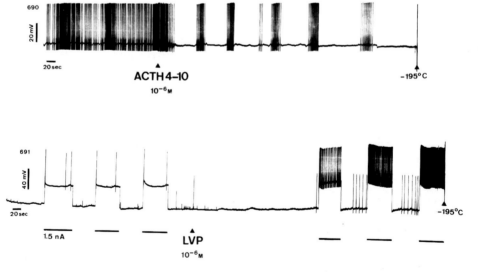

FIG. 2. Top: Rhythmic pattern of spontaneous activity of a GDN after administration of ACTH 4–10 *(arrow)*. At the point "−195°C," the cell was frozen. *Bottom:* Enhanced firing in response to depolarization (which is itself slightly increased) after LVP *(arrow)*. In this experiment, current *(bar)* was injected for 60 sec in order to obtain a period of prolonged activation of the cell for subsequent microfluorimetric analysis.

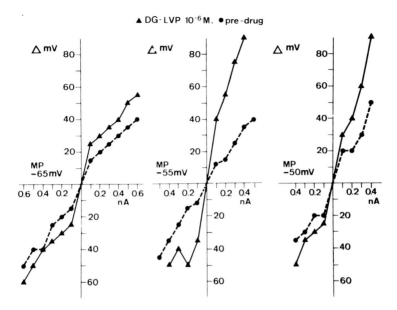

FIG. 3. Effect of DG-LVP on changes in membrane potential (ΔmV) induced by injection of depolarizing or hyperpolarizing current (nA) into the GDN. The effect of DG-LVP is of the same type as seen after LVP, but considerably more pronounced. Current was again injected for 5 sec. MP, resting membrane potential of the cell.

to give a concentration of 10^{-6} M (5.2 IU/12 ml), spontaneous activity increased in most GDNs (increase 4, decrease 1, no change 1). A similar tendency to increased spontaneous firing was also noted in some of the neurons studied with current injection. In order to obtain additional information on the mechanisms underlying the peptide effect, we analyzed the response of GDNs to injection of depolarizing or hyperpolarizing current. When tested about 2 min after administration of LVP (10^{-6} M), the current-induced change in membrane potential was consistently increased (Fig. 1) and firing in response to depolarization was enhanced (Fig. 2b; increased firing 9, decrease Ø, no change 2 GDNs; ref. 7). The specificity of this effect cannot be definitely judged at present, but it may be pointed out that an even greater increase in membrane resistance was noted with a potent analogue of LVP, desglycinamide-lysine vasopressin (DG-LVP, 10^{-6} M) (Fig. 3). This compound exerts central actions in mammals (3) and influences also mammalian DA systems (7). Firing upon depolarization was enhanced also after DG-LVP.

ELECTRICAL ACTIVITY OF GDN AFTER TREATMENT WITH ACTH 4–10

Spontaneous activity was influenced by ACTH 4–10 (5×10^{-7}–1×10^{-6} M) in a characteristic way: In four-fifths of the GDNs, the preexisting, often

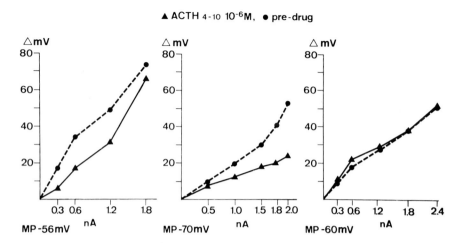

FIG. 4. ACTH 4–10 reduces the current-induced changes in membrane potential (ΔmV) in some but not all GDNs studied. MP, resting membrane potential of the cell.

slightly rhythmic but continuous activity was changed into a clearly rhythmic pattern with periods of silence or markedly reduced activity (7) (Fig. 2 top). ACTH 4–10 (10^{-6} M) also affected membrane resistance of GDN, but with this peptide the resistance was reduced (Fig. 4). The effect was not as consistent as that of LVP or DG-LVP where all GDNs responded, but it was observed in about three-fourths of the GDNs studied. In the remaining neurons, membrane resistance remained largely unchanged. An increase as with LVP has not been seen so far. Firing in response to depolarization remained unchanged in the majority of GDNs.

CORRELATION OF FIRING RATE AND INTENSITY OF NEURONAL DA FLUORESCENCE

The intensity of DA fluorescence emitted by the cell body of GDN was found to be correlated with the firing rate (4,5) in the same way as that of mammalian (rat) DA neurons (6). As far as can be judged from the available data, neither LVP nor ACTH 4–10 changed the basic relationship between spontaneous activity and histofluorescence (Fig. 5). Slight quantitative changes of the relation (regression function) could not be excluded on the basis of the limited number of neurons studied so far. The data appear to indicate that in the acute situation, the two peptides affect neuronal DA metabolism mainly through their effect on electrical activity. For a detailed analysis of these findings, more information is required on the biochemical background of cellular histofluorescence which is presently being investigated.

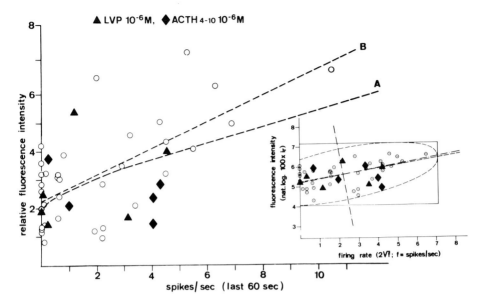

FIG. 5. Fluorescence intensity of GDNs as a function of their spontaneous firing rate. When compared with data from a previous correlative study (*open symbols*, values taken from ref. 5), the intensities of peptide-treated GDNs (LVP or ACTH 4–10) are in the range to be expected from their spontaneous firing rate. The peptide-treated cells are all found within the 99% confidence ellipse of the regression between intensity and firing rate **(inset).** Firing rate represents the mean value of the last 60 sec before freezing to −195°C. Fluorescence intensity is expressed in relation to the intensity of a noradrenaline-containing standard (= 1.0). The mean intensity of each cell is calculated from about 40 measurements (i_r) per GDN; the individual values i_r are obtained from the equation $i_r = (c - \bar{t})/(\overline{NA} - \bar{t})$, where c = absolute intensity in the measuring field, $\bar{t}$ = mean nonspecific background fluorescence outside GDN, $\overline{NA}$ and $\bar{t}$ = mean intensities of noradrenaline-containing and noradrenaline-free gelatin standards, respectively, in the corresponding tissue section. **Inset:** Regression function between the two parameters after normalization of the skew distributions of values, assuming a lognormal distribution of intensities and a Poisson distribution of firing rates (5). Only GDNs on which effects on spontaneous activity were studied, are shown here. Curve A shows the correct non-linear regression function. As indicated by line B, a linear regression function would also provide an acceptable approximation of the data observed so far (cf. ref. 5).

CONCLUSIONS

It remains to be elucidated whether the peptide effects on the GDN mimic physiological mechanisms existing in *Planorbis*. Electrophysiological actions of LVP have been reported for different types of neurons in another snail species (1), where there is some evidence for the existence of a related peptide. In contrast, effects of a peptide of the ACTH family appear not to have been observed in snails so far. The changes we found in the GDN, an increase (in the case of LVP or DG-LVP) or a decrease in membrane resistance (in the case of ACTH 4–10), might be seen as representing typical modulatory actions, as they would tend to reinforce or reduce responses to activating as well as inhibitory inputs, although possibly to different extents.

ACKNOWLEDGMENTS

We thank Prof. D. de Wied (Utrecht) for a gift of DG-LVP and Dr. H. M. Greven (Organon, Oss) for ACTH 4–10. The excellent technical assistance of Miss F. Boller, R. Böswald, and U. Frangi is gratefully acknowledged. The study was supported by grants from the Swiss National Science Foundation (3.231–0.77 and 3.271–0.78), the Hartmann-Müller-Stiftung, and the Dr. Eric Slack-Gyr Foundation.

REFERENCES

1. Barker, J. L., and Smith, T. G., Jr. (1977): Peptides as neurohormones. In: *Society for Neuroscience Symposia, Vol. II,* edited by W. M. Cowan and J. A. Ferrendelli, pp. 340–373. Society for Neuroscience, Bethesda, Maryland.
2. Cottrell, G. A. (1977): Identified amine-containing neurones and their synaptic connections. *Neuroscience,* 2:1–18.
3. de Wied, D., Greven, H. M., Lande, S., and Witter, A. (1972): Dissociation of the behavior and endocrine effects of lysine vasopressin by tryptic digestion. *Br. J. Pharmacol.,* 45:118–122.
4. Lichtensteiger, W., Felix, D., and Hefti, F. (1978): Correlation of firing rate and histochemical fluorescence intensity in individual giant dopamine neurons of the water snail *Planorbis corneus. Experientia,* 34:901.
5. Lichtensteiger, W., Felix, D., and Hefti, F. (1979): Spike activity and histofluorescence correlated in the giant dopamine neuron of *Planorbis corneus. Brain Res.,* 170:231–245.
6. Lichtensteiger, W., Felix, D., Lienhart, R., and Hefti, F. (1976): A quantitative correlation between single unit activity and fluorescence intensity of dopamine neurones in zona compacta of substantia nigra, as demonstrated under the influence of nicotine and physostigmine. *Brain Res.,* 117:85–103.
7. Lichtensteiger, W., Monnet, F., and Felix, D. (1979): Peptide effects on mammalian and invertebrate dopamine (DA) neurons. In: *Catecholamines: Basic and Clinical Frontiers,* Vol. 2., edited by E. Usdin, I. J. Kopin, and J. Barchas, pp. 1086–1088. Pergamon, Oxford.
8. Osborne, N. N., Priggemeier, E., and Neuhoff, V. (1975): Dopamine metabolism in characterised neurones of *Planorbis corneus. Brain Res.,* 90:261–271.

Neuropeptides and Neural Transmission,
edited by C. Ajmone Marsan and W. Z. Traczyk.
Raven Press, New York © 1980.

Action of Neuropeptides on Self-stimulation Behavior in Rats

H. Schwarzberg, K. Betschen, and H. Unger

*Institute of Physiology, Medical Academy,
DDR-301 Magdeburg, German Democratic Republic*

In recent years several workers have demonstrated with sufficient certainty that information processing events of the central nervous system (CNS) are influenced by the neuropeptides vasopressin and oxytocin. As a result of a specific functional status of the CNS, intracerebral self-stimulation lends itself as an indicator in assaying the neuroactive efficacy of substances. The course of self-stimulation is similar to addiction phenomena; however, the physiological background has not yet been satisfactorily clarified. Nevertheless, more recently the self-stimulation approach has been increasingly accepted as a measuring principle since it is a suitable means to record the excitation status in the CNS. Therefore, the present investigation was undertaken to induce endogenously and exogenously born changes in vasopressin and oxytocin contents and assay the effects on hypothalamic self-stimulation in rats.

MATERIAL AND METHODS

Thirty male Wistar rats weighing 250 g were used for the experiments. One pair each of enamel-insulated steel electrodes were chronically implanted in the lateral hypothalamus for intracranial stimulation, and a sealable cannula was inserted in the right lateral brain ventricle.

Pressing a lever provided in the experimental cage the rats could initiate an electric stimulator to apply to themselves trains of 40 to 50 square pulses through the connected electrodes (pulse width 0.1–0.4 msec; frequency 100 Hz; amplitude 3–9 V; current 0.7–4 mA). Lever operations per minute were recorded by an electronic counter. Synthetic lysine-vasopressin (first subseries) or oxytocin (second subseries) in a liquid volume of 5 μl was applied to the animals through the ventricle cannula. The self-stimulation rate was recorded at selected times during the following 48 hr. In a separate series, the rats were deprived of drinking water for 6 days and the self-stimulation rate assayed daily for 30 min.

Statistical significance of the results was computed by means of the nonparametric rank test according to Wilcoxon et al. (see ref. 2).

TABLE 1. *Changes in self-stimulation rats after intraventricular application of lysine-vasopressin, oxytocin, and artificial CSF (control)*

Substance	\multicolumn{8}{c}{Time after application (min)}							
	0	30	60	90	120	150	24 hr	48 hr
Artificial	100	98	98	96	97	94	100	103
CSF		(10)	(10)	(10)	(9)	(8)	(8)	(7)
Vasopressin	100	94	90[a]	86[b]	80[c]	84[a]	90[c]	97
(50 μU)		(7)	(7)	(7)	(6)	(6)	(5)	(5)
Oxytocin	100	104[b]	106[a]	102	103	—	115[d]	111[b]
(500 μU)		(6)	(6)	(4)	(4)		(8)	(7)

[a] $p < 0.05$.
[b] $p < 0.01$.
[c] $p < 0.005$.
[d] $p < 0.001$.
Data as percentage; number of experiments in parentheses; Wilcoxon test for significance.

RESULTS

Intraventricular injection of 500 μU oxytocin enhanced the self-stimulation rate, which diminished after a similar application of 50 μU vasopressin. The effect was long-lasting and could be demonstrated with certainty over at least 24 hr (Table 1).

Deprivation of drinking water caused a clear reduction of the self-stimulation rate by an average of 10%, with the adjustment to a steady value being particularly striking during the first days of the thirst experiment. It was only after

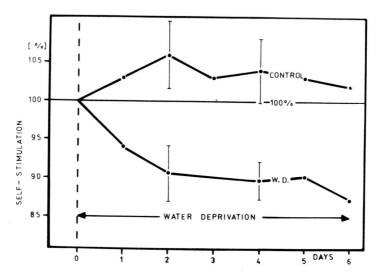

FIG. 1. Changes in self-stimulation rate during water deprivation (M ± SEM).

6 to 7 days, even though initial weakening phenomena were observed on the rats, that the onset of a further reduction of the self-stimulation rate was noted (Fig. 1).

DISCUSSION

The marked changes in the self-stimulation rate after intraventricular application of the neuropeptides vasopressin and oxytocin suggest a direct influence on the processes involved in the development of this phenomenon. Indirect hormone effects through a modification of peripheral autonomous functions were greatly avoided by using the smallest dose possible. Therefore, the hormone dose applied in each of the present investigations was selected in accordance with today's knowledge about its occurrence in the cerebrospinal fluid.

The catecholamine systems seem to be the most essential neural substrate for intracranial self-stimulation (1). Obviously, these may be the site of action of vasopressin and oxytocin since both hormones were found to alter the content and the turnover rate of catecholamines in different brain regions (3,6).

It is remarkable that the self-stimulation rate diminished while the animals were deprived of water. The same effect was observed after intraventricular and intramuscular vasopressin application (5). While in the state of thirst, rats revealed an increased vasopressin content in the blood (4).

Thus, it is reasonable to conclude that the decrease of the self-stimulation rate during deprivation of water may be due to the concurrently increased vasopressin content in blood. However, utmost care should be exercised in this context since deprivation of water probably affects a great number of systems in the organism which are assumed to influence CNS function. Final assessment of the relationships will be possible only after further investigations.

ACKNOWLEDGMENT

This work was supported by the G.D.R. Ministry of Science and Technology.

REFERENCES

1. German, D. C., and Bowden, D. M. (1974): Catecholamine systems as the neural substrate for intracranial self-stimulation: A hypothesis. *Brain Res.,* 73:381–419.
2. Sachs, L. (1969): *Statistische Auswertungsmethoden.* Springer, Berlin, Heidelberg, New York.
3. Schulz, H., Kovács, G. L., and Telegdy, G. (1979): The effect of posterior pituitary peptides on avoidance learning in correlation with the brain catecholamine content in rats. In: *Biological Aspects of Learning, Memory Formation and Ontogeny of the CNS,* edited by H. Matthies, M. Krug, N. Popov, pp. 319–324, Akademie Verlag, Berlin.
4. Schwarzberg, H. (1968): Untersuchungen über den Einfluss des Wasserentzuges auf das periphere und zentralnervöse Geschehen der Ratte. *Acta Biol. Med. Germ.,* 21:23–49.
5. Schwarzberg, H., Betschen, K., Unger, H., and Schulz, H. (1979): Beziehungen zwischen peptidergen Neurohormonen und der hypothalamischen Selbststimulation bei Ratten. *Verh. Ges. Exp. Med. (in press).*
6. Tanaka, M., de Kloet, E. R., de Wied, D., and Versteeg, D. H. G. (1977): Arginine[8]-vasopressin affects catecholamine metabolism in specific brain nuclei. *Life Sci.,* 20:1799–1808.

Neuropeptides and Neural Transmission,
edited by C. Ajmone Marsan and W. Z. Traczyk.
Raven Press, New York © 1980.

The Action of Vasopressin and Oxytocin on the Nigro-striatal Dopaminergic System

Horst Schulz, Gábor L. Kovács, and Gyula Telegdy

Institute of Physiology, Medical Academy Magdeburg, DDR-301 Magdeburg, German Democratic Republic; and Department of Pathophysiology, School of Medicine, Szeged, Hungary

Neurohypophyseal hormones vasopressin (LVP) and oxytocin (OXT) are synthesized in mammals predominantly in the cell bodies of the supraoptic and paraventricular nuclei. Extrahypothalamic vasopressinergic and oxytocinergic fibres are also present in the dorsal and ventral hippocampus, the nuclei of amygdala, the substantia nigra and substantia grisea, the nucleus tractus solitarii, the nucleus ambiguous, and the substantia gelatinosa of the spinal cord (3). The presence of LVP and OXT in the CSF argues for a direct central release of these peptides (8). The CSF might also serve as a vehicle for these neuroactive peptides. On the other hand, a direct transport of these peptides to CNS target sites via peptidergic neurosecretory fibres is also possible under physiological conditions. Both peptides modify the electrical activity of the brain (16,21,27) and are physiologically involved in the regulation of memory processes in laboratory animals (2,6,7,30). LVP also improves disturbances of memory and affective disorders in humans (15,17). Biochemically, LVP and OXT affect dopaminergic and noradrenergic activities in certain brain regions after peripheral and/or intracerebroventricular administration (12,14,20,23–25).

Neurochemical lesioning of different transmitter pathways in the brain, as well as pharmacological blockade of catecholamine synthesis, show that the peptide-induced changes in the brain catecholamine metabolism are essential for the effects of these peptides on memory (13,14). Although indirect behavioral evidence indicates a presynaptic effect of LVP on limbic-midbrain terminals of the dorsal noradrenergic bundle (13), such a presynaptic interaction has not yet been proved directly. For the separation of pre- and postsynaptic components of neuroactive peptides, rotational behavior following unilateral lesion of the substantia nigra has been used (1,26). With this model system, the effects of LVP, OXT, and prolyl-leucyl-glycinamide (PLG), the C-terminal tripeptide of oxytocin, have been tested.

METHODS

Male rats of an inbred CFY strain (150–200 g) were anaesthetized with sodium pentobarbital (Nembutal®) in a dose of 40 mg/kg. A guiding cannula was stereotaxically implanted into the right cerebral ventricle using the stereotaxic coordinates (AP + 1.0, L 1.5, V 3.0) of Fifková and Maršala (9). Unilateral lesioning of the substantia nigra was made by injection of 6-hydroxydopamine (6-OHDA) into the right nigral area (AP + 4.5, L 1.8, V 8.8). For intranigral applications a cannula was implanted into the left (intact) substantia nigra. For drug- or peptide-induced rotational behavior animals were tested in a glass cylinder (24 cm diameter) immediately after treatment. The number of turnings to the ipsi- or contralateral side (referred to the lesioned right substantia nigra) was counted during 60 min, and expressed as the relative asymmetry (RA).

$$RA\ (\%) = \left[\left[\frac{T_i - T_c}{T_t}\ \text{pep} \right] - \left[\frac{T_i - T_c}{T_t}\ \text{contr} \right] \right] \times 100$$

Where T = number of turnings, i = ipsilateral, c = contralateral, t = total number of turnings, pep = peptide treatment, and contr = controls with saline.

Neuropeptides were tested in a randomized sequence at 3-day intervals 7 days after surgery, following intracerebroventricular or intranigral application. For intracerebroventricular administration LVP (Organon, 232 IU/mg) was given to alert and free-moving rats over a period of 2 min in a dose of 50 ng, OXT (Richter, 371 IU/mg) in a dose of 50 or 100 ng, PLG (Organon) in a dose of 50 ng, dissolved in 2 μl saline. Peptides also were injected into the substantia nigra in the following doses: LVP 2.5 ng, OXT 5 ng, and PLG 2.5 ng, in a volume of 1 μl. At the end of the behavioral studies, each rat was given dl-amphetamine (2.5 mg/kg) and apomorphine hydrochloride (1 mg/kg) intraperitoneally for pharmacological control. The localization of the lesions and the positions of the ventricular cannulae were histologically controlled. Forebrains were immediately frozen and the dopamine contents of the left and right striata were separately measured by the fluorimetric method of Shellenberger and Gordon (22). The one-tailed t-test was used, and probability level of .05 was accepted as a significant difference.

RESULTS

After intracerebroventricular administration LVP induced a significant ipsilateral relative asymmetry (RA) of approximately 50% ($p < 0.01$). Likewise, the same effect on rotational behavior was observed after intracerebroventricular OXT treatment (100 ng) with an RA of approximately 45% in the same direction ($p < 0.01$). The lower dose of OXT (50 ng) caused an RA of 25% ($p < 0.01$). Experiments with PLG showed a significant RA to the ipsilateral side of approximately 35% ($p < 0.05$) (Fig. 1).

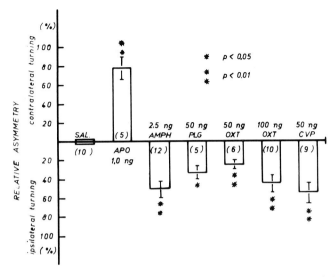

FIG. 1. Changes of the rotational behavior after i.c.v. administration of PLG, OXT, LVP and of i.p. injection of *dl*-amphetamine (AMPH) and apomorphine (APO). SAL, saline control.

Intraperitoneal injection of apomorphine in a dose of 1 mg/kg induced an RA of 80% to the contralateral side of the nigral lesion ($p < 0.01$), while intraperitoneal administration of amphetamine (2.5 mg/kg) resulted in an ipsilateral turning of approximately 50% ($p < 0.01$) (Fig. 1).

Measurements of the contra- and ipsilateral striatal dopamine contents after unilateral injection of 6-OHDA into the substantia nigra showed a significant decrease on the lesioned side ($p < 0.001$) (Fig. 2).

No significant changes were observed after intranigral treatment of LVP, OXT, or PLG in the rotational behavior of the animals. That the ascending

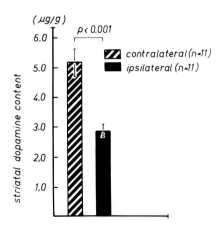

FIG. 2. Contralateral and ipsilateral dopamine contents of the striatum after unilateral 6-OHDA induced lesion of the substantia nigra in rats.

TABLE 1. *The effect of intranigral administration of neuroactive peptides on rotational behavior in rats*

Treatment	Dose	RA (%)	Direction	No. animals	Significance
Amphetamine	2.5 mg/kg[a]	34.5 ± 7.7[b]	Ipsilateral	6	$p < 0.01$
LVP	2.5 ng	14.0 ± 24.0	Ipsilateral	5	ns[c]
OXT	5 ng	10.4 ± 18.3	Contralateral	7	ns
PLG	2.5 ng	0.6 ± 12.9	Contralateral	7	ns

[a] Mean ± SE.
[b] Not significant (ns).
[c] Intraperitoneal treatment for pharmacological control.

dopaminergic nigro-striatal pathways was not lesioned by implanting the nigral cannula per se, is shown by the normal ipsilateral turning after intraperitoneal amphetamine administration (Table 1).

DISCUSSION

Lesioning of the dopaminergic cell bodies in the substantia nigra on one side results in a degradation of the ascending dopaminergic pathways on the ipsilateral side, with a concomitant decrease in the striatal dopamine content, and in development of supersensitivity of striatal dopaminergic receptors. This striatal dopaminergic imbalance does not cause spontaneous asymmetry in rat extrapyramidal motor coordination.

Rotational behavior can be induced, however, by administration of amphetamine or apomorphine. Systemic administration of amphetamine causes activation of the presynaptic nigro-striatal neurons and the dominance of the presynaptic terminals on the intact side results in an ipsilateral rotation. On the other hand, apomorphine stimulates dopaminergic receptors on both sides, and the stimulation of the dominant supersensitive receptors of the lesioned side will cause contralateral turning. In this way, the direction of turning can be used as an index of pre- or postsynaptic activation (1,5,18,26).

In this behavioral model, intracerebroventricular treatment with LVP, OXT, or PLG caused ipsilateral rotation, indicating presynaptic activation of the nigrostriatal dopaminergic system. Local injection of the peptides into the intact substantia nigra failed to cause asymmetry in movement.

It is deemed of interest that the effect of LVP on memory consolidation processes is also related to an interaction of the neuropeptide with presynaptic catecholaminergic terminals, i.e., with limbic-midbrain terminals of the dorsal noradrenergic bundle (13). No data indicate activation of the dopaminergic nigro-striatal system by oxytocin. The effect of OXT on rotational behavior might be indirect because PLG can be produced from OXT by brain tissue (4,29). The tripeptide has been shown to increase brain catecholamine turnover, including striatal dopamine disappearance (11,28). It is possible, therefore, that the OXT-induced ipsilateral turning behavior is related to the *in vivo* conversion of the neuropeptide to PLG.

In our observations PLG seemed to have activated the presynaptic dopaminergic terminals, as indicated by the ipsilateral rotation behavior. The effect of PLG on striatal dopaminergic neurotransmission, however, might be a more complex one. Recently Kostrzewa et al. (10) showed that PLG potentiates apomorphine-induced contralateral turning and hence concluded that the peptide interacts with postsynaptic dopaminergic receptors. A complex pre- and postsynaptic mechanism of action would explain the diverse conclusions. Theoretically, it cannot be excluded that in our model the tripeptide activates postsynaptic dopaminergic receptors on the ipsilateral side, but affects presynaptic dopaminergic terminals more potently on the contralateral side. This would also result in ipsilateral turning. With apomorphine pretreatment (10) the presynaptic mechanism of action cannot be revealed and the peptide potentiates the effect of apomorphine by its postsynaptic mechanism of action. Such a combined pre- and postsynaptic mechanism of action is not likely in the case of LVP treatment: LVP caused an asymmetry of the same magnitude as amphetamine in a dose of 2.5 mg/kg. To induce this asymmetry by a combined pre- and postsynaptic mechanism, LVP ought to have activated the presynaptic terminals more potently than the maximally effective dose of amphetamine.

Memory processes are oppositely affected by LVP and OXT (2,13,19). In contrast, as regards rotational behavior, both peptides act in the same direction. In conclusion, our data present behavioral evidence for a presynaptic interaction of these neuropeptides with nigro-striatal dopaminergic neurons. The presynaptic action might be one of the mechanisms by which PLG or the other neuropeptides affect information processing in the central nervous system.

ACKNOWLEDGMENTS

The authors wish to acknowledge the expert technical assistance of Mrs. Katalin Kovács and Miss Ágnes Szöke. Lysine[8]-vasopressin and PLG were kindly donated by Prof. David de Wied (Utrecht, The Netherlands), and oxytocin was a gift of the Richter Chem. Co., Budapest (Hungary). The work was supported by the Scientific Research Council, Ministry of Health, Hungary (Grant No. 4–08–0302–03–O/T).

REFERENCES

1. Anden, N. E., Dahlström, A., Fuxe, K., and Larsen, K. (1966): Functional role of the nigro-striatal dopamine neuron. *Acta Pharmacol. Toxicol.*, 24:263–274.
2. Bohus, B., Kovács, G. L., and de Wied, D. (1978): Oxytocin, vasopressin and memory: Opposite effects on consolidation and retrieval processes. *Brain Res.*, 157:414–418.
3. Buijs, R. M. (1978): Intra- and extrahypothalamic vasopressin and oxytocin pathways in the rat. *Cell Tiss. Res.*, 192:423–435.

4. Celis, M. E., Taleisnik, S., and Walter, R. (1971): Release of pituitary melanocyte-stimulating hormone by the oxytocin-fragment H-Cys-Tyr-Ile-Gln-Asn-OH. *Biochem. Biophys. Res. Commun.,* 45:564–569.
5. Creese, J., Burt, D. R., and Snyder, S. H. (1977): Dopamine receptor binding enhancement accompanies lesion-induced behavioral supersensitivity. *Science,* 197:596–598.
6. de Wied, D. (1976): Behavioral effects of intraventricularly administered vasopressin and vasopressin fragments. *Life Sci.,* 19:685–690.
7. de Wied, D., and Bohus, B. (1966): Long term and short term effects on retention of a conditioned avoidance response in rats by treatment respectively with long acting pitressin or α-MSH. *Nature,* 212:1484–1488.
8. Dogterom, J., Wimersma Greidanus, Tj. B. van, and Swaab, D. F. (1977): Evidence for the release of vasopressin and oxytocin into cerebrospinal fluid: Measurements in plasma and CSF of intact and hypophysectomized rats. *Neuroendocrinology,* 24:108–118.
9. Fifková, E., and Maršala, J. (1967): Stereotaxic atlases for the cat, rabbit and rat. In: *Electrophysiological Methods in Biological Research,* edited by J. Bureš, M. Petrán, and J. Zachar. Publishing House of the Czechoslovak Academy of Science, Prague.
10. Kostrzewa, R. M., Kastin, A. J., and Sobrian, S. K. (1978): Potentiation of apomorphine action in rats by l-prolyl-l-leucyl-glycin amide. *Pharmacol. Biochem. Behav.,* 9:375–378.
11. Kostrzewa, R. M., Kastin, A. J., and Spirtes, M. A. (1975): α-MSH and MIF-I effects on catecholamine levels and synthesis in various rat brain areas. *Pharmacol. Biochem. Behav.,* 3:1017–1023.
12. Kovács, G. L., Bohus, B., and Versteeg, D. H. G. (1979): Facilitation of memory consolidation by vasopressin: Mediation by terminals of the dorsal noradrenergic bundle? *Brain Res.,* 172:73–85.
13. Kovács, G. L., Bohus, B., Versteeg, D. H. G., de Kloet, E. R., and de Wied, D. (1979): Effect of oxytocin and vasopressin on memory consolidation: Sites of action and catecholaminergic correlates after local microinjection into limbic-midbrain structures. *Brain Res.,* 175:303–314.
14. Kovács, G. L., Vécsei, L., Szabó, G., and Telegdy, G. (1977): The involvement of catecholaminergic mechanisms in the behavioral action of vasopressin. *Neurosci. Lett.,* 5:337–344.
15. Legros, J. L., Gilot, P., Seron, X., Claessens, J., Adams, A., Moeglen, J. M., Audibert, A., and Berchier, P. (1978): Influence of vasopressin on learning and memory. *Lancet,* 1:41–42.
16. Moss, R. L., Dyball, R. E., and Cross, B. A. (1972): Excitation of antidromically identified neurosecretory cells of the paraventricular nucleus by oxytocin applied iontophoretically. *Exp. Neurol.* 34:95–102.
17. Oliveros, J. C., Jandali, M. K., Timsit-Bertier, M., Remy, R. R., Benghezal, A., Audibert, A., and Moeglen, J. M. (1978): Vasopressin in amnesia. *Lancet,* 1:42.
18. Pert, A. (1978): The effect of opiates on nigrostriatal dopaminergic activity. In: *Characteristics and Function of Opioides,* edited by J. van Ree and L. Terenius. Elsevier, Amsterdam.
19. Schulz, H., Kovács, G. L., and Telegdy, G. (1974): The effect of physiological doses of vasopressin and oxytocin on avoidance and exploratory behaviour in rats. *Acta Physiol. Acad. Sci. Hung.,* 45:211–215.
20. Schulz, H., Kovács, G. L., and Telegdy, G. (1979): The effect of posterior pituitary peptides on avoidance learning in correlation with the brain catecholamine content in rats. In: *Biological Aspects of Learning, Memory Formation and Ontogeny of the CNS,* edited by H. Matthies, M. Krug, and N. Popov. Akademie Verlag, Berlin.
21. Schulz, H., Unger, H., Schwarzberg, H., Pommrich, G., and Stolze, R. (1971): Neuronenaktivität hypothalamischer Kerngebiete von Kaninchen nach intraventrikulärer Applikation von Vasopressin und Oxytocin. *Experientia,* 27:1482–1483.
22. Shellenberger, M. K., and Gordon, J. H. (1971): A rapid simplified procedure for simultaneous assay of norepinephrine, dopamine, and 5-hydroxytryptamine from discrete brain areas. *Anal. Biochem.,* 39:356–372.
23. Tanaka, M., de Kloet, E. R., de Wied, D., and Versteeg, D. H. G. (1977): Arginine⁸-vasopressin affects catecholamine metabolism in specific brain nuclei. *Life Sci.,* 20:1799–1808.
24. Tanaka, M., Versteeg, D. H. G., and de Wied, D. (1977): Regional effect of vasopressin on rat brain catecholamine metabolism. *Neurosci. Lett.,* 4:321–325.
25. Telegdy, G., and Kovács, G. L. (1979): The role of monoamines in mediating the action of hormones in learning and memory. In: *Brain Mechanisms in Memory and Learning: From Single Neuron to Man,* edited by M. A. B. Brazier. Raven Press, New York.

26. Ungerstedt, U. (1971): Striatal dopamine release after amphetamine or nerve degeneration revealed by rotational behavior. *Acta Physiol. Scand. (Suppl.),* 367:69–93.
27. Urban, I., and de Wied, D. (1975): Inferior quality of RSA during paradoxical sleep in rats with hereditary diabetes insipidus. *Brain Res.,* 97:362–366.
28. Versteeg, D. H. G., Tanaka, M., de Kloet, E. R., Ree, J. M. van, and de Wied, D. (1978): Prolyl-leucyl-glycinamide (PLG): regional effects on α-MPT-induced catecholamine disappearance in rat brain. *Brain Res.,* 142:561–563.
29. Walter, R., Griffith, E. C., and Hooper, K. C. (1973): Production of MIF by a particulate preparation of hypothalami: Mechanisms of oxytocin inactivation. *Brain Res.,* 60:449–457.
30. Wimersma Greidanus, Tj. B. van, Dogterom, J., and de Wied, D. (1975): Intraventricular administration of anti-vasopressin serum inhibits memory consolidation in rats. *Life Sci.,* 16:637–644.

Neuropeptides and Neural Transmission,
edited by C. Ajmone Marsan and W. Z. Traczyk.
Raven Press, New York © 1980.

Effects of Pro-Leu-Gly-NH₂ (MIF) on the Central Nervous System Responses to Morphine

Ronald F. Ritzmann, Roderich Walter, and *Hemendra N. Bhargava

*Department of Physiology and Biophysics, and *Department of Pharmacognosy and Pharmacology, University of Illinois at the Medical Center, Chicago, Illinois 60612*

During the past several years, it has become evident that mammalian neurohypophyseal peptides have effects on the central nervous system (CNS) which are not directly related to their classic effects as hormones. Since these CNS effects are observed following the intraventricular administration of low doses of these compounds, it has been postulated that such effects are mediated by the interaction of these peptides with specific receptors in the CNS.

The isolation of peptides with opiate-like activity in the brain has led to the hypothesis that these compounds may mediate the response to pain (1). It has been reported that there is a positive correlation between the analgesic potency of many of these compounds and their ability to alter body temperature (8). We have recently found Pro-Leu-Gly-NH₂ (melanocyte release-inhibiting factor; MIF) as well as several fragments and analogs of MIF to have the ability to block the hypothermic response observed during withdrawal in morphine-dependent mice if the peptides are administered concomitantly with morphine (11). These same peptides also prevent the development of tolerance to the analgesic properties of morphine (12). Since tolerance and physical dependence are typically considered to be two aspects of a single phenomenon (3,13), these two pieces of data were considered to be indicative of a blockage of the development of the "addictive" state. However, we have recently demonstrated that for ethanol, another drug to which dependence and tolerance develop, these two states can be dissociated (10). It has also been shown that the rate of the development of tolerance to morphine is contingent upon the dependent variable used to assess tolerance. Furthermore, different agonists and antagonists for various neurotransmitters have been shown to differently alter various types of tolerance. Dopaminergic systems, for example, have been shown to be involved in the analgesic response to morphine, but not involved in the respiratory depression produced by morphine (7). We have, therefore, decided to further investigate the effectiveness of MIF (also known as melanocyte-stimulating hormone–release-inhibiting factor; MSH-RIF) and cyclo(Leu-Gly) in preventing the development of various aspects of tolerance to and physical dependence on morphine.

MATERIALS AND METHODS

Morphine and Peptide Treatment in Mice

MIF and cyclo(Leu-Gly) used in these studies were synthesized in our laboratories (6,11). Male Swiss Webster mice weighing 26 ± 4 g (SD) were randomly divided into three groups: one group received a subcutaneous injection of water (vehicle); the remaining two groups received a subcutaneous injection of either MIF or cyclo(Leu-Gly) at the appropriate dose. All subcutaneous injections were 0.1 ml in volume. Two hours post injection, mice were further subdivided, each subgroup was implanted with either a placebo or morphine (75 mg free base) pellet (12). The pellets were removed 72 hr later.

Brain levels of morphine were measured in mice that had received peptide or vehicle injection. For these studies, 3 days after morphine pellet implantation, the mice were then sacrificed by decapitation and the brains were rapidly removed, frozen on dry ice, and stored at $-80°$ until assayed for morphine content. Brain morphine concentrations were determined fluorometrically (2).

Assessment of Physical Dependence and Tolerance in Mice

To determine the effects of peptide treatment on development of physical dependence, the abstinence syndrome was precipitated by using the morphine antagonist naloxone (Endo Laboratories Inc., N.Y.) (0.1 mg/kg) injected intraperitoneally 1 hr after removal of the morphine and placebo pellets. These mice were monitored for changes in body temperature and body weight at 15-min intervals for 1 hr after the naloxone injection. Effects of removing the pellets (withdrawing morphine) were also assessed by utilizing body temperature and weight as physical dependence parameters; these measurements were made at 2-hr intervals for 10 hr after the removal of the pellets. Placebo-implanted mice were treated in the same manner as the morphine pellet-implanted mice (12). Temperature was measured by using a lubricated rectal probe (inserted 2.5 cm into the rectum) and telethermometer (model 43TA, Yellow Springs Instrument Co., Yellow Springs, Ohio).

Stereotyped jumping was also measured 1 hr after pellet removal. Mice were injected with naloxone (0.1 mg/kg) and placed on a platform 33 cm in diameter. Four mice were tested at a time, and the total number of jumps off the platform during a 10-min period was recorded. Tolerance to the analgesic effects of morphine was measured by injecting morphine (40 mg/kg) intraperitoneally 24 hr after the removal of the pellets from a separate group of mice (12). The analgesic response was determined by measuring the jump threshold to an increasing electric current on an electrified grid attached to a BRS/LVE shock generator/scrambler. The level of analgesia was determined by comparing the change in threshold just prior to, and 30 min after, the injection of morphine (12).

Determination of Tolerance in Isolated Guinea Pig Ileum

Male guinea pigs, 250 to 400 g, were killed by cervical dislocation. The ileum was removed from a point approximately 10 cm above the caecum and thoroughly cleaned of any contents (4,5). A 3-cm length of ileum was used for each assay. One end of the tissue was tied to a platinum electrode, while the other end was attached directly to a Harvard Smooth Muscle Transducer. The tissue was suspended in a 10 ml jacketed tissue bath in Krebs-Ringers solution maintained at 37°C. The tissue bath had been siliconized with 1% Dri-Film Sc-87 in heptane to prevent absorption of morphine to the glass and was allowed to dry thoroughly before use (2). Thirty minutes prior to the start and during testing, 95% O_2–5% CO_2 was bubbled through the bathing medium (9). Tissue was allowed to equilibrate for 30 min before beginning stimulation. The tissue was stimulated with a modified Grass SD9B stimulator with a square wave pulse of 1 msec duration, 0.4 msec delay, 80 V, with 4 pulses/min. Contractions were recorded on a Grass model 79D Polygraph calibrated to 0.5 g/cm. The experiment with the ileum was started when the tissue contraction became uniform and at least 2 cm in size. Morphine (50 ng, 4.69×10^{-9} M) in 0.1 cc was added to the tissue bath at 10-min intervals without intervening rinses. Injections were repeated until tolerance was evident. Ten minutes later a large challenge dose of 350 ng of morphine (3.28×10^{-8} M) was injected. Cyclo(Leu-Gly) treatment was performed by pretreating ileum with 10 to 60 µg injected into the bathing medium 10 min prior to morphine treatment.

RESULTS

As in our previous studies the peptide treatment did not alter any of the acute responses to morphine tested (12). Both peptide- and the vehicle-treated mice which received chronic morphine treatment exhibited tail straub and stereotyped running during the morphine treatment. All three groups also lost an equal amount of body weight during the 3-day morphine treatment: vehicle 1.95 ± 0.96, MIF 1.85 ± 0.88, cyclo(Leu-Gly) 1.99 ± 0.90. There was no difference among the three groups in the amount of morphine in the brains of 3-day morphine-pelleted mice: vehicle, 295 ng/g, MIF, 303 ng/g, cyclo(Leu-Gly), 285 ng/g.

The effect of administering MIF or cyclo(Leu-Gly) 2 hr prior to pellet implantation on the hypothermia which occurs during abrupt withdrawal is illustrated in Fig. 1. Vehicle-injected mice which received morphine exhibited a loss in body temperature (−1.5°C) 6 to 8 hr after pellet removal, which was significantly different from placebo-implanted mice regardless of peptide treatment ($p < 0.05$). Peptide-treated mice, on the other hand, did not differ in body temperature from placebo-implanted mice at any of the time points ($p < 0.05$). Body weight loss, however, appeared to be equal in each of the morphine-treated groups: vehicle −2.75 ± 0.95, MIF −1.95 ± 0.88, and cyclo(Leu-Gly) −1.99 ± 0.90.

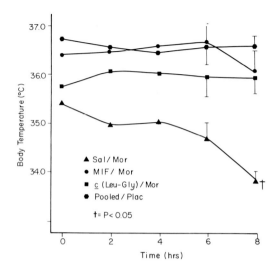

FIG. 1 Inhibition of the development of physical dependence (abrupt withdrawal). Mice were pretreated with either vehicle (Sal), MIF, or cyclo(Leu-Gly); 2 hr later half of each group was implanted with placebo pellets, the remaining half received morphine pellets (75 mg free base). Pellets were removed after 72 hr and body temperature was recorded for the next 8 hr. Since there was no significant difference among any of the placebo-implanted mice, they were pooled.

A similar relationship was found during naloxone-induced withdrawal. Peptide-treated mice which received the chronic morphine treatment did not exhibit any hypothermic response to the injection of naloxone (0.1 mg/kg), while vehicle-injected chronic morphine-treated mice showed significant hypothermia both at 15 ($-1.35°C$) and 30 ($-1.25°C$) min after the naloxone injection. At equimolar doses cyclo(Leu-Gly) was found to be more potent than MIF. The peptides were effective at doses of 0.07 and 0.18 μmoles/mouse, respectively (Fig. 2). In agreement with our previous findings, the injection of either of these peptides after physical dependence had already developed did not alter the response to the injection of naloxone (Fig. 2). The vehicle and the two peptide (0.18 μmole/mouse)-treated groups did not differ in the amount of body weight lost 1 hr after injection of naloxone. The weight loss for the three groups was: vehicle 1.75 ± 0.85 g, MIF 1.50 ± 0.65 g, and cyclo(Leu-Gly) 1.45 ± 0.50 g. Placebo-implanted mice lost neither body weight nor body temperature subsequent to the injection of naloxone. The number of jumps off a platform was not altered by peptide treatment. The number of jumps during the 10-min period was: vehicle 8.4 ± 4.4, MIF 7.3 ± 2.5, and cyclo(Leu-Gly) 8.7 ± 4.3 (Mean ± SEM). Naloxone did not produce any jumping in the placebo-implanted mice regardless of peptide treatment.

Similar to our findings, with the continuous treatment with these peptides, the single injection of either MIF or cyclo(Leu-Gly) at a dose of 0.18 μmole/

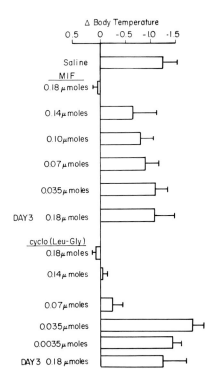

FIG. 2. See legend to Fig. 1 for morphine treatment. Two hours prior to morphine treatment, or on day 3 of morphine treatment, mice were injected with various doses of either MIF or cyclo(Leu-Gly). One hour after the removal of pellets mice were injected with naloxone (0.1 mg/kg i.p.). Body temperature was recorded just prior to and 30 min after the injection of naloxone.

mouse prevented the development of tolerance to the analgesic effects of morphine. The lack of differences in the jump threshold in chronic morphine-treated mice just prior and subsequent to the injection of morphine is indicative of the tolerance which developed during the chronic morphine treatment ($\Delta = 0.24$). The injection of MIF or cyclo(Leu-Gly) prior to chronic morphine treatment resulted in a difference of MIF ($\Delta = 1.46$) and cyclo(Leu-Gly) ($\Delta = 1.56$) in pre- and postmorphine injection jump threshold. These differences were not significantly different from the analgesia produced by morphine in placebo-implanted mice: vehicle ($\Delta = 1.26$), MIF ($\Delta = 1.00$), and cyclo(Leu-Gly) ($\Delta = 1.20$). The development of tolerance in the guinea pig ileum was not altered by the presence of cyclo(Leu-Gly) in the bathing medium. The initial reduction in the contraction of the ileum produced by morphine was 41% compared with 37% in the presence of cyclo(Leu-Gly). After seven injections of morphine the amount of reduction produced by morphine was only 5%, while in the presence of cyclo(Leu-Gly) the reduction was 7%. There was no significant difference in the amount of reduction produced by morphine at any of the intervening injections. The challenge dose of morphine (350 ng 3.28×10^{-8} M) produced a 36% reduction in the morphine exposed group without cyclo(Leu-Gly) and a 38% reduction in the presence of cyclo(Leu-Gly). These data indicate that the peptide did not alter the development of tolerance in the isolated guinea pig ileum.

DISCUSSION

A single injection of either MIF or cyclo(Leu-Gly) 2 hr prior to chronic morphine treatment significantly inhibited the development of tolerance and physical dependence on morphine. This was accomplished without altering the acute effect of the opiate or changing the disposition of morphine in the brain. Since the peptide treatments given after tolerance and dependence had already developed were not effective in altering the display of these states, it would appear that MIF and cyclo(Leu-Gly) are acting by altering the genesis of tolerance and dependence process. The recent finding that ethanol tolerance and dependence may be dissociated, led us to investigate in more detail the scope of these alterations. These studies show that these peptides prevent the hypothermic response which occurs in chronic morphine-treated mice either during abrupt or naloxone-induced withdrawal. On the other hand, the peptides did not alter either the loss of body weight or naloxone-induced stereotyped jumping behavior. These findings indicate that some aspects of dependence are prevented from developing by these peptides while the development of others appear unaltered.

A similar relationship exists for the tolerant state. The tolerance which develops to the analgesic properties of morphine appears to be blocked by peptide treatment. We have previously shown that the structurally related peptide Z-Pro-D-Leu also blocks the tolerance that develops to the hypothermic response to morphine (12). On the other hand, the tolerance that develops to morphine-induced reduction in the electrically stimulated contraction of the isolated guinea pig ileum is not altered by cyclo(Leu-Gly).

The correlation between the ability to produce alterations in body temperature and analgesia has also been reported for several endogenous neuropeptides (2). These data suggest that analgesia and thermoregulation may have some common neurochemical mechanism which is altered by morphine, and this alteration is prevented by peptides such as MIF and cyclo(Leu-Gly). It also appears that these same neurochemical mechanisms may be involved in some aspects of the genesis of morphine tolerant and dependent states.

ACKNOWLEDGMENT

This work was supported by U.S. Public Health Service Grant AM-18399, by National Science Foundation Grant GB-42758, and by the Illinois Department of Mental Health and Development Disabilities Grant 904–02. The authors thank Mr. Gerald Skala for his excellent technical assistance.

REFERENCES

1. Akil, H., Richardson, D. E., Hughes, J., and Barchus, J. P. (1978): Enkephalin-like material elevated in ventricular cerebrospinal fluid of patients after analgesic focal stimulation. *Science,* 201:463–465.
2. Bhargava, H. N. (1977): Improved recovery of morphine from biological tissue using siliconized glassware. *J. Pharm. Sci.,* 66:1044–1045.
3. Cheney, D. L., and Goldstein, A. (1971): Tolerance to opium narcotics: Time course and reversibility of physical dependence in mice. *Nature,* 232:447–448.
4. Ehrenpreis, S. (1975): Determination of actions of narcotic analgesics and their antagonists on electrically stimulated guinea pig ileum. In: *Methods in Narcotics Research,* edited by S. Ehrenpreis and A. Neidle, pp. 111–125. Dekker, New York.
5. Ehrenpreis, S., Light, I., and Schonbuch, G. H. (1972): Use of the electrically stimulated guinea pig ileum to study potent analgesics. In: *Addiction: Experimental Pharmacology,* edited by J. M. Singh, L. H. Miller, and H. Lal, pp. 319–342. Futura Publishing Co., Mount Kisco, N.Y.
6. Koida, M., and Walter, R. (1976): Post-proline cleaving enzyme. Purification of this endopeptidase by affinity chromatography. *J. Biol. Chem.,* 251:7593–7599.
7. McGillard, K. L., and Takemori, A. E. (1979): The effect of dopaminergic modifiers on morphine-induced analgesia and respiratory depression. *Eur. J. Pharmacol.,* 54:61–68.
8. Nemeroff, C., Osbahr, A., Ervin, G., and Prange, A. (1979): Evaluation of the analgesic effect of centrally administered neuropeptides. *Trans. Am. Soc. Neurochem.,* 10:105.
9. Rang, H. P. (1964): Stimulant actions of volatile anesthetics on smooth muscle. *Br. J. Pharmacol.,* 22:356–365.
10. Ritzmann, R. F., and Tabakoff, B. (1976): Dissociation of alcohol tolerance and dependence. *Nature,* 263:418–420.
11. Walter, R., Ritzmann, R. F., Bhargava, H. N., and Flexner, L. B. (1979): Prolyl-leucyl-glycinamide, cyclo (leucyl-glycine), and derivatives block development of physical dependence on morphine in mice. *Proc. Natl. Acad. Sci. USA,* 76:518–520.
12. Walter, R., Ritzmann, R. F., Bhargava, H. N., Flexner, L. B., and Krivoy, W. A. (1978): Inhibition by Z-Pro-D-Leu of development of tolerance to and physical dependence on morphine. *Proc. Natl. Acad. Sci. USA,* 75:4573–4576.
13. Way, E. L., Loh, H. H., and Shen, F. (1969): Simultaneous quantitative assessment of morphine tolerance and physical dependence. *J. Pharmacol. Exp. Ther.,* 167:1–8.

Neuropeptides and Neural Transmission,
edited by C. Ajmone Marsan and W. Z. Traczyk.
Raven Press, New York © 1980.

The Hypothalamic and Neurohypophyseal Vasopressin Content in Pinealectomized Male Rats

Irmina Szczepańska-Szyburska, Jan W. Guzek, and Krystyna Kmieć

Department of Pathophysiology, University School of Medicine, 90–136 Lodz, Poland

The vertebral pineal gland is someway involved in the control of hypothalamic centers. The connections of an epithalamo-pineal complex with the hypothalamus have been described by Roussy and Mosinger as early as 1938 (see ref. 12). Possible functional interactions between the pineal and hypothalamo-neurohypophyseal systems have been suggested as well. The hypothalamic neurosecretory function has been found to change following administration of pineal extracts or melatonin (see ref. 4); supraoptic and paraventricular nuclei, too, were thought to be of some importance for neuroendocrinological interrelations of the pineal (17). As the pineal function is known to be dependent on the environmental light cycle, it is noteworthy that alterations of the neurosecretory hypothalamo-neurohypophyseal activity have been found in rats (7) and rabbits (9,10) kept in continuous light or darkness.

There is a surprising resemblance between the neurohypophyseal hormones and epiphyseal peptides. The pineal contains some peptides with antidiuretic and oxytocic potencies. These activities reported for mammalian pineal extracts are thought to be mainly due to a compound that is a neurohypophyseal hormone in several nonmammalian vertebrates: arginine vasotocin (lysine vasotocin in porcine pineal), which is supposed to be a peptidergic antigonadotropic hormone modifying the release of some hypothalamic neurohormonal transducers (13). However, a discordance has recently been found between the biological vasotocin activity in the rat pineal and the immunoreactivity of this material (6,14,15). It was therefore assumed that, instead of arginine vasotocin, a structurally similar peptide occurs in the rat pineal (6,15). Moreover, evidence has been obtained in a radioimmunological system that both arginine vasopressin and oxytocin are present in the pineal of the rat (5,6,15) and of cattle (6). Lastly, the pineal of some species (rat, ox, and human) has been shown to contain neurophysins as well (16).

Following pinealectomy a decrease of neurosecretory activity in the magnocellular hypothalamic nuclei in rats has been reported (3,4) and the suggestion has been made that this occurs via the gonadal regulatory system (4). The uptake of ^{3}H-leucine—a direct precursor of oxytocin and neurophysins—by supraoptic and paraventricular neurones was found to increase following pineal-ectomy in female prepuberal and mature rats (1). So the studies of the effects caused by pinealectomy in the hypothalamo-neurohypophyseal system have so far been limited to indirect evaluation of neurosecretory activity or of synthetic processes. It was therefore thought possible that pinealectomy, being found effective in such a way, could also alter the amount of hormones stored within the hypothalamo-neurohypophyseal sytem. This chapter presents results of pre-liminary studies comparing vasopressor activity of the hypothalamus and neuro-hypophysis in groups of pinealectomized, sham-operated, and intact control male rats.

MATERIAL AND METHODS

Animals

Male rats of the Wistar strain, born in this Department, were used. They were housed at a room temperature of about 22°C and a 14-hr light, 10-hr dark cycle was provided (artificial illumination from 6.00 A.M. to 8.00 P.M.). Animals were allowed free access to standard pelleted chow and tap water throughout the experiment.

Experimental Design

Complete experimental protocol was followed in a total of 39 animals divided into three groups (see Table 1): (a) animals subjected to pinealectomy at 2 months of age and decapitated after survival period of another 2 months; (b)

TABLE 1. *The hypothalamic and neurohypophyseal vasopressin content in pinealectomized male rats*

	Hypothalamus[a]	Neurohypophysis[a]
Experimental group[b]		
a. Pinealectomy (10)	36 ± 7.1	332 ± 21
b. Sham operation (19)	27 ± 3.3	514 ± 46
c. Intact control (10)	34 ± 4.8	520 ± 67
Significance[c]		
a vs b	NS	$p < 0.005$
a vs c	NS	$p < 0.05$
b vs c	NS	NS

[a] Values expressed in milliunits per whole hypothalamus and neurohypophysis; mean ± SEM.
[b] Number of animals in parentheses.
[c] Determined by Student's *t*-test. NS, not significant.

animals sham-operated at the same age and decapitated after a survival period of 1–2 months; and (c) intact controls, born and killed at the same time as the animals in group a.

Pinealectomy

The rats of the group a, pinealectomized under hexobarbital anaesthesia following the procedure of Kuszak and Rodin (11), responded well to surgery; only few animals were lost as a consequence of intervention. The effectiveness of operation has been verified histologically in a pilot experimental series. Sham operation consisted of an identical surgical trauma including ligation and resection of superior sagittal vein, without removal of pineal body.

Experimental Procedure

All rats were sacrificed by rapid decapitation between 10.00 A.M. and 12.00 A.M. The brain with intact pituitary was quickly removed, the infundibular stalk cut up under stereomicroscope, and the neurohypophysis separated within 3 min and immediately homogenized in 0.25% acetic acid in 0.9% saline. The sample was heated for 5 min on a boiling water bath, centrifuged, and the supernatant removed and adjusted to a constant volume. From the brain, hardened on dry ice, the hypothalamus was rapidly dissected and the extracts were prepared in a similar manner, except that tissue samples were homogenized in 0.5% acetic acid in 0.9% saline. The final extracts were frozen and stored at −6°C until assayed for their vasopressor potency.

Bioassay of Vasopressor Activity

Bioassay of the vasopressor activity was processed according to the method of Dekański (2). Male Wistar rats weighing 320 to 380 g were pretreated intravenously with 0.1% solution of phenoxybenzamine hydrochloride, 1.0 ml/100 g body weight. After 18 hr they were anaesthetized by an intraperitoneal injection of 10% urethane, 1.0 ml/100 g body weight, and the changes of arterial blood pressure were recorded on a smoked drum. Unknown extracts were assayed against synthetic lysine vasopressin (Sandoz, Basle, batch no. 01113). The four-point assay procedure of Gaddum (8) was followed.

RESULTS

The mean vasopressor potency in the hypothalamus (Table 1) did not change significantly in pinealectomized animals, as compared with sham-operated respectively intact control rats.

The mean vasopressor activity in the neurohypophysis (Table 1) diminished significantly in animals killed 2 months following pinealectomy, down to about

64% when compared with the intact controls. The mean value in sham-operated rats did not differ significantly from that found in the intact controls.

DISCUSSION

The hypothalamic vasopressin content is known to be a function of two variables: the hormonal synthesis rate as well as the intensity of infundibular axonal transport towards neurohypophysis. Similarly, the neurohypophyseal supply is a resultant of the vasopressin amount transported down the fibers of hypothalamo-neurohypophyseal tract and/or the amount released into the blood. In our experiments, failure to show any changes in the hypothalamic vasopressin storage suggests that the rate of hormonal synthesis and axonal transport were quite well balanced. The depletion of vasopressin reserves in the neural lobe following pinealectomy may be due to an increased release into the blood and/ or a diminished infundibular transport. However, the present data give no direct information about either the synthesis and turnover rate of vasopressin or its liberation into the blood.

The sham-operated animals did not show, on the average, any significant difference when compared with the neurohypophyseal vasopressin content found in the intact rats. The decrease in the vasopressin storage in the neurohypophysis seems therefore to be a specific effect of pineal removal. In this respect, the findings reported here are in accord with previous data (1,3,4) indicating alterations in the function of neurosecretory neurones following pinealectomy.

Thus, the following conclusion appears justified from the results of the present preliminary studies: The pineal body seems to be of some importance in determining the activity of the vasopressinergic neurones, the actual vasopressin storage in the neurohypophysis being chosen as the functional index.

ACKNOWLEDGMENT

The authors wish to thank Doc. dr hab. med. M. Karasek for his help in the histological verification of pinealectomy effectiveness.

REFERENCES

1. Chazov, M. A., Veselova, S. P., Krivosheev, O. G., and Isachenkov, V. A. (1976): Interrelationship between the pineal gland and the hypothalamo-hypophysial complex. Report 1: The effect of pinealectomy, blinding and continuous illumination on the ^{3}H-leucine incorporation into the nuclei of the anterior, middle and the posterior hypothalamus of the prepubertal and mature rats. *Probl. Endokrinol.,* 22(1):33–39 (in Russian).
2. Dekański, J. (1952): The quantitative assay of vasopressin. *Br. J. Pharmacol.,* 7:567–572.
3. de Vries, R. A. C. (1972): Influence of pinealectomy on hypothalamic magnocellular neurosecretory activity in the female rat during normal light conditions, light-induced persistent oestrus, and after gonadectomy. *Neuroendocrinology,* 9:244–249.
4. de Vries, R. A. C., and Ariëns-Kappers, J. (1971): Influence of the pineal gland on the neurosecretory activity of the supraoptic hypothalamic nucleus in the male rat. *Neuroendocrinology,* 8:359–366.

5. Dogterom, J., Snijdewint, F. G. M., Pevet, P., and Buijs, R. M. (1978): On the presence of neuropeptides in the mammalian pineal gland. In: *EPSG Newsletter, Suppl. 1: First Colloquium of the European Pineal Study Group,* edited by P. Pevet and E. Tapp, pp. 15–16.
6. Dogterom, J., Snijdewint, F. G. M., Pevet, P., and Swaab, D. F. (1979): Studies on the presence of vasopressin, oxytocin and vasotocin in the pineal gland, subcommissural organ and foetal pituitary gland: Failure to demonstrate vasotocin in mammals. *J. Endocrind., (in press).*
7. Fiske, V. M., and Greep, R. O. (1959): Neurosecretory activity in rats under continuous light and darkness. *Endocrinology,* 64:175–185.
8. Gaddum, J. H. (1953): Bioassay and mathematics. *Pharmacol. Rev.,* 5:87–134.
9. Guzek, J. W. (1959): The exclusion of daylight and the endocrine glands. VI: The pituitary. *Patol. Pol.,* 10:137–149 (in Polish).
10. Guzek, J. W. (1959): The exclusion of daylight and the endocrine glands. VII: The hypothalamus. *Patol. Pol.,* 10:307–316 (in Polish).
11. Kuszak, J., and Rodin, M. (1977): A new technique of pinealectomy for adult rats. *Experientia,* 33:283–284.
12. Mosinger, M. (1954): Neuro-endocrinologie et neuro-ergonologie. Masson, Paris; Coimbra Editora, Coimbra.
13. Pavel, S. (1978): Arginine vasotocin as a pineal hormone. In: *J. Neural Transmission, Suppl. 13: The Pineal Gland,* edited by I. Nir, R. J. Reiter, and R. J. Wurtman, pp. 135–155. Springer-Verlag, Wien, New York.
14. Pevet, P., Dogterom, J., Buijs, R. M., Ebels, I., Swaab, D. F., and Arimura, A. (1980): Presence of alpha-MSH-, AVT, and LHRH-like compounds in the mammalian pineal and subcommissural organ and their relationship with the UMO5R pineal fraction. Xth Conference of European Comparative Endocrinologists, Sorrento (Italy) 21–25.05.1979. *Gen. Comp. Endocrinol., (in press).*
15. Pevet, P., Dogterom, J., Buijs, R. M., and Reinharz, A. (1979): Is the vasotocin or a vasotocin-like peptide which is present in the mammalian pineal and subcommissural organ? *J. Endocrinol.,* 80:49P.
16. Reinharz, A. C., and Vallotton, M. B. (1978): Evidence for the presence of neurohormone, neurophysins and peptidases in the pineal gland. In: *J. Neural Transmission, Suppl. 13: The Pineal Gland,* edited by I. Nir, R. J. Reiter, and R. J. Wurtman, p. 393. Springer-Verlag, Wien, New York.
17. Thiéblot, L. (1965): Physiology of the pineal body. In: *Progress in Brain Research, Vol. 10: Structure and Function of the Epiphysis Cerebri,* edited by J. Ariëns-Kappers and J. P. Schadé, pp. 479–488. Elsevier, Amsterdam, London, New York.

Author Index

Numbers in parentheses before page of citation are reference numbers; italicized numbers represent the page on which the reference appears.

Subject Index